DNA PROBES

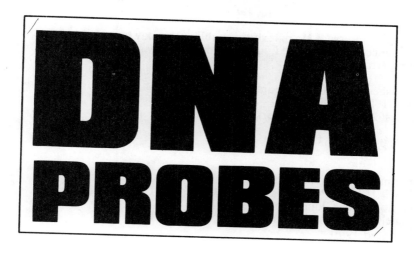

WITHDRAWN

George H. Keller
Mark M. Manak

M
stockton
press

Published in the United States and Canada by
STOCKTON PRESS, 1989
15 East 26th Street, New York, N.Y. 10010

ISBN 0-935859-63-2

First published in the United Kingdom by
MACMILLAN PUBLISHERS LTD (Journals Division), 1989
Distributed by Globe Book Services Ltd
Brunel Road, Houndmills, Basingstoke, Hants RG21 2XS
Reprinted 1990

British Library Cataloguing in Publication Data

Keller, George H.
DNA probes.
     1. Organisms. DNA. Structure
     I. Title II. Manak, Mark M.
     574.87'3282

ISBN 0-333-47659-X

Printed in Great Britain

Table of Contents

Preface   xv

SECTION 1 - BACKGROUND   1

MOLECULAR HYBRIDIZATION TECHNOLOGY   1
The Probe-Target Interaction   1
Advances in Hybridization Technology   5

GENERAL CONSIDERATIONS   11
Probe Selection and Specificity   11
Hybridization Rate   12
Probe Concentration   14
Stringency   15
Hybridization Accelerators   16

TYPES OF APPLICATIONS   18
Recombinant DNA Laboratory Techniques   18
Bacterial Detection   18
Viral Detection   20
Mammalian Sequences   22

REFERENCES   23

SECTION 2 - SAMPLE PREPARATION   29

INTRODUCTION   29

EXTRACTION AND PRECIPITATION OF NUCLEIC ACIDS   30
Procedure 2.1   Phenol Extraction of DNA   31
Ethanol Precipitation   32
Procedure 2.2   Ethanol Precipitation of DNA   33
Ethanol Precipitation of High Molecular Weight DNA   34
Procedure 2.3   Spooling of High Molecular Weight DNA   35
Alternatives to Ethanol Precipitation   35
Determining the Yield and Purity of DNA   36

EXTRACTION OF DNA FROM BLOOD   36
Procedure 2.4   Separation of Mononuclear Lymphocytes   37
   from Heparinized Whole Blood
   Rapid Isolation of White Cell Nuclei from Blood   38
   Extraction of DNA from Serum   39
Procedure 2.5   Extraction of HBV DNA from Human Serum   39

EXTRACTION OF DNA FROM TISSUES   40
Procedure 2.6   Extraction of DNA from Fresh or Frozen Tissues   41
Procedure 2.7   Extraction of DNA from Paraffin-Embedded Tissues   42

EXTRACTION OF DNA FROM BACTERIA   43
Procedure 2.8   Extraction of DNA from Bacterial Cells   43

EXTRACTION OF RNA   44
   Precautions for Working with RNA   44
   Ribonucleoside Vanadyl Complex-Phenol Extraction Method   45
Procedure 2.9   Preparation of Ribonucleoside Vanadyl Complex   45
Procedure 2.10   Isolation of Cytoplasmic RNA   46
   Isolation of RNA using Guanidinium Thiocyanate   47
Procedure 2.11   Guanidinium Thiocyanate Method for
                 RNA Isolation I   48
Procedure 2.12   Guanidinium Thiocyanate Method for
                 RNA Isolation II   49
Procedure 2.13   Urea-Lithium Chloride Method for Extraction
                 of RNA   50
Procedure 2.14   Purification of Poly (A$^+$) RNA   53

EXTRACTION OF NUCLEIC ACID FROM OTHER SOURCES   54
   Stool   54
Procedure 2.15   Stool Specimen Preparation I - DNA Extraction   55
Procedure 2.16   Stool Specimen Preparation II - Direct Spot
                 Blotting Procedure   55
   Urine   56
Procedure 2.17   Extraction of CMV from Urine Samples   57
   Other Samples   58

PREPARATION OF CELLS AND TISSUES FOR IN SITU
   HYBRIDIZATION   59
   Pretreatment of Slides Before Mounting Cells or Tissues   59
Procedure 2.18   Acid Washing of Slides   60
Procedure 2.19   Pretreatment of Slides with APES   60
Procedure 2.20   Pretreatment of Slides with Poly-L-Lysine   61

Preparation of Cells for *In Situ* Hybridization 61

Fixation of Cells for *In Situ* Hybridization 62

Procedure 2.21 Ethanol/Methanol Based Fixation 62

Procedure 2.22 4% Paraformaldehyde Fixation 63

Procedure 2.23 Formalin Fixation of Slides 63

Preparation of Tissues for *In Situ* Hybridization 64

Procedure 2.24 Preparation of Frozen Tissue Sections 64

Procedure 2.25 Formalin Fixation and Paraffin Embedding of Tissues 65

In Situ Hybridization on Chromosomes 66

Procedure 2.26 Preparation of Metaphase Spreads 66

Procedure 2.27 Giemsa Banding 67

REFERENCES 68

SECTION 3 - RADIOACTIVE LABELING PROCEDURES 71

INTRODUCTION 71

General Considerations 71

LABELING OF DNA BY ENZYMATIC MODIFICATION 76

Nick-Translation of DNA 76

Procedure 3.1 Labeling of DNA with Radioactive Nucleotides
by Nick-Translation 78

Optimization of DNase I Digestion 79

Labeling of DNA by Random Priming 80

Procedure 3.2 Labeling of DNA with Radioactive Nucleotides
by Random Priming 82

Synthesis of Probes from M13 Templates 83

Radiolabeled RNA Probes 85

Procedure 3.3 Transcription of ^{35}S-Labeled RNA Probes 88

OLIGONUCLEOTIDE PROBES 89

Production of RNA Probes from Oligodeoxynucleotide
Templates 89

Procedure 3.4 Transcription of [^{35}S]RNA Probes from
Synthetic Single-Stranded Oligonucleotides 89

Preparation of 'Tailed' Oligonucleotide Probes 91

Procedure 3.5 Oligonucleotide Tailing with Terminal Deoxynucleotidy
Transferase 92

Labeling of Oligonucleotides at the 5' end 93

Procedure 3.6 5' End Labeling with T4 Polynucleotide Kinase 93

Other Labeling Methods 94

Procedure 3.7 Estimation of Specific Activity by TCA Precipitation 95

PURIFICATION OF RADIOLABELED PROBES   96
  Gel Filtration Methods   96
Procedure 3.8   Purification of Labeled Probes on Sephadex
           Columns   97
Procedure 3.9   DNA Purification on QuickSpin Columns   97
  Ethanol Precipitation of Labeled Probes   98
Procedure 3.10   Purification of Labeled Probes by
           Ethanol Precipitation   98
Procedure 3.11   Denaturing Polyacrylamide Gels   99
  Hydrophobic Chromatography - NENSorb Columns   100
Procedure 3.12   Purification of Cloned DNA on Nensorb Columns   100
Procedure 3.13   Purification of Tritylated Oligonucleotide Probes 101

REFERENCES   103

SECTION 4 - NON-RADIOACTIVE LABELING PROCEDURES   105

INTRODUCTION   105

ENZYMATIC MODIFICATION   107
Procedure 4.1   Labeling of DNA with Modified Nucleotides
           by Nick-Translation   109
  Probe Testing   112
Procedure 4.2   Preparation of Target Test Strips   112
Procedure 4.3   Labeling of Cloned DNA with Modified
           Nucleotides by Random Priming   113
  Tailing of Cloned DNA Fragments   114
Procedure 4.4   Tailing of Cloned DNA Fragments with
           Modified Nucleotides   114
Procedure 4.5   Synthesis of 8-Aminohexyl dATP (AH-dATP)   117
  Biotinylated RNA Probes   119
Procedure 4.6   Incorporation of Biotinylated Nucleotides into
           RNA Transcripts   119

CHEMICAL MODIFICATION   120
  Chemical Labeling with Biotin   120
Procedure 4.7   Photo-Biotin Labeling of DNA   122
  Chemical Labeling with a Hapten   123
Procedure 4.8   Photo-DNP Labeling of DNA   124
Procedure 4.9a   Synthesis of Photo-DNP   125
Procedure 4.9b   Synthesis of DNP-Diaminohexane   127
  Linker Arm Modification of DNA   128

Procedure 4.10   Modification of DNA with Bisulfite and
                     Diaminohexane   128
        Bromine-Mediated DNA Modification   130
Procedure 4.11   Modification of DNA with Bromine
                     and Diaminohexane   131

OLIGONUCLEOTIDE PROBES   134
Procedure 4.12   Enzymatic Tailing of Oligonucleotide Probes   135
Procedure 4.13   Synthesis and Purification of Amino-
                     Oligonucleotide Probes   136
        Adding Detectable Groups to Amino-Oligonucleotides   137
Procedure 4.14   Biotin Labeling of Oligonucleotide Probes   138
        Enzyme Conjugation I   140
Procedure 4.15   Enzyme Labeling of Oligonucleotide Probes
                     using a Homobifunctional Linker Arm   141
        Enzyme Conjugation II   143
Procedure 4.16   Enzyme Labeling of Oligonucleotide Probes
                     using a Heterobifunctional Linker Arm   144

REFERENCES   145

**SECTION 5 - HYBRIDIZATION FORMATS
AND DETECTION PROCEDURES**   149

INTRODUCTION   149

FILTER HYBRIDIZATION   150
        Spot Blot Hybridization   151
Procedure 5.1   Slot Blotting of DNA   152
Procedure 5.2   Slot Blotting of RNA   153
        Cytoplasmic Dot Hybridization   154
Procedure 5.3   Cytoplasmic Dot Hybridization   154
        Dot Blotting of Intact Cells   155
Procedure 5.4   Rapid Screening of Cell Cultures for DNA
                     Sequences by Dot Blotting   155

SOUTHERN BLOT HYBRIDIZATION   157
        Agarose Gel Electrophoresis   157
Procedure 5.5   Agarose Gel Electrophoresis   158
Procedure 5.6   Southern Blot Transfer to Nitrocellulose   159
        Southern Transfer to Nylon Membranes   160
Procedure 5.7   Transfer of DNA from Agarose Gels to
                     Nylon Membranes   161

NORTHERN BLOTTING OF RNA   162
Procedure 5.8   RNA Electrophoresis in Methyl Mercury
                    Hydroxide Gels and Transfer Conditions   162
Procedure 5.9   RNA Electrophoresis in Formaldehyde Gels and
                    Transfer Conditions   164

COLONY AND PLAQUE SCREENING   165
Procedure 5.10   Lifting Colonies from Plates   166
Procedure 5.11   Lysing Cells and Fixing DNA onto Filters   167

FILTER HYBRIDIZATION PROCEDURES   168
Procedure 5.12   Hybridization of Filters with Radiolabeled Probes   169
    Autoradiography   170
Procedure 5.13   Autoradiography   171
    Reprobing of Filters   172
Procedure 5.14   Stripping Radiolabeled Probes from Membranes   172
    Non-Radioactive Filter Hybridization Conditions   173
Procedure 5.15   General Filter Hybridization Conditions for
                     Non-Radioactive Probes   173
    Hapten Detection   175
Procedure 5.16   Colorimetric Detection of Hapten-Labeled Probes
                     on Filters   175
    Biotin Detection   177
Procedure 5.17   One-Step Colorimetric Detection of Biotin-Labeled
                     Probes on Filters   177
    Alternative Protocol   178
Procedure 5.18   Two-Step Colorimetric Detection of Biotin-Labeled
                     Probes on Filters   178
    Chemiluminescent Detection   179
Procedure 5.19   Chemiluminescent Detection on Filters   179
    Detection of Peroxidase   179
    Detection of Alkaline Phosphatase   180
Procedure 5.20   Stripping Biotin-Labeled Probes from Nylon
                     Membranes   180

IN SITU HYBRIDIZATION   181
Procedure 5.21   Pretreatment of Slides with Denhardt's Solution   184
Procedure 5.22   Pretreatment of Formalin-Fixed Paraffin-Embedded
                     Slides for Use with Non-Radioactive Probes   185
Procedure 5.23   *In Situ* Hybridization using ^{35}S-Radiolabeled Probes   186
    Prehybridization   186
    Hybridization   186

Post-hybridization Steps   187
Autoradiography   188
Staining of Slides   188
Procedure 5.24   Staining Slides with Hematoxylin after *In Situ*
                  Hybridization   189
Procedure 5.25   *In Situ* Hybridization with Hapten or
                  Biotin-Labeled Probes   189
Procedure 5.26   Visualization of Hapten-Labeled Probes   190
Procedure 5.27   Visualization of Biotin-Labeled Probes   191

HYBRIDIZATION FORMATS FOR DETECTION OF
SOLUBLE TARGETS   192
Affinity Capture   192
Homogeneous Solution Hybridization Assays   195
         Strand Displacement   196
         Acridinium Esters   198
Sandwich Hybridization   198
         Solid-Phase Sandwich Hybridization   198
Procedure 5.29 Sandwich Hybridization in Microtiter Wells   200
Microtiter Well Preparation   201
Prehybridization (8 wells)   203
Sandwich Hybridization   203
Well Strip Development   204
         Solution-Phase Sandwich Hybridization   204
Other Formats   208
         Immobilized Probes   208

REFERENCES   210

SECTION 6 - PROBE AND TARGET AMPLIFICATION
SYSTEMS   215

INTRODUCTION   215

TARGET AMPLIFICATION   215
Polymerase Chain Reaction   215
Procedure 6.1   Standard Sample Preparation Method for the PCR   219
Procedure 6.2   Rapid PCR Sample Preparation from Whole Blood   220
Procedure 6.3   Enzyme Amplification of Target DNA using
                 the PCR   221
Hybridization Analysis of Products   222
Transcription-Based Amplification System   223

PROBE AMPLIFICATION   225
    Qß-Replicase System   225
    Probe Networks   229

REFERENCES   230

APPENDIX A - REAGENTS   233

BUFFERS AND REAGENTS   233

PROCEDURES   236
Procedure A.1 Large-scale Preparation of Hybridization Buffer   236
Procedure A.2 NBT and BCIP Substrate Solutions for
                        Alkaline Phosphatase   238
Procedure A.3 INT and BCIP Substrate Solutions for
                        Alkaline Phosphatase   239
Procedure A.4 Fast Red Substrate for Alkaline Phosphatase   240
Procedure A.5 Preparation of Acetylated BSA   241
Procedure A.6 Preparation of 5x Tailing Buffer   241

REFERENCES   242

DNA CONVERSION TABLES   243
    Conversion Factors   243
    Coding Capacity of DNA   243
    Quantitation of DNA and RNA   243
    Metric Prefixes   244

NUCLEOTIDE EXTINCTION COEFFICIENTS   244
    Conversion Formula   244

LIST OF ABBREVIATIONS   245

APPENDIX B - ADDITIONAL PROTOCOLS   247

PROCEDURES   247
Procedure B.1 Preparation of Rabbit Anti-DNP Antibody   247
    Synthesis of NHS-aminocaproic acid-DNP   247
    Preparation of DNP-BSA   249
    Immunization of Rabbits   249
    Processing of Serum   249
Procedure B.2 Conjugation of Alkaline Phosphatase to an Antibody 250

Procedure B.3 Synthesis of FITC-Diaminohexane   251
Procedure B.4 Conjugation of FITC to BSA   252

REFERENCES   253

APPENDIX C - SUPPLIERS   255

Preface

DNA Probes was undertaken to serve as a tutor and reference manual to all persons, from college undergraduate to corporate vice president, who are interested in the development and use of nucleic acid hybridization assays. This manual differs from other books devoted to nucleic acid probes in two respects. First, it is hopefully a coherent and integrated manual, incorporating background material, advice and specific protocols, in contrast to other books composed of a collection of chapters written by various authors. Second, this book contains a great deal of information on non-radioactive DNA probes in contrast to one or two pages as found in other books. Since the use of nucleic acid probes as cloning tools has been extensively covered in previous works, the emphasis in this book is on the potential commercial uses of such probes, as in diagnostic applications.

Radioactively labeled nucleic acid probes have seen wide use for two decades. However, DNA probes modified with non-radioactive labels are revolutionizing molecular biology and clinical diagnostics. Not only because they eliminate the inherent problems of working with radioisotopes (exposure, disposal, short working life, long detection times, record keeping and monitoring), but because they are generally easier to use and they can often be employed in assays that would not be practical with radioactive DNA probes. Development of these probes required an understanding of techniques from molecular biology, biochemistry, organic chemistry, immunochemistry and cytology. Since few individuals have the time to survey these disciplines, much less feel comfortable with them, this book should be a valuable aid.

Although the labeling and detection procedures are the heart of the manual, the other sections should provide extra insight and stimulation for those individuals unfamiliar with nucleic acid hybridization assays. This extra material also makes the manual a valuable reference for those who wish to understand commercial DNA probe assays which they may use 'as is' or modify for a special purpose.

If you simply want to get an experiment started (like most of us), first choose a labeling procedure and hybridization format suitable for your specific sample. Next select a compatible detection system. Finally, order the components using the list of suppliers and get going. Later, when time is available, read the rest of the manual to get an idea of the vast combination of labels, detection procedures and hybridization formats that are possible with nucleic acid probes. You may find a combination that greatly simplifies your work or one which allows you to detect nucleic acid in a way you never previously considered. The choice is yours.

It is our pleasure to acknowledge our colleagues, past and present, whose work has contributed to many of the protocols in this book. They are: Cecilia Cumming, Kate Moore and Cathy Overholt for their help in developing non-radioactive labeling techniques, detection techniques and hybridization formats; Tony Moore and Brad Sisson for their work with *in situ* hybridization assays and Dao-Pei Huang, Dave Petersen and Michael Fisher for their contributions to the development of PCR-based diagnostic assays.

We would also like to acknowledge and thank the people who helped us to complete this book: Sandra Dusing for her significant contributions to Section 3, Linda Jagodzinski for advice on PCR primer selection, Dao-Pei Huang for advice on PCR sample preparation and optimization, Sharon Vogel for typing much of the manuscript and Lee Sanders for his expert computer graphics assistance. In addition, we thank Cathy Overholt for her excellent proofreading and suggestions and Rosemary Foster, our publisher, for the opportunity to write this book and the encouragement to finish it.

Section 1: Background

Molecular hybridization technology

THE PROBE-TARGET INTERACTION

A probe, in the chemical or biological sense, is a molecule having a strong interaction only with a specific target and having a means of being detected following the interaction. Examples of such strong and specific probe-target interactions are: antibody-antigen, lectin-carbohydrate, avidin-biotin, receptor-nucleic acid and interactions between complementary nucleic acids. Protein probes (i.e., antibodies) interact with their specific target through a mixture of forces: hydrophobic, ionic and hydrogen bonding, at only a few specific sites. By contrast, nucleic acid probes interact with their complement primarily through H-bonding, at tens, hundreds or thousands of sites, depending on the length of the hybrid. Hydrophobic interactions also play a role, as evidenced by the reduction of hybrid stability by organic solvents, but probably contribute little to specificity.

The specificity of base pairing lies in the size of the nucleotide bases and placement of the amino (NH_2) and carboxyl ($C=O$) moieties on the rings (Figure 1.1). Only the purine-pyrimidine pair can be incorporated into the double helix at the proper H-bonding distance and only guanine-cytosine or adenine-thymine purine-pyrimidine pairs have moieties in the proper locations for H-bonding to occur. Purine-purine ring pairs would be too bulky to fit into the helix; pyrimidine-pyrimidine ring pairs would be too far apart. G-C pairs are more stable than A-T pairs because G and C form three H-bonds as opposed to two between A and T. For this reason, double-stranded DNA rich in G and C will have a higher melting temperature (more energy required to separate the strands) than A-T rich DNA. Figure 1.2 illustrates this effect of G-C content on melting temperature (T_m) for a number of DNAs The calculation of T_m is discussed under General Considerations in this section.

Base pairing is also possible for nucleotides modified with single atoms, functional groups or long side chains, depending on the site of attachment and the nature of the side chain. This property is important to understand for the

1

FIGURE 1.1   Diagram of H-Bond Location in G-C and A-T Base Pairs. R represents deoxyribose-phosphate backbone.

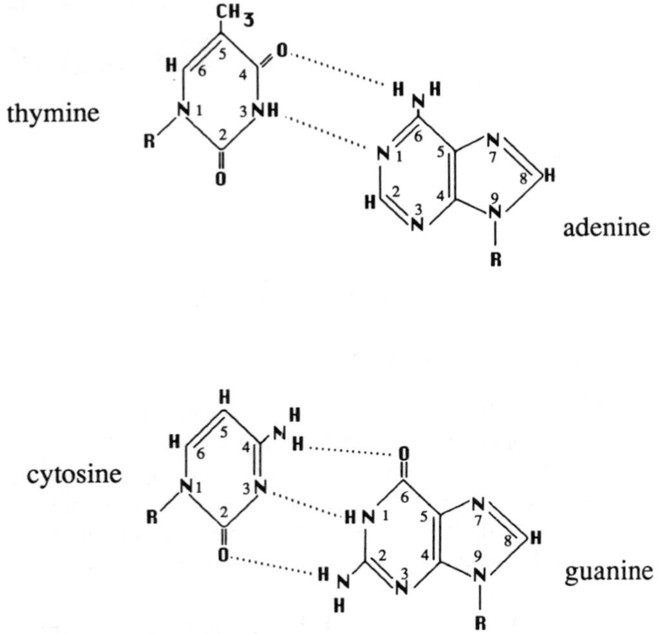

design of non-radioactive nucleic acid probes and for the chemical attachment of ^{125}I to DNA probes. Examples of single atoms capable of coupling to nucleic acid bases are mercury (Dale and Ward, 1975), bromine (Jones and Woodhouse, 1959) and iodine (Commerford, 1971). These elements react with the C-5 position of pyrimidines (except thymine) or the C-8 position of purines (Figure 1.3). Bromine may also react with the C-6 position of thymine (Keller *et al.*, 1988).

Figure 1.3 illustrates the most convenient modification sites on the five common bases encountered in nucleic acid probes. The C-5 position of cytosine and uracil, the C-6 of thymine and the C-8 of guanine and adenine are sites not involved in H-bonding and so are useful attachment sites. However, the N-4 position of cytosine (Viscidi *et al.*, 1986) and the N-6 position of adenine (Gebeychu et al., 1987) are also practical sites, even though they are involved in H-bonding. The explanation for this apparent discrepancy is that it is necessary to incorporate only 10-30 modified bases per 1,000 bases in order to obtain a useful probe (Keller *et al.*, 1988), corresponding to only 4 to 12% of an individual base being replaced by its modified analog. Although there may be weak or non-existent base pairing at the site of incorporation, the hybrid molecule usually loses very little stability overall. One way to avoid the disruption of H-bonding

FIGURE 1.2   Effect of G-C Content on the Melting Temperature of DNA. Double-stranded DNA from the sources indicated was heated in temperature increments and denaturation of the DNA was monitored by measuring the change in absorbance at 260 nm (data of Marmur and Doty, 1959).

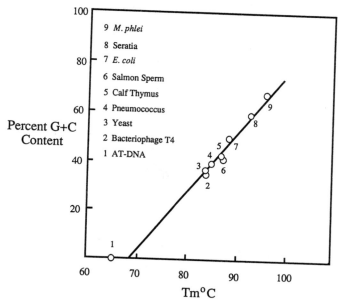

is to modify probes, cloned into a vector such as M13, exclusively in the vector region, leaving the insert bases unmodified. When labeling nucleic acids with the radioactive isotopes ^{32}P and ^{35}S, there is no modification of the bases since the isotopes are incorporated into the phosphodiester "backbone" of the nucleic acid. Chemical modification is possible at the 5' terminal phosphate moiety (Chu *et al.*, 1983; Chu and Orgel, 1985), and is most effective with oligonucleotide probes. This site is generally not useful on long, cloned probes because only one detectable group is introduced per probe molecule.

It is also possible to *enhance* hybrid stability or specificity by using modified bases. 2-Aminoadenine has been incorporated into oligonucleotide hybridization probes where it enhanced hybrid stability by forming three H-bonds with thymine instead of the usual two (Chollet and Kawashima, 1988). In addition, inosine has been used as a replacement for guanine in a G-C rich RNA probe (Varshney *et al.*, 1988) to obtain better hybridization specificity. This was achieved because I-C base pairs contain only two H-bonds instead of three for G-C pairs, effectively lowering the T_m of the hybrids. Since the melting temperature and the hybridization temperature were brought closer together, hybridization stringency was increased, thus increasing specificity.

Considering the variety of attachment sites and taking into account the various detectable groups and detection systems, it is clear that there are many ways to label a nucleic acid probe. These options are discussed in detail among the labeling procedures in Sections 3 and 4.

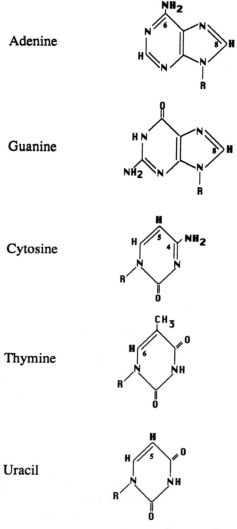

FIGURE 1.3 Potential Base Modification Sites. The C-8 sites of adenine and guanine and the C-5 sites of cytosine and uracil can potentially be modified without interfering with the base pair pair H-bonding. The C-4 position of cytosine and the N-6 of adenine are sites that can no longer form base-pair H-bonds when modified.

ADVANCES IN HYBRIDIZATION TECHNOLOGY

Nucleic acid hybridization technology essentially began with the work of Hall and Spiegelman (1961). Probe and target were hybridized in solution and hybrids were isolated by equilibrium-density gradient centrifugation. This procedure was slow, labor-intensive and inaccurate. Bolton and McCarthy (1962) developed the first simple solid phase hybridization method called the DNA-agar technique. Denatured DNA was immobilized in agar where it could not renature, but could hybridize with other complementary nucleic acid sequences. Typically, short, pulse-labeled DNA or RNA molecules were hybridized overnight to the gel-trapped DNA, after which the gel was placed in a column and washed to remove unbound probe. Bound probe was eluted with high temperature and low salt; eluted radioactivity was proportional to the amount of probe bound (McCarthy and Bolton, 1963). This format was well-suited for probe-excess saturation hybridization experiments. Another early attempt to analyze cellular genomes involved DNA reassociation studies in solution (DNA-DNA hybridization) to compare nucleic acid complexity from divergent sources (Britten and Kohne, 1968). This approach allowed detailed kinetic analysis of the DNA annealing reaction. Typically, DNA was isolated from different organisms (bacteria, yeast, fish, mammals) and sheared to fragments about 450 nucleotides in length, using a hydraulic pressure cell. The sheared DNA solution, containing 0.12 M phosphate buffer or 0.18 M Na$^+$, was boiled to separate the DNA strands, then cooled to about 60°C. The extent of reassociation of the complementary strands was monitored during incubation at 60°C by measuring the decrease in light absorbance by the solution at 260 nm (hypochromicity), over a period of hours to days. By this approach, the reassociation rates of DNA from widely different organisms could be compared and the relationship between *sequence complexity* and *kinetic complexity* was established.

The sequence complexity of a DNA molecule can be defined as the total length of unique sequences, while the kinetic complexity of the molecule is a function of its reassociation rate. Figure 1.4 beautifully illustrates the relationship between sequence complexity and reassociation rate. Various DNAs, ranging in sequence complexity from 1 to 10^9, were denatured and then allowed to reassociate to the Cot values indicated. The degree of reassociation was plotted as Cot (same as $C_o t$) values, where C_o is the initial DNA concentration in moles/liter and t is the incubation time in seconds.

Reassociation rate was defined as the Cot value where one half of the DNA had reassociated, or $Cot_{1/2}$. This figure illustrates how reassociation rate is inversely proportional to sequence complexity; as sequence complexity increases, the reassociation rate decreases. The difference in reassociation rate between poly(U):poly(A) and calf unique sequence DNA is about 10^9, paralleling the 10^9-fold difference in sequence complexity.

FIGURE 1.4   Reassociation Rates of Various DNAs. Denatured DNAs from mouse, *E. coli*, T4 and calf were renatured in 0.12 M phosphate buffer at 60°C and the change in A260 was plotted versus Cot value. Calf non-repetitive DNA was isolated by the hydroxylapatite chromatography. The poly(U)-poly(A) curve was estimated by calculation and the bacteriophage MS-2 curve was based on RNase resistance of the duplexes (data of Britten and Kohne, 1968).

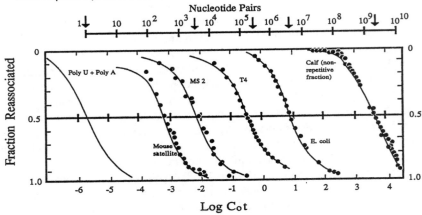

Thus, the $Cot_{1/2}$ value for a given DNA is its *kinetic* complexity and is inversely proportional to its *sequence* complexity. The term kinetic component is used to describe a group of different sequences, all present at about the same cellular concentration. One kinetic component may consist of unique sequences, present at two copies per cell while another component may consist of repeated sequences, each present at 10-50 copies per cell. DNA containing only one kinetic component reassociates within 2 orders of magnitude of Cot values. This is the case for all of the DNAs in Figure 1.4; none of the curves spans more than two log Cot values.

In the experiment illustrated in Figure 1.5, Britten and Kohne (1968) followed the reassociation of unfractionated calf thymus DNA by hydroxylapatite chromatography. *E. coli* DNA was included as an example of DNA containing a single kinetic component. Hydroxylapatite specifically binds double-stranded nucleic acid molecules under low salt conditions; these molecules can be eluted with high salt and quantitated by UV absorption. Unlike hypochromicity which measures the fraction of hybridized bases, hydroxylapatite chromatography measures the fraction of hybridized molecules, providing a more accurate view of the reaction results.

As illustrated in this experiment, unfractionated mammalian DNA requires at least seven orders of magnitude of Cot for complete reassociation, corresponding to at least three kinetic components. These kinetic components consist of a rapidly reassociating component (highly repetitive sequences), moderately rapidly

FIGURE 1.5   Reassociation of Unfractionated Calf Thymus DNA. The reactions were as described in Figure 1.4. Reassociation was monitored by hydroxylapatite chromatography (data of Britten and Kohne, 1968).

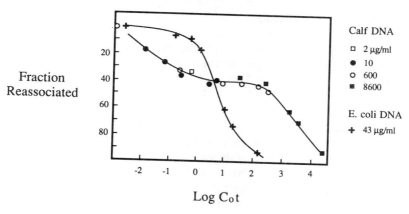

reassociating component (middle repetitive sequences) and a slowly reassociating component (unique sequences) (Davidson and Britten, 1973). This type of experiment provided the first hint that mammalian DNA was structurally different from and more complex than microbial DNA. As determined by modern cloning and hybridization techniques, examples of these families of components are: satellite DNA (highly repetitive), Alu family sequences (moderately repetitive) and structural or protein coding sequences (non-repetitive or unique).

The next set of advances in hybridization technology were tied to another immobilization procedure. The combined work of Nygaard and Hall (1964), Gillespie and Spiegelman (1965) and Denhardt (1966) made it possible to detect DNA sequences immobilized on nitrocellulose, using labeled DNA or RNA probes. For example, Brown and Weber (1968) used this technique to estimate the gene copy numbers for Xenopus ribosomal RNAs (rRNAs). RNA was metabolically-labeled with [^{3}H] uridine and hybridized in excess to filter bound genomic DNA. Following RNase treatment to digest non-specifically bound RNA, filters were washed and counted to determine the amount of probe hybridized. By calculating the amount of RNA (from its specific activity) that could hybridize to a known amount of DNA, the number of rRNA genes could be estimated. The expression of other specific genes could not be studied by these methods, because of a lack of specific probes. These early probe-excess, filter hybridization experiments eventually led to modern filter-based assays.

Hybridization technology was next enhanced by a number of significant developments, permitting the analysis of transcription products of specific genes and causing a renewed interest in kinetic hybridization experiments. Immobilized ligands such as poly(U)-Sepharose and oligo(dT)-cellulose made it possible to isolate poly(A)$^+$ RNA (a representative portion of messenger RNA (mRNA)) away from its major contaminant, ribosomal RNA (Aviv and Leder, 1972). In turn, mRNA purification allowed the preparation of a mixture of alpha and beta globin mRNAs from total reticulocyte RNA. These globin mRNA preparations were used as a template in the first synthesis of a gene-specific probe (Weiss *et al.*, 1976) for the analysis of globin gene expression. The probe was prepared by using an oligo(dT) primer and an RNA-dependent DNA polymerase (reverse transcriptase) resulting in a radioactively-labeled complementary DNA (cDNA) probe.

Measurement of the degree of hybridization became more accurate because strand-specific nucleases replaced hydroxylapatite chromatography. Nucleases were also more convenient because dozens of reactions (time points) could be processed simultaneously. Physical and immunological techniques (sucrose gradients and polysome immunoprecipitation) for the isolation of relatively abundant mRNAs (>1% of total mRNA) combined with reverse transcriptase, led to the preparation of other specific DNA probes, complementary to a few additional mammalian genes (Taylor and Tse, 1976; Innis and Miller, 1977; Buell *et al.*, 1978; Robson *et al.*, 1982). These probes were typically used to quantitate specific mRNA levels and total RNA complexity (Keller and Taylor, 1979). Figure 1.6 is an example of a target-excess RNA:cDNA hybridization experiment. The hybridization rate of liver RNA from different sources to labeled albumin cDNA was compared with that of pure albumin mRNA in order to determine the albumin mRNA concentration in the samples. Rot is analogous to Cot, where R_o is the initial RNA concentration.

Despite these significant advances, molecular hybridization could still not be applied to problems of more commercial or diagnostic interest, so long as the only DNA probes available were against relatively abundant mRNAs. Probe synthesis procedures were tedious because purified mRNA was required for each reaction. The reliance on multiple mRNA preparations and enzymatic copying of the template meant that cDNA purity and length were variable and this significantly affected the solution hybridization kinetics. In addition, target-excess solution hybridization required large amounts of excess ('driver') nucleic acid which was virtually impossible to obtain from sources of diagnostic interest. These problems were overcome by yet another set of complementary techniques which appeared within a short period of time.

Restriction endonucleases (Nathans and Smith, 1975; Smith, 1979), molecular cloning (Cohen *et al.*, 1973), genomic DNA libraries (Maniatis *et al.*, 1978), Southern blotting (Southern, 1975) and high specific activity radioactive labeling techniques such as nick-translation (Rigby *et al.*, 1977) allowed investigators to exploit the probe-excess filter hybridization technology developed a decade before. Cloned probe sequences are homogeneous in length and purity

FIGURE 1.6 Hybridization Kinetics of Rat Liver RNA with Albumin cDNA. Excess RNA was hybridized to ^{3}H-labeled albumin cDNA to various Rot values. The degree of hybridization was determined by measuring trichloroacetic acid-precipitable radioactivity following S1-nuclease digestion of single-stranded molecules. Sources of RNA: albumin mRNA, affinity purified rat liver albumin mRNA; poly(A), polyadenylated liver RNA; total, total liver RNA; unbound, liver RNA which does not bind to poly(U)-Sepharose. Closed circles, RNA from normal rats; open circles, RNA from hypophysectomized rats. The experiment shows that albumin mRNA comprises about 9% of poly(A)$^+$ RNA in normal rat liver and about 4% in hypophysectomized (growth hormone deprived) liver. The same trend was also seen in total mRNA and in mRNA that did not bind to poly(U)-Sepharose (unbound) (data of Keller, 1978).

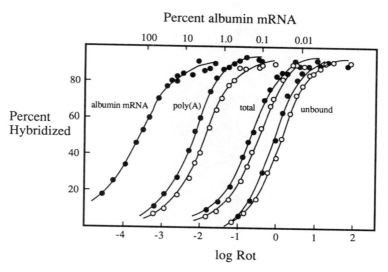

and easy to prepare in quantity. With the introduction of efficient, immobilized chemistries and automated synthesizers, synthesis of oligomer probes of 18-100 bases is now simple and large quantities are routinely obtained. Using restriction enzymes and Southern blotting, specific genes can be analyzed in a few micrograms of DNA. Both the *quantity* and *size* of specific DNA or mRNA sequences can be measured by Southern and northern (Alwine *et al.*, 1977) blotting, greatly enhancing the information level and confidence level of hybridization data, compared with previous techniques. In addition, the advances in sequencing technology (Maxam and Gilbert, 1977; Sanger *et al.*, 1977) mean that DNA probes can be analyzed, base by base, so that probe sequences and end-points are well defined. Figure 1.7 illustrates a typical application which depends on many of these techniques: detection of the sickle beta-globin allele in total human DNA. The normal beta-globin locus generates an *Mst* II restriction endonuclease fragment of 1.15 kilobases (kb). The sickle beta-globin locus generates a 1.35 kb fragment, because the sickle point mutation inactivates the *Mst* II site in the first exon, marked by an arrow. Note that the control DNA, from an individual with two normal beta-globin alleles, shows a 1.25 kb band in addition to the normal 1.15 kb band, presumably due to a mutation in the upstream *Mst* II site marked with an asterisk.

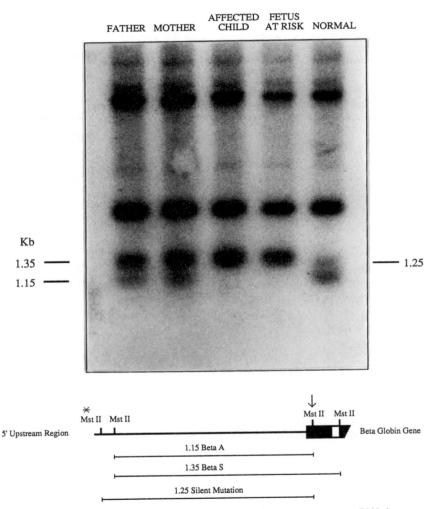

FIGURE 1.7 Detection of the Sickle Beta-Globin Allele. Lymphocyte DNA from normal, sickle cell carrier and sickle cell affected individuals was digested with *Mst* II, separated by agarose gel electrophoresis and transferred to nitrocellulose. The transfer was hybridized with a ^{32}P-labeled 4.4 kb *Pst* I DNA fragment containing the entire human beta-globin coding sequence. The hybridized probe was visualized by autoradiography (Keller, G.H. and Ladda, R.L., unpublished data).

By now, a huge number of specific DNA probes have been cloned and characterized, but a specific probe is only one requirement for developing a useful nucleic acid detection system. Laboratory research would benefit from the sensitivity to measure rare target molecules and the elimination of radioactive labeling to decrease the cost of isotope purchase, isotope disposal and frequent relabeling of probes. In order to bridge the gap between laboratory research and practical applications (clinical assays), DNA probe tests must be simple, rapid and inexpensive. In other words, speed, complexity and cost must be similar to existing antibody-based assays and sensitivity should be superior to provide the incentive to purchase and become familiar with a new assay. Thus, current efforts to simplify and extend hybridization technology have three main goals: 1) Perfecting non-radioactive DNA probes, 2) amplifying target, probe or signal and 3) developing simplified hybridization formats. These topics are discussed along with specific procedures, in the appropriate sections of this book.

General considerations

PROBE SELECTION AND SPECIFICITY

The process of selecting a specific hybridization probe depends on whether a biologically amplified (cloned) probe or a synthetic (oligomer) probe is desired. Cloned probes are normally used when a specific clone is available or when the DNA sequence is unknown and must be cloned first in order to be mapped and sequenced. Cloned probes generally provide greater specificity than oligomers because of their longer sequence and thus greater complexity. Statistically speaking, the complement of a long sequence is less likely to be encountered at random than the complement of a short sequence. Another advantage of cloned probes is that stronger hybridization signals are typically obtained, because more detectable groups per probe molecule can be incorporated into cloned probes than into oligomers.

Synthetic oligonucleotide probes possess some complementary advantages. First, owing to their short length, oligonucleotide probes have a low sequence complexity and low molecular weight. These factors mean shorter hybridization times are required to cover an equivalent number of target sites as compared with cloned probes. For example, an oligonucleotide probe of 20 nucleotides (nt) will require 10 min to reach its maximum percent hybridization at a concentration of 100 ng/ml (assuming 1-100 pg of a 1 kilobase (kb) target or 3×10^{-18} to 3×10^{-16} moles). A cloned probe of 2 kb at the same concentration (100 ng/ml) will require 161 hours to hybridize to the same number of target sites. These calculations are explained under the subsection 'Hybridization Rate.' Second, oligonucleotide probe specificity can be tailored to recognize single-base changes in target sequences since a single-base mismatch in a short probe can greatly decrease the T_m of the hybrid. Third, large quantities (1-10 mg) of oligonucleotide probe can be obtained from a single synthesis making these probes very cost-effective. Like cloned probes, oligonucleotide probes can be enzymatically and chemically modified to allow attachment of non-radioactive reporter groups. Although cloned probes are generally more specific, very specific oligonucleotide probes can be designed by careful sequence selection and/or by selecting a relatively long sequence ($\geq$ 30 nt). The most common oligonucleotide probes contain 18-30 bases, but current synthesizers allow efficient synthesis of probes containing at least 100 bases.

The selection of oligonucleotide probe sequences can be done manually using the following guidelines.

1. Probe length should be between 18-50 bases. Longer probes will result in longer hybridization times and low synthesis yields, shorter probes will lack specificity.
2. Base composition should be 40-60% G-C. Non-specific hybridization may increase for G-C ratios outside of this range.
3. Be certain that no intra-probe complementary regions are present. These may result in the formation of "hairpin" structures which will inhibit hybridization of the probe.
4. Avoid sequences containing long stretches (more than four) of a single base (i.e., -GGGGG-).
5. Once a sequence meeting the above criteria has been identified, computerized sequence analysis is highly recommended. The probe sequence should be compared with the sequence region or genome that it was derived from, as well as to the reverse complement of the region. If homologies to non-target regions greater than 70% or 8 or more bases in a row are found, that probe sequence should not be used.

Following these guidelines does not guarantee that a useful oligonucleotide probe will result, but it greatly enhances the chance of success. The final test is to synthesize, label and hybridize the probe to specific and non-specific target nucleic acids over a range of hybridization temperatures.

HYBRIDIZATION RATE

Traditional analysis of hybridization rate was based on DNA reassociation studies. Under those conditions, probe and target strands were present in solution and at equal concentrations. Modern hybridization experiments are conducted in probe excess whether they involve solution hybridization or solid phase hybridization to immobilized targets (filters, beads). In fact, since the solid phase targets are not in solution, realistic concentrations cannot be calculated for the target nucleic acid. For these reasons, the traditional second order rate formulas usually cited for hybridization reactions will not be discussed, only first order kinetic relationships will be described.

In probe excess situations, the hybridization rate is mainly dependent upon probe length (complexity) and probe concentration. The first order formulas presented below are descriptive of single-stranded probes present in excess over target sequences. Double-stranded probes exhibit similar kinetics at short (1-4 hours) hybridization times, but not at longer times because of reassociation of the probe, which decreases the available probe concentration with time. Equation [1.1] (Meinkoth and Wahl, 1984) can be used to estimate the time required to hybridize half of the probe to its immobilized target sequences:

$$t_{1/2} = \frac{\ln 2}{kC} \qquad [1.1]$$

k = rate constant for hybrid formation (mol liters/nucleotides sec)
C = probe concentration in solution (moles of probe molecules/liter)

The rate constant, k, is dependent upon probe length (L), probe complexity (N), temperature, ionic strength, viscosity and pH. L=N for probes which contain no repeated sequences. For example, for a 40-mer that contains two copies of a 20 nt sequence, L=40 and N=20. The relationship of k to these variables is:

$$k = \frac{k_n L^{0.5}}{N} \qquad [1.2]$$

k_n is the nucleation constant and is 3.5×10^5 for Na^+ concentrations of 0.4-1.0M, pH values of 5-9 and hybridization temperatures 25°C below the T_m of the probe-target hybrids (Wetmur and Davidson, 1968). To calculate the rate, in seconds, for hybridization of half of the probe to its target, equations [1.1] and [1.2] can be combined to give:

$$t_{1/2} = \frac{N \ln 2}{3.5 \times 10^5 \, (L^{0.5}) \, C} \qquad [1.3]$$

For a probe 500 bases in length, the numbers would be:

$$t_{1/2} = \frac{500 \, (0.693)}{3.5 \times 10^5 \, (22) \, 6 \times 10^{-10}} = 75,000 \text{ sec or 20 hours}$$

FIGURE 1.8 Effect of Probe Length on Hybridization Rate at Constant Molar Probe Concentration. Data points were calculated using equation [1.3] and a constant *molar* probe concentration (6.1×10^{-10} M) equivalent to a 500 nucleotide probe at 100 ng/ml.

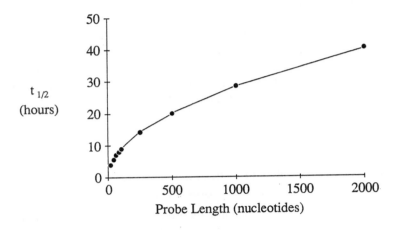

Figure 1.8 graphically shows the relationship between $t_{1/2}$ and probe length for a range of probe sizes and a constant *molar* concentration of probe. The very long times for probes longer than 500 bases illustrate the importance of using relatively short probes and the usefulness of hybridization accelerators (see below), since hybridization times exceeding 18 hours are impractical. These times must be considered estimates because the increase in rate with probe length predicted in equation [1.3] is probably not always valid. This is due to the wide range of possible probe sizes (the factor L may not adequately compensate for probes >1 kb because of diffusion and viscosity effects), as well as the fact that all of the immobilized target may not be available for hybridization.

PROBE CONCENTRATION

In general, hybridization rate increases with probe concentration. Also, within narrow limits, sensitivity increases with increasing probe concentration. In our experience, the concentration limits for sensitivity are approximately 5-100 ng/ml for ^{32}P-labeled probes in filter hybridizations, 25-1,000 ng/ml for non-radioactively-labeled probes in filter hybridizations and 0.5-5.0 µg/ml for *in situ* hybridizations with either type of label. The concentration limit is not determined by any inherent physical property of nucleic acid probes, but by the type of label and non-specific binding properties of the immobilization medium involved.

STRINGENCY

Factors that affect the stability of hybrids determine the stringency of the hybridization conditions. Since hybridization occurs most readily at 25°C below the T_m of the hybrids, the calculation of T_m is a necessary first step. Equation [1.4] illustrates the relationship between factors which determine T_m. The stringency can be adjusted as required by changing salt concentration, temperature or formamide concentration. For DNA:DNA hybridization using probes of more than 20 bases:

$$T_m = \frac{81.5°C + 16.6 \log M + 0.41(\%G+C) - 500}{n - 0.61(\%formamide)}$$

$M = [Na^+]$ in moles/liter
$n = $ length of shortest chain in duplex   [1.4]

Thus for a probe of 500 bases, containing 42% G+C, in 5x SSC (0.75M Na^+) and 50% formamide:

$$T_m = 81.5 + (-2.07) + 17.22 - 1 - (30.5) = 65°C$$

$$T_{hyb} = 65°C - 25°C = 40°C$$

Other factors which affect T_m:
1. T_m decreases 1.5°C for each 1% decrease in homology (cloned probes). This effect is much more pronounced for oligonucleotide probes of 15-150 bases.
2. The T_m of RNA:DNA hybrids is 10-15°C higher.
3. The T_m of RNA:RNA hybrids is 20-25°C higher.

Clearly formamide is necessary when using RNA as probe or target to keep the hybridization temperature reasonably low. When performing filter hybridizations with cloned probes, the most stringent conditions are applied during the final washes of the filter. The typical final wash conditions of 0.1x SSC (0.015M Na^+) at 55°C with a 500 base probe can be plugged into equation [1.4]:

$$T_m = 81.5 + (-30.3) + 17.22 - 1 - 0 = 67°C$$

$$67°C - 55°C = 12°C$$

Thus, these wash conditions are 12°C below T_m, considerably more stringent than the hybridization conditions of 25°C below T_m.

For oligonucleotides, the hybridization temperature is usually 5°C below the T_m. Thus, for a 30'mer containing 50% G+C:

$$T_m = \frac{81.5 + (-30.3) + 20.5 - 500}{30 - 0} = 55°C$$

$$T_{hyb} = 55°C - 5°C = 50°C$$

A different and more empirical formula is required for oligonucleotides of 14-20 bases:

$$T_m = 4°C \text{ per GC pair} + 2°C \text{ per A-T pair.}$$

In practice, the optimum hybridization temperature for oligonucleotides must be empirically determined. A convenient method is to prepare a filter containing dilutions of specific target DNA (complementary to the probe) and non-specific target DNA (i.e., salmon sperm or *E. coli* DNA). The filters are each hybridized with the oligonucleotide probe at a different temperature. The optimum is the temperature at which the specific target binds the probe strongly, but the non-specific target does not. Under certain conditions, dimethylsulfoxide (DMSO) can be used as a replacement for formamide to lower T_m. One example is in the polymerase chain reaction (Section 6), where it can be used to obtain complete denaturation of DNA at 93°C, the highest temperature that the thermostable polymerase can tolerate. In this reaction, formamide can inhibit the enzyme while DMSO is well tolerated.

Bear in mind that the estimation of T_m is more complex in hybridization systems employing more than one probe, such as sandwich hybridization (Section 5). The same expressions can be used to predict the behavior of each probe individually, but conditions will have to be selected that are a compromise between the requirements of each probe.

HYBRIDIZATION ACCELERATORS

Inert polymers can be used to accelerate the hybridization rate of probes longer than about 250 bases. The rate enhancement is about 3-fold for single-stranded probes and up to 100-fold for double-stranded, randomly nicked or primed probes (Wahl *et al.*, 1979). The importance of using a rate accelerator with cloned probes can be appreciated by examining Figure 1.9, which shows a more practical analysis of the type presented in Figure 1.8. In this figure, $t_{1/2}$ versus probe length is again plotted, but the *weight* concentration of probe is held constant rather than the *molar* concentration. Thus, all probes are at 100 ng/ml so that the short probes are present at a greater molar concentration than the longer probes, proportional to their difference in length. This means that when a 50-mer and a 500 nt probe are present in solution at 100 ng/ml, the molar concentration of the 50-mer is 10-fold greater. The point of this analysis is to demonstrate that short probes do not need accelerating agents. They have endogenously high hybridization rates due to their low complexity and low molecular weight.

Dextran sulfate is the most widely used hybridization accelerator with longer, double-stranded probes. It is a polyanion with an average molecular weight of 500,000 and is used at a final concentration of 5-10%. The disadvantage of using dextran sulfate is the presence of a significant concentration of a high molecular weight polymer which greatly increases the viscosity of hybridization solutions. Another common accelerator is polyethylene glycol (PEG, Amasino, 1986). It has the advantages of low cost and low viscosity (M.W.= 6,000-8,000), but it can not automatically be substituted for dextran sulfate. In our experience, there are some situations where 5-10% dextran sulfate works well, but 5-10% PEG causes very high backgrounds. It is imperative to optimize your own conditions. Another accelerating polymer is polyacrylic acid (Miller *et al.*, 1988). It is used as the sodium salt at a concentration of 2-4% and has a molecular weight of 90,000. Advantages are its low cost and lower viscosity compared with dextran sulfate.

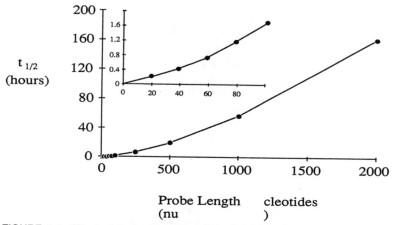

FIGURE 1.9 Effect of Probe Length on Hybridization Rate at Constant Weight Probe Concentration. Data points were calculated using equation [1.3] and a constant *weight* concentration of probe (100 ng/ml). Under these conditions, the effect of length on rate is more pronounced than under the conditions in Figure 1.8.

Two accelerating agents which are not polymers are phenol and guanidine thiocyanate. They may act by rendering water more hydrophobic and lowering the energy difference between double and single-stranded DNA. Phenol was described as a hybridization accelerator by Kohne *et al.* (1977), who termed their approach the 'phenol emulsion reassociation technique.' The accelerating effect was observed on DNA renaturation in solution and only at low DNA concentrations. It cannot be applied to hybridization reactions where the probe or target is immobilized (because it causes non-specific sticking of nucleic acid to the filter) and probably is of limited use even for solution hybridization formats. Of more practical use are chaotropic salts, first described by Hamaguchi and Geiduschek (1962), for their ability to lower the T_m of DNA duplexes. Thompson and Gillespie (1987) showed that one of these salts, 4M guanidine thiocyanate, enhances RNA hybridization in addition to lysing cells and inhibiting RNase. Dextran sulfate and polyethylene glycol are the most commonly used hybridization accelerating agents, presumably because they are compatible with filter formats.

Types of Applications

RECOMBINANT DNA LABORATORY TECHNIQUES

Recombinant DNA techniques incorporate a number of different hybridization schemes. Bacterial colony and phage plaque screening on filters as well as plasmid DNA screening on Southern and slot blots are examples of target-excess hybridization since there is usually more target DNA than probe nucleic acid. A low probe concentration and short hybridization time work best under these conditions, since specificity is more important than sensitivity. Genomic Southern, northern and slot blots are examples of probe-excess hybridization where high probe concentration and overnight hybridization times provide the best results, since sensitivity is most critical. Target RNA-excess hybridization is also employed and an example is the Berk-Sharp S1 nuclease method used for mapping RNA transcripts (Berk and Sharp, 1977).

BACTERIAL DETECTION

A variety of hybridization formats are being employed in the detection of bacterial infections and some examples are presented in Table 1.1. While most research laboratories use classical filter hybridization methods, commercially developed tests generally employ novel formats chosen to provide sensitivity, speed, convenience or patent protection. These formats and the probe labeling and detection procedures are discussed in detail in the appropriate sections of

DEVELOPER	TARGET	FORMAT	HYBRIDIZATION	LABEL	SENSITIVITY	REFERENCE
Research lab	Mycobacterium tuberculosis genomic DNA	filter probe-excess	direct	^{32}P	10^6 cells	Eisenach et al. (1988)
Gen-Probe	Mycoplasma pneumoniae	tube	soln. hybrid. HAP capture	^{125}I	40 pg rRNA 2500 cells	Dular et al. (1988)
Gen-Probe	Gonorrhea rRNA	tube	soln. hybrid. mag bead capture	acriflavin luminescent	25 pg RNA 1500 cells	Harper et al. (1988)
Chiron	Gonorrhea plasmid DNA	microwell	sandwich hybrid 3 det. probes 1 capture probe	alkaline phosphatase (luminescent)	50,000 cells	Sanchez-Pescador et al. (1988)
Orion	Chlamydia genomic and plasmid DNA	sandwich	probe-excess	^{32}P	10^5 molecules	Palva et al. (1988)
Miles	E. coli and B.subtilis rRNA	bead immobilized probe	direct	alkaline phosphatase (colorimetric)	500 cells	Miller et al. (1988)

Table 1.1 Examples of Nucleic Acid Hybridization Assays for the Detection of Specific Bacterial Infections.

this book. For those researchers unfamiliar with commercial DNA probe assays, Table 1.1 can provide a hint as to the creativity and effort focused on this area. Note that many tests take advantage of rRNA as the target nucleic acid. At about 10,000 copies per cell, this allows for far greater sensitivity than single-copy gene detection. Ribosomal RNA also has the advantage of being single-stranded, so denaturation is not required prior to hybridization. Another amplified target is the plasmid-borne sequence which may also be an antibiotic-resistance gene. This approach has been used by Sanchez-Pescador et al. (1988) to detect penicillin-resistant gonorrhea. DNA probes are also frequently used to identify (rather than detect) bacterial colonies. Here it is specificity rather than sensitivity which is important, since a single bacterial colony usually contains large quantities of DNA. One example is the identification of enterotoxin producing E. coli (a major cause of diarrheal disease) following culture (Sommerfelt et al., 1988). Those bacteria producing heat-stable toxins must be differentiated from producers of heat-labile toxins and their non-toxic counterparts in order to study the epidemiology and etiology of the resulting disease as well as evaluating the effectiveness of any vaccines. Along these same lines, DNA probes have also been used to detect Shiga-like toxins in E. coli (Newland and Neill, 1988), which are associated with hemorrhagic colitis. Another way in which DNA probes are used for identification is the separation of cultured mycoplasmas into species and strains using genomic DNA 'fingerprints' generated by Southern blotting with a rRNA-specific probe (Yogev et al., 1988).

VIRAL DETECTION

There are no amplified sequences within viruses, so other strategies must be employed for maximum detection sensitivity. A number of examples are presented in Table 1.2. One strategy is to detect infected cells directly by in situ hybridization. Each cell will contain hundreds or thousands of copies of viral genomic nucleic acid when virus replication is occurring. In some cases, in situ hybridization is sensitive enough to detect virus directly in clinical specimens, such as human papilloma virus (HPV) detection in cervical biopsies (Beckmann et al., 1985). In other situations, in situ hybridization is used as a culture confirmation assay, analogous to the identification of bacterial colonies. For instance, clinical samples suspected of containing cytomegalovirus (CMV) are used to inoculate tissue culture cells. After 1 to 30 days, a sample of the cells is fixed on a coverslip and the presence of CMV is monitored by in situ hybridization (Scott et al., 1988).

A second method for detecting virus directly in clinical samples relies on probes labeled to high specific activity ($>10^9$ cpm/µg) with ^{125}I (Richards et al., 1988; Kuhns et al., 1988). This high energy radioactive isotope provides good sensitivity, but its shelf life is short and there can be considerable radioactive exposure to the user. A third method employs probe amplification using large

DEVELOPER	TARGET	FORMAT	HYBRIDIZATION	LABEL	SENSITIVITY	REFERENCE
Research Lab	CMV viral DNA	filter	direct probe excess	^{32}P	10^6 viral particles	Buffone *et al.* (1988)
Enzo Biochem	CMV viral DNA	*in situ*	direct probe excess	biotin (colorimetric)	one infected cell (200-500 copies)	Scott *et al.* (1988)
Molecular Biosystems	CMV viral DNA	*in situ*	direct probe excess	alkalineone phosphatase (colorimetric)	infected cell (500-1,000 copies)	Kerschner *et al.* (1988)
	Rotavirus RNA	filter	direct probe excess	alkaline phosphatase (colorimetric)	10^6 copies	Roszak *et al.* (1988)
ENZO	HPV viral DNA	*in situ*	direct probe excess	biotin (colorimetric)	one infected cell (200-500 copies)	Goltz *et al.* (1987)
Gene-Trak	HIV-1 viral RNA	magnetic bead	sandwich capture	^{125}I	1,000 cells	Richards *et al.* (1988)
Abbott	HBV viral DNA	tube and column	direct probe excess	^{125}I	0.1 pg 60,000 molecules	Kuhns *et al.* (1988)

Table 1.2 Examples of Nucleic Acid Hybridization Assays for the Detection of Specific Viral Infections.

secondary branched probes and tertiary enzyme-labeled probes (Urdea *et al.*, 1988). The result is that 60-300 enzyme molecules are bound to each immobilized primary probe molecule, providing a very strong non-radioactive hybridization signal. The system is also designed to minimize non-specific interactions among the various detection probes, the sample and the microtiter well where the reaction takes place. Still, none of these techniques permits the direct detection of very low levels of viruses, such as human immunodeficiency virus type 1 (HIV-1) in peripheral blood lymphocytes.

A strategy that does permit detection of single infected cells without a microscope or radioactive isotopes, is target or probe amplification. Probe or target sequences can be amplified 10^6-fold or more, making final detection relatively simple (Saiki *et al.*, 1988; Lizardi *et al.*, 1988; Kwoh *et al.*, 1988). However, these techniques introduce new problems of contamination and background which must be understood. Details of these amplification methods are presented in Section 6.

MAMMALIAN SEQUENCES

In the vast majority of cases, the analysis of mammalian genomic sequences is done by Southern blotting. Simple detection and quantification, as done with bacteria and viruses, is usually not sufficient. The endpoint of these analyses is often the detection of a restriction fragment of a specific size. In addition to the detection of a specific gene, this type of experiment provides information about the sequences surrounding that gene, such as restriction site mutations, which can be used to follow the inheritance pattern of specific chromosomes. One example was the ß-globin restriction fragment polymorphism illustrated in Figure 1.7. Another example is DNA fingerprinting analysis to determine parentage or to compare cell lines (Jeffreys *et al.*, 1985). In this technique, cellular DNA is digested with a specific restriction endonuclease, separated by size and transferred to a membrane. Low-copy polymorphic repetitive sequences are visualized on the membrane by hybridization with a labeled DNA probe specific for the repetitive sequence family of interest. The pattern of bands generated will be essentially unique to that DNA sample and is a very accurate way to compare human and many other mammalian DNA samples.

There are now over 4,000 cloned human DNA sequences, which include 1,000 different protein coding sequences, pseudogene sequences, repetitive sequences and uncharacterized DNA segments (Schmidtke and Cooper, 1988). With so many potential human hybridization probes, certain regions of the human genome can be analyzed in great detail. Using the sequence information of such clones, it is also possible to analyze specific alleles without Southern blotting. Using a combination of target amplification and allele-specific oligonucleotides on slot blots, analysis of HLA genes (Higuchi *et al.*, 1988), for example, can be performed rapidly using very small quantities of DNA.

REFERENCES

1. Alwine, J.C., Kemp, D.J. and Stark, G.R. (1977): Method for detection of specific RNAs in agarose gels by transfer to diazobenzyloxymethyl paper and hybridization with DNA probes, Proc. Natl. Acad. Sci. USA **74**, 5350-5354.

2. Amasino, R.M. (1986): Acceleration of nucleic acid hybridization rate by polyethylene glycol, Anal. Biochem. **152**, 304-307.

3. Aviv, H. and Leder, P. (1972): Purification of biologically active globin mRNA by chromatography on oligothymidylic acid cellulose, Proc. Natl. Acad. Sci. USA **69**, 1408-1412.

4. Beckmann, A.M., Myerson, D., Daling, J.R., Kiviat, N.B., Fenoglio, C.M. and McDougall, J.K. (1985): Detection and localization of human papillomavirus DNA in human genital condylomas by *in situ* hybridization with biotinylated probes, J. Med. Virol. **16**, 265-273 .

5. Berk, A.J. and Sharp, P.A (1977): Sizing and mapping of early adenovirus mRNAs by gel electrophoresis of S1 endonuclease digested hybrids, Cell **12**, 721-732.

6. Bolton, E.T. and McCarthy, B.J. (1962): A general method for the isolation of RNA complementary to DNA, Proc. Nat. Acad. Sci. Wash. **48**, 1390-1397.

7. Britten, R.J. and Kohne, D.E. (1968): Repeated sequences in DNA, Science **161**, 529-540.

8. Brown, D.D. and Weber, C.S. (1968): Gene linkage by RNA-DNA hybridization. I. Unique DNA sequences homologous to 4S RNA, 5S RNA and ribosomal RNA, J. Mol. Biol. **34**, 661-680.

9. Buell, G.N., Wickens, M.P., Payvar, F. and Schimke, R.T. (1978): Synthesis of full length cDNAs from four partially purified oviduct mRNAs, J. Biol. Chem. **253**, 2471-2482.

10. Buffone, G.J., Demmler, G.J., Schimbor, C.M. and Yow, M.D. (1988): A hybridization assay for congenital cytomegalovirus infection, J. Clin. Microbiol. **26**, 2184-2186.

11. Chollet, A. and Kawashima, E. (1988): DNA containing the base analogue 2-aminoadenine: Preparation, use as hybridization probes and cleavage by restriction endonucleases, Nucleic Acids Res. **16**, 305-317.

12. Chu, B.C.F., Wahl, G.M. and Orgel, L.E. (1983): Derivatization of unprotected polynucleotides, Nucleic Acids Res. **11**, 6513-6529.

13. Chu, B.C.F. and Orgel, L.E. (1985): Detection of specific DNA sequences with short biotin-labeled probes, DNA **4**, 327-331.

14. Cohen, S.N., Chang, A.C.Y., Boyer, H.W. and Helling, R.B. (1973): Construction of biologically functional bacterial plasmids *in vitro*, Proc. Natl. Acad. Sci. USA **70**, 3240-3244.

15. Commerford, S.L. (1971): Iodination of nucleic acids *in vitro*, Biochemistry **10**, 1993-1999.

16. Dale, R.M.K. and Ward, D.C. (1975): Mercurated polynucleotides: New probes for hybridization and selective polymer fractionation, Biochemistry **14**, 2458-2469.

17   Davidson, E.H. and Britten, R.J. (1979): Regulation of gene expression: Possible role of repetitive sequences, Science **204**, 1052-1059.

18. Denhardt, D.T. (1966): A membrane filter technique for the detection of complementary DNA, Biochem. Biophys. Res. Commun. **23**, 641-646.

19. Dular, R., Kajioka, R. and Kasatiya, S. (1988): Comparison of Gen-Probe commercial kit and culture technique for the diagnosis of *Mycoplasma pneumoniae* infection, J. Clin. Microbiol. **26**, 1068-1069.

20. Eisenach, K.D., Crawford, J.T. and Bates, J.H. (1988): Repetitive DNA sequences as probes for *Mycobacterium tuberculosis*, J. Clin. Microbiol. **26**, 2240-2245.

21. Gebeychu, G., Rao, P.Y., SooChan, P., Simms, D.A. and Klevan, L. (1987): Novel biotinylated nucleotide analogs for labeling and colorimetric detection of DNA, Nucleic Acids Res. **15**, 4513-4534.

22. Gillespie, D. and Spiegelman, S. (1965): A quantitive assay for DNA-RNA hybrids with DNA immobilized on a membrane, J. Mol. Biol. **12**, 829-842.

23. Goltz, S.P., Todd, J.A. and Yang, H.L.(1987): A rapid DNA probe test for detecting HPV in biopsy specimens, American Clinical Products Review, December, 16-19.

24. Hall, B.D. and Spiegelman, S. (1961): Sequence complementarity of T2-DNA and T2-specific RNA, Proc. Nat. Acad. Sci. Wash. **47**, 137-146.

25. Hamaguchi, K. and Geiduschek, E.P. (1962): The effect of electrolytes on the stability of the deoxyribonucleate helix, J. Amer. Chem. Soc. **84**, 1329-1338.

26. Harper, M.E., Gonzalez, C., You, M.S., Gegg, C.V., Kranig-Brown, D., Yang, Y.Y., Respess, R.A. and Roeder, P.R.(1988): A rapid non-isotopic DNA probe test for the direct detection of *Neisseria gonorrhoeae* in clinical specimens, Abstracts of the American Society for Microbiology Annual Meeting, p 338.

27. Higuchi, R., von Beroldingen, C.H., Sensabaugh, G.F. and Erlich, H.A. (1988): DNA typing from single hairs, Nature **332**, 543-546.

28. Innis, M.A. and Miller, D.L. (1977): Quantitation of rat alpha-fetoprotein mRNA with a cDNA probe, J. Biol. Chem. **252**, 8469-8475.

29. Jeffries, A.J., Wilson, V. and Thein, S.L. (1985): Hypervariable minisatellite regions in human DNA, Nature **314**, 67-73.

30. Jones, A.S. and Woodhouse, D.L. (1959): Bromination of nucleic acids and their derivatives, Nature **183**, 1603-1605.

31. Keller, G.H. (1978): Effects of hypophysectomy and growth hormone treatment on albumin mRNA and total rat liver poly(A)-containing RNAs, Ph.D. thesis, the Pennsylvania State University.

32. Keller, G.H. and Taylor, J.M. (1979): Effect of hypophysectomy and growth hormone treatment on albumin mRNA levels in the rat liver, J. Biol. Chem. **254**, 276-278.

33. Keller, G.H., Cumming, C.U., Huang, D.P., Manak, M.M. and Ting, R. (1988): A chemical method for introducing haptens onto DNA probes, Anal. Biochem. **170**, 441-450.

34. Kerschner, J.H., Eastman, P.S., Hirata, K.K., Waller, D.B., Marich, J.E. and Ruth, J.L. (1988): Colorimetric detection of cytomegalovirus by *in situ* hybridization using enzyme-labeled synthetic DNA probes, Abstracts of the American Society for Microbiology annual meeting, p 320.

35. Kuhns, M.C., Mcnamara, A.L., Cabal, C.M., Decker, R.H., Theirs, V., Brechot,

C. and Tiollais, P. (1988): A new assay for the quantitative detection of hepatitis B viral DNA in human serum, in *Viral Hepatitis and Liver Disease*, Zuckerman, A.J., (ed.), Alan Liss, Inc., New York, N.Y.

36. Kohne, D.E., Levinson, S.A. and Byers, M.J. (1977): Room temperature method for increasing the rate of DNA reassociation by many thousandfold: The phenol emulsion reassociation technique, Biochemistry **16**, 5329-5341.

37. Kwoh, D.Y., Davis, G.R., Whitfield, K., Chapelle, H., DiMichele, L. and Gingeras, T.R. (1988): Transcription-based amplification system and detection of amplified HIV-1 sequences in infected cells using a bead-based sandwich hybridization format, in abstracts of The Third San Diego Conference 'Practical Aspects of Molecular Probes.'

38. Lizardi, P.M., Guerra, C.E., Lomeli, H., Tussie-Luna, I. and Kramer, F.R. (1988): Exponential amplification of recombinant RNA hybridization probes, Biotechnology **6**, 1197-1202.

39. Maniatis, T., Hardison, R.C., Lacy, E., Lauer, J., O'Connel, C., Quon, D., Sim, G.K. and Efstradiadis, A. (1978): The isolation of structural genes from libraries of eukaryotic DNA, Cell **15**, 687-701.

40. Marmur, J. and Doty, P. (1959): Heterogeneity in DNA. I. Dependence on composition of the configurational stability of deoxyribonucleic acids, Nature **183**, 1427-1428.

41. Maxam, A. and Gilbert, W. (1977): A new method for sequencing DNA, Proc. Natl. Acad. Sci. USA, **74**, 560-564.

42. McCarthy, B.J. and Bolton, E.T. (1963): An approach to the measurement of genetic relatedness among organisms, Proc. Nat. Acad. Sci. USA, **50**, 156-164.

43. Meinkoth, J. and Wahl, G. (1984): Hybridization of nucleic acids immobilized on solid supports, Anal. Biochem. **138**, 267-284.

44. Miller, C.A., Patterson, W.L., Johnson, P.K., Swartzell, C.T., Wogoman, F., Albarella, J.P. and Carrico, R.J. (1988): Detection of bacteria by hybridization of rRNA with DNA-latex and immunodetection of hybrids, J. Clin. Microbiol. **26**, 1271-1276.

45. Nathans, D. and Smith, H.O. (1975): Restriction endonucleases in the analysis and restructuring of DNA molecules, Ann. Rev. Biochem. **44**, 273-293.

46. Newland, J.W. and Neill, R.J. (1988): DNA probes for shiga-like toxins I and II and for toxin-converting bacteriophages, J. Clin. Microbiol. **26**, 1292-1297.

47. Nygaard, A.P. and Hall, B.D. (1963): A method for the detection of RNA-DNA complexes, J. Mol. Biol. **9**, 125-142.

48. Palva, A., Korpela, K., Lassus, A. and Ranki, M. (1987): Detection of *Chlamydia trachomatis* from genito-urinary specimens by improved nucleic acid sandwich hybridization, FEMS Microbiol. Lett. **40**, 211-217.

49. Richards, J., Collins, M., Groody, P., Pritchard, C., Thompson, J. and Gillespie, D. (1988): Development of a sensitive hybridization assay for detection of human immunodeficiency virus RNA, Abstracts of the American Society for Microbiology annual meeting, p 331.

50. Rigby, P.W.S., Dieckman, M., Rhodes, C. and Berg, P. (1977): Labeling deoxyribonucleic acid to high specific actuvuty *in vitro* by nick translation with DNA polymerase I, J. Mol. Biol. **113**, 237-251.

51. Robson, K.J.H., Chandra, T., MacGillivray, R.T.A. and Woo, S.L.C. (1982):

Polysome immunoprecipitation of phenylalanine hydroxylase mRNA from rat liver and cloning of its cDNA, Proc. Natl. Acad. Sci. USA **79**, 4701-4705.

52. Roszak, E.J., Freier, S.M., Driver, D.A., Bridge, C.L., Cerny, D.J. and Schmidt, L.M. (1988): Rapid testing of diarrheal agents: non-radioactive DNA probe tests for the direct detection of Campylobacter and Rotavirus in stool, Abstracts of the American Society for Microbiology Annual Meeting, p348.

53. Saiki, R.K., Gelfand, D.H., Stoffel, S., Scharf, S.J., Higuchi, R., Horn, G.T., Mullis, K.B. and Erlich, H.A. (1988): Primer-directed enzymatic amplification of DNA with a thermostable DNA polymerase, Science **239**, 487-494.

54. Sanchez-Pescador, R., Stempien, M.S. and Urdea, M.S. (1988): Rapid chemiluminescent nucleic acid assays for the detection of TEM-1 beta-lactamase-mediated penicillin resistance in *Neisseria gonorrhoeae* and other bacteria, J. Clin. Microbiol. **26**, 1934-1938.

55. Sanger, F., Nicklen, S. and Coulson, A.R. (1977): DNA sequencing with chain terminating inhibitors, Proc. Natl. Acad. Sci. USA, **74**, 5463-5467.

56. Schmidtke, J. and Cooper, D.N. (1988): A comprehensive list of cloned human DNA sequences, Nucleic Acids Res. **16**, 403-480.

57. Scott, A.A., Walker, K.A., Hennigar, L.M., Williams, C.H., Manos, J.P. and Gansler, T. (1988): Detection of cytomegalovirus in shell vial cultures by using a DNA probe and early nuclear antigen monoclonal antibody, J. Clin. Microbiol. **26**, 1895-1897.

58. Smith, H.O. (1979): Nucleotide sequence specificity of restriction endonucleases, Science **205**, 455-462.

59. Sommerfelt, H., Svennerholm, A., Kalland, K.H., Haukanes, B. and Bjorvatn, B. (1988): Comparative study of colony hybridization with synthetic oligonucleotide probes and enzyme-linked immunosorbent assay for identification of enterotoxigenic *Escherichia coli*, J. Clin. Microbiol. **26**, 530-534.

60. Southern, E.M. (1975): Detection of specific sequences among DNA fragments separated by gel electrophoresis, J. Mol. Biol. **98**, 503-517.

61. Taylor, J.M. and Tse, T.P.H. (1976): Isolation of rat liver albumin messenger RNA, J. Biol. Chem. **251**, 7461-7467.

62. Thompson, J. and Gillespie, D. (1987): Molecular hybridization with RNA probes in concentrated solutions of guanidine thiocyanate, Anal. Biochem. **163**, 281-291.

63. Urdea, M.S., Running, J.A., Horn, T., Clyne, J., Ku, L. and Warner, B.D. (1988): A novel method for the rapid detection of specific nucleotide sequences in crude biological samples without blotting or radioactivity: Application to the analysis of hepatitis B virus in human serum, Gene **61**, 253-264.

64. Varshney, U., Jahroudi, N., van de Sande, J.H. and Gedamu, L. (1988): Inosine incorporation in GC rich RNA probes increases hybridization sequence specificity, Nucleic Acids Res. **16**, 4162.

65. Viscidi, R.P., Connelly, C.J. and Yolken, R.H. (1986): Novel chemical method for the preparation of nucleic acids for nonisotopic hybridization, J. Clin. Microbiol. **23**, 311-317.

66. Wahl, G.M., Stern, M. and Stark, G.R. (1979): Efficient transfer of large DNA fragments from agarose gels to diazobenzyloxymethyl-paper and rapid hybridization by using dextran sulfate, Proc. Natl. Acad. Sci. USA **76**, 3683-3687.

67. Weiss, G.B., Wilson, G.N., Steggles, A.W. and Anderson, W.F. (1976): Importance of full size cDNA in nucleic acid hybridization, J. Biol. Chem. **251**, 3425-3431.
68. Wetmur, J.G. and Davidson, N. (1968): Kinetics of renaturation of DNA, J. Mol. Biol. **31**, 349-370.
69. Yogev, D., Halachmi, D., Kenny, G.E. and Razin, S. (1988): Distinction of species and strains of mycoplasmas (mollicutes) by genomic DNA fingerprints with an rRNA gene probe, J. Clin. Microbiol. **26**, 1198-1201.

Section 2:
Sample Preparation

Introduction

Hybridization methods have provided powerful tools for the detection of specific genes and the analysis of gene function. The advances in recombinant DNA technology and the availability of procedures for chemical synthesis of nucleic acids have made it possible to produce specific hybridization probes. This technology has applications in a variety of areas including the diagnosis of viral, bacterial and parasitic infections, the detection of human genetic diseases and cancers and for forensic uses. The nucleic acids required for analysis can be recovered from a variety of biological samples including blood, saliva, urine, stool, nasopharyngeal secretions, tissues and other sources. The sample preparation procedure selected must provide nucleic acids in a form compatible with the chosen hybridization format (Section 5).

In many applications, such as spot blot hybridization, sample preparation procedures yielding crude nucleic acid extracts are adequate. For example, in the preliminary screening of samples with radioactive probes, crude lysates containing protein or other contaminants are suitable. Whole cells or body fluids can be lysed directly on nylon or nitrocellulose filters followed by denaturing and fixing the nucleic acids to the filter. These procedures are suitable for quickly screening large numbers of samples, but poor sensitivity and background problems limit their use to samples containing large concentrations of target nucleic acid.

Other applications require purified nucleic acid which is free of protein, lipid, carbohydrate and other cellular impurities. Clean nucleic acid samples are needed when they are used as a substrate for specific enzymes, such as: reverse transcriptase for cDNA synthesis, Taq DNA polymerase for the polymerase chain reaction, restriction endonucleases for assays requiring size determination, or reactivity with immunochemical reagents for the detection of non-radioactive probes. These applications require conventional isolation procedures, including organic extraction and purification of the nucleic acid from the cells or tissues.

Furthermore, concentrating the purified nucleic acids increases the potential sensitivity. This can be accomplished by additional fractionation of the purified nucleic acids by size separation on agarose gels (Southern and northern blotting) or selective chromatography (oligo(dT) columns for isolation of poly(A)$^+$mRNA). Detection of RNA rather than DNA sequences permits the analysis of specific gene expression. Also, the sensitivity is usually increased when detecting RNA owing to the abundance of RNA transcripts over DNA coding sequences. Whenever working with RNA, precautions must be taken to prevent degradation of the RNA by nucleases.

In situ hybridization formats allow even greater sensitivity since the nucleic acids are already concentrated within the fixed cells. The microscopic enlargement of the site of hybridization allows detection of even a small number of hybrids, without dilution by nucleic acid from cells not expressing the sequence of interest. The sample preparation and fixation conditions needed to obtain optimum *in situ* results must balance nucleic acid immobilization and the retention of cellular morphology while allowing for diffusion of the probe and detection reagents into the cells.

Extraction and Precipitation of Nucleic Acids

The most commonly used procedure for DNA extraction makes use of the differential susceptibility of nucleic acids and proteins to the denaturing effects of organic solvents like phenol and chloroform. Following extraction with phenol and centrifugation, the protein component of a sample is denatured, or rendered insoluble, while the nucleic acids remain in solution in the aqueous phase (Brawerman *et al.*, 1972; Blobel and Potter, 1966). Nucleic acids are readily prepared from washed, single cell suspensions such as cultured cells or lymphocytes. Tissues, however, require additional pretreatments before the nucleic acids can be extracted (see Extraction of DNA from Tissues). Adherent cultured cells are washed with PBS in culture flasks and trypsinized or scraped into PBS and collected by centrifugation. To aid in the complete extraction of DNA, treatment of cells with sodium dodecyl sulfate (SDS) and proteinase K helps to lyse the cells and nuclei and liberates the DNA which is tightly bound in chromatin. Phenol extractions are usually performed using mixtures of phenol, chloroform and isoamyl alcohol. This mixture is a more effective protein denaturant than straight phenol and it helps to stabilize the RNA. Upon centrifugation, the phenol layer containing some protein and lipids moves toward the bottom of the tube, while the aqueous layer containing the nucleic acids remains on top. The denatured protein forms an insoluble layer at the interphase.

Note that when extracting concentrated salt solutions, such as those used in CsCl centrifugation, the phases may be reversed! A large interphase between the phenol and aqueous layers indicates incomplete extraction of the nucleic acid. Additional rounds of extraction of the aqueous layer and the interphase may be required. Following the extraction, the residual phenol must be removed from the aqueous layer (containing the nucleic acids) by extraction with chloroform:isoamyl alcohol (24:1). The DNA is then precipitated with ethanol, which also removes any traces of chloroform.

For some applications, such as Southern blotting, genomic analysis and cloning, where large molecular weight (>10 kb) DNA molecules are required, additional precautions should be taken to avoid the shearing forces that are produced by vigorous vortexing or rapid pipetting through narrow gauge pipettes. For all mixing steps, rock the sample gently. Use only large bore pipettes for transferring DNA containing solutions from one tube to another. Following the extraction steps, high molecular weight DNA molecules can be precipitated in cold ethanol and collected by spooling onto a glass rod. After ethanol precipitation, the DNA should be slowly redissolved in TE buffer (see Appendix A) with gentle rocking or mixing. This procedure leaves RNA, low molecular weight DNA and fragmented DNA behind, resulting in a preparation enriched for large DNA molecules (Procedure 2.3)

For most applications such as probing small stretches of DNA or slot blotting, precautions for maintaining large molecular weight DNA are not required. More vigorous extraction procedures will provide greater recoveries of DNA and can be completed in less time. Extracted nucleic acids should also be treated with RNase because the presence of RNA may mask small molecular weight DNAs on agarose gels or lead to overestimation of the quantity of DNA by the measurement of UV absorbance.

The following procedure is optimized for the extraction of small numbers of cells (5×10^5 to 5×10^7) which can easily be processed in microfuge tubes. For larger numbers of cells, the procedure can be scaled up and carried out in tightly capped 15 or 50 ml polypropylene tubes.

PROCEDURE 2.1

PHENOL EXTRACTION OF DNA

Caution: Phenol is poisonous and caustic. It will burn the skin and can be absorbed into the blood by skin contact. All work with phenol should be carried out in a fume hood, and gloves, safety glasses and lab coat should be worn. Use only glass or polypropylene tubes or pipettes. Dispose of phenol and chloroform waste in an appropriate container in accordance with guidelines for the disposal of toxic waste.

Reagents:
a)   Phosphate buffered saline (PBS, Appendix A)
b)   Cell Lysis Buffer
     10 mM Tris-HCl, pH 7.4
     10 mM sodium chloride
     10 mM EDTA
c)   10% sodium dodecyl sulfate (SDS)
d)   25 mg/ml Proteinase K (BoehringerMannheim).
     Store aliquoted at -20°C.
e)   Phenol:chloroform:isoamyl alcohol (25:24:1) (Appendix A)
f)   Chloroform:isoamyl: alcohol (24:1)
g)   TE Buffer
     10 mM Tris HCl, pH 7.6
     1 mM EDTA

Procedure:
1.   Wash fresh cells with 1-10 ml of cold PBS and centrifuge at 1,000 xg for
     10 minutes.
2.   Resuspend the pelleted cells to 1×10^8 cells/ml in cold cell lysis buffer. A
     minimum volume of 100 µl of lysis buffer should be used.
3.   Add SDS to a final concentration of 1%. If SDS is added directly to the
     cell pellet prior to resuspension, large clumps of cells may form which are
     difficult to break up and may reduce the total yield of DNA. This may be
     a problem, especially when $>10^7$ cells are to be extracted.
4.   Add Proteinase K to a final concentration of 200 µg/ml.
5.   Incubate the reaction for 1 hour at 50°C or overnight at 37°C with gentle
     rocking.
6.   Extract with an equal volume phenol:chloroform:isoamyl alcohol
     (25:24:1). Centrifuge for 10 minutes in a microfuge. The phases should
     be well separated, otherwise recentrifuge the sample.
7.   Transfer the aqueous layer to a new tube. If the interphase is large, add an
     additional 1/4 volume of cell lysis buffer to the tube containing the phenol
     and the interphase and reextract as in step 6. Combine the aqueous layers.
8.   Extract with an equal volume of chloroform:isoamyl alcohol (24:1).
     Centrifuge for 10 minutes in a microfuge.
9.   Transfer the aqueous layer containing the DNA to a new tube.

ETHANOL PRECIPITATION

Traces of phenol and chloroform must be removed from the DNA before it is
used in enzymatic reactions or applied to filters. The most common method for
removing these solvents is precipitation of the nucleic acids with cold ethanol, in
the presence of high salt. The precipitated DNA is recovered by centrifugation

and the pellet washed in 70% ethanol to remove residual salt, which may make the DNA difficult to dissolve and can inhibit enzymatic reactions.

When small amounts of DNA (<1 μg) or dilute solutions (<10 μg/ml) are precipitated, use 3 volumes of absolute ethanol for the initial precipitation and incubate for 1 hour in a dry ice bath or overnight at -20°C before centrifugation. Centrifuge at 4°C at maximum rotor speed for 15-20 minutes. Small quantities of DNA can also be recovered efficiently by coprecipitation with a carrier nucleic acid , such as tRNA from *E. coli*, yeast or bovine liver or salmon sperm DNA. The carrier nucleic acid should be added to the sample prior to the addition of ethanol and its presence will not interfere with hybridization assays, but some enzymatic reactions are inhibited by tRNA.

The procedures outlined below are designed for ethanol precipitation of small volumes of DNA (50-200 μl) using microfuge tubes. For larger volumes, use 15-50 ml polypropylene tubes or siliconized Corex tubes (see Alternatives to Ethanol Precipitation).

PROCEDURE 2.2

ETHANOL PRECIPITATION OF DNA

Reagents:
a)   2 M sodium acetate, pH 6.5
b)   Cold 100% ethanol
c)   Cold 70% ethanol
d)   <u>TE Buffer</u>
      10 mM Tris HCl, pH 7.6
      1 mM EDTA
e)   25 mg/ml Proteinase K (Boehringer-Mannheim)
f)   5 mg/ml RNase A
g)   Phenol:chloroform:isoamyl alcohol (25:24:1) (Appendix A)
h)   Chloroform:isoamyl: alcohol (24:1)

Procedure:
1. Add 1/10 volume of 2 M sodium acetate and 2 volumes of cold 100% ethanol to the DNA solution and mix. Incubate for periods from 1 hour to overnight at -20°C. For more rapid precipitation, incubate for 10 minutes on an ethanol:dry ice bath.
2. Centrifuge the solution for 10 minutes in a microfuge.
3. Carefully aspirate or pour the ethanol from the DNA pellet, being careful not to disturb the pellet.
4. Wash the pellet with 500 μl of cold 70% ethanol. Centrifuge for 5 minutes in a microfuge.

5. Carefully aspirate or pour off the ethanol, being careful not to disturb the pellet. Wash the pellet with 500 µl of cold 100% ethanol. Centrifuge for 5 minutes in a microfuge. Note: Nucleic acids are very stable when stored precipitated in ethanol at -20°C.

6. Carefully aspirate or pour off the ethanol, then drain off excess ethanol by inverting the tube on a paper towel. Allow the pellet to air-dry for about 10-15 minutes to evaporate the surface ethanol. Do not allow pellet to dry completely, because it will be more difficult to redissolve.

7. Resuspend the DNA pellet in a small volume of TE or water. Vortex at low speed or pipette up and down, gradually adding additional TE and mixing until the DNA is completely in solution. Use about 1 µl TE per extract of $1-5 \times 10^6$ cells.

Optional: Steps 8-13 are necessary only to obtain DNA free from RNA contamination. Otherwise, proceed to step 14.

8. Add RNase A to the DNA solution to a final concentration of 100 µg/ml and incubate at 37°C for 30 minutes.

9. Add SDS to a final concentration of 0.5% and Proteinase K to a final concentration of 100 µg/ml and incubate at 37°C for 30 minutes.

10. Extract the reaction with an equal volume of phenol:chloroform:isoamyl alcohol (25:24:1). Centrifuge in a microfuge for 10 minutes.

11. Carefully remove the aqueous layer and re-extract it with an equal volume of chloroform:isoamyl alcohol (24:1). Centrifuge in a microfuge for 10 minutes.

12. Carefully remove the aqueous layer and add 1/10 volume of 2 M sodium acetate followed by 2.5 volumes of cold ethanol. Mix and incubate the tube at -20°C for 1 hour.

13. Wash the pellet with 70% ethanol and 100% ethanol, air-dry and resuspend the nucleic acid as in Steps 3-6.

14. Determine the purity and yield of the DNA by measuring its absorbance at 260 nm and 280 nm (see Determining Yield and Purity of DNA).

15. Store the DNA in aliquots at -20°C, but do not use a frost-free freezer to avoid repeated freezing and thawing of the DNA.

ETHANOL PRECIPITATION OF HIGH MOLECULAR WEIGHT DNA

For ethanol precipitation of high molecular weight DNA (>10 kb), the DNA is spooled onto a glass rod rather than centrifuged. This procedure enriches for high molecular weight DNA, leaving the RNA, small molecular weight DNA and fragmented DNA behind.

PROCEDURE 2.3

SPOOLING OF HIGH MOLECULAR WEIGHT DNA

1. Adjust the DNA solution to 0.2 M sodium acetate and chill on ice. Carefully layer 2 volumes of cold (-20°C) 100% ethanol on top of the solution. The DNA will form a cloudy precipitate at the interphase.
2. Gently swirl an autoclaved glass rod at the interphase until the DNA begins to adhere to the rod. Continue winding the DNA around the rod until all of the DNA is recovered.
3. Gently press the rod with its attached DNA against the side of the tube to remove excess ethanol. Place the rod into TE buffer cooled to 4°C, allow the DNA to rehydrate for 20 minutes and unwind the DNA from the rod.
4. Store the solution at 4°C and occasionally mix by inverting. The DNA may take as long as two days to completely redissolve.
5. When it has dissolved, determine its UV absorbance as described in Procedure 2.2. Store the DNA solution at 4°C with a few drops of chloroform added to inhibit bacterial growth. Sodium azide (0.02%) may also be used as a stabilizer if it does not interfere with subsequent assays.

ALTERNATIVES TO ETHANOL PRECIPITATION

Several alternatives to ethanol precipitation are available to recover the DNA following phenol extraction. Isopropanol can be substituted for ethanol in the first precipitation step. An equal volume of cold isopropanol is added to the aqueous DNA solution instead of two volumes of cold ethanol. This smaller volume of alcohol may be convenient because a single microfuge tube can be used to precipitate up to 700 µl of DNA solution. The pellet should still be washed with 70% ethanol to remove the residual salt.

Dilute solutions of DNA can be concentrated by extraction with sec-butanol (2-butanol). The DNA is mixed with an equal volume of sec-butanol and centrifuged briefly at room temperature. The butanol absorbs water from the aqueous layer, leaving the DNA and salts behind in a smaller aqueous volume at the *bottom* of the tube. The butanol layer can be drawn off from the top with a pipette and the process repeated, if desired. If too much sec-butanol is added, the water phase may disappear completely. The DNA can still be recovered by adding water, mixing and recentrifuging. Sec-butanol extractions also concentrate any salts present in the DNA solution. This salt can be removed by ethanol precipitation, traditional dialysis, rapid dialysis (Centricon Microconcentrator, Amicon) or molecular seive columns (Quick Spin, Boehringer-Mannheim).

Traces of organic solvents can also be removed from a DNA solution by extraction with ether. The DNA solution is mixed well with an equal volume of ether. The phases are allowed to separate for about 5 minutes and the top ether phase is drawn off and discarded. The extraction can then be repeated a second or third time. Residual ether is removed by leaving the tube open under a hood for 10-20 minutes. Extreme caution should be exercised when working with ether since it is highly flammable and can cause drowsiness. All work with ether should be carried out in a well ventilated fume hood.

DETERMINING THE YIELD AND PURITY OF DNA

The yield and purity of a DNA solution can best be determined by spectrophotometric measurement of the absorbance of the DNA at 260 and 280 nm. The ratio of A_{260} to A_{280} measurements for pure DNA should be about 1.8. Ratios lower than 1.6 indicate significant contamination with protein or phenol and such samples will require further purification. To remove the residual protein, the sample should be redigested with SDS/Proteinase K, then re-extracted with phenol and reprecipitated with ethanol (Procedures 2.1 and 2.2). A 50 μg/ml solution of pure double-stranded DNA should give a reading of 1 A_{260} (using a 1 cm path length cell). One A_{260} unit of single-stranded DNA represents a 33 μg/ml solution, or a 40 μg/ml solution of RNA.

Extraction of DNA from Blood

Blood samples are frequently used as a source of DNA in the diagnosis of infectious agents or for genetic analysis. Peripheral blood lymphocytes (PBLs) provide a rich and easily accessible source of nucleated cells which contain the genomic DNA. These cells are also the source of many viruses or bacteria that replicate in blood cells. For isolation of the human lymphotropic viruses HIV-1 and HTLV-I, for example, it is convenient to isolate the PBLs before extraction. Other viruses, such as hepatitis B virus, are usually not cell-associated, but exist free in plasma or serum, where they can be isolated in the absence of contaminating genomic DNA from nucleated cells.

The DNA prepared from isolated lymphocytes is much cleaner than DNA extracted from whole blood. A variety of procedures have been developed for the isolation of lymphoid cells from blood. As the initial step in their isolation, peripheral blood mononuclear cells (PBMC) are often separated from the bulk erythrocytes by centrifugation of anticoagulant-treated blood in a narrow tube. The erythrocytes form a pellet, with the leukocytes (buffy coat cells) forming a layer on top. This buffy coat layer is carefully removed, washed with PBS and used for further processing. For cleaner separation of mononuclear cells from erythrocytes and granulocytes, blood samples can be centrifuged through Ficoll-

FIGURE 2.1 Isolation of Lymphocytes on Ficoll-Hypaque Gradients. A) Whole blood is diluted with PBS and layered on top of a Ficoll-Hypaque solution. B) Following centrifugation at 400 xg for 30 minutes, the granulocytes and erythrocytes pellet to the bottom of the tube, leaving the lymphocytes in a thin band on top of the Ficoll-Hypaque. C) The upper layer containing the plasma and platelets is removed and the lymphocyte band is collected.

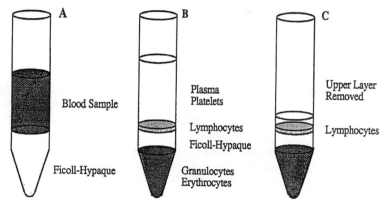

Hypaque or plasmagel (Boyum, 1968; Miller and Phillips, 1969). In these gradients, the red cells pellet, the plasma and platelets remain on top and the lymphocytes form a discrete band at the interphase (Figure 2.1).

The yield of lymphocytes from blood varies depending on a number of factors. The blood must be processed within 24 hours of collection, otherwise aggregates will form which trap the lymphocytes before they can be separated. The optimum results are achieved by storing blood at 18-20°C and processing it as soon as possible after collection. There are several sources of commercially prepared lymphocyte separation solutions.

PROCEDURE 2.4

SEPARATION OF MONONUCLEAR LYMPHOCYTES FROM HEPARINIZED WHOLE BLOOD

Reagents:
a) Lymphocyte separation medium (LSM, Organon Teknika Corporation)
b) Phosphate buffered saline (PBS, Appendix A)

Procedure:
1. Collect blood in an anticoagulant-coated (heparin, citrate) tube. The blood should be stored at room temperature and processed as soon as possible, preferably within 24 hours of collection.

2. Dilute the whole blood with two volumes of PBS (i.e. if 12 mls of whole blood are collected, this blood should be transferred to a 50 ml polypropylene conical tube and diluted with PBS up to 36 mls).
3. Underlay the diluted blood with a volume of LSM equal to that of the original blood sample (12 ml in this example). Place the tip of the pipette containing LSM at the bottom of the conical tube and *slowly* release the LSM, making sure that the layers do not mix.
4. Centrifuge the tube in a table-top centrifuge at 1,500 rpm (400 xg) for 30 minutes at room temperature. Be careful to slowly accelerate up to speed.
5. Following centrifugation, there should be a clearly defined interface, with lymphocytes on the top of the LSM layer. First, remove the upper layer containing the plasma and platelets, moving the pipette downward along the side of the tube as the solution is removed. Stop just above the lymphocyte layer (Figure 2.1).
6. Using a fresh pipette, slowly draw up the lymphocytes, being careful not to disturb the red cells on the bottom of the tube. Transfer the lymphocytes to a new conical tube.
7. Dilute the lymphocytes to 50 mls with PBS and mix. Centrifuge the diluted cells at 1,500 rpm for 10 minutes.
8. Decant the supernatant and resuspend the pellet in 10 mls of PBS.
9. Count the cells using a hemocytometer or Coulter Counter, if necessary.
10. Centrifuge the cells at 1,500 rpm for 10 minutes and remove the PBS by aspiration. The washed cells are ready for DNA extraction, or they can be stored frozen as a pellet at -70°C. If the cells are to be used for RNA extraction, do not freeze them. Extract the RNA immediately after isolation.

RAPID ISOLATION OF WHITE CELL NUCLEI FROM BLOOD

Buffone and Darlington (1985) described a rapid procedure for the isolation of total white blood cell nuclei from whole blood. The red and white blood cell membranes are lysed by a hypotonic buffer in the presence of the non-ionic detergent Triton X-100, while the white blood nuclei are stabilized by the presence of $MgCl_2$ and sucrose. After centrifugation to pellet the nuclei, plasma and lysed red cells are removed with the supernatant. The cytoplasmic DNA and RNA of the lymphocytes are also lost in the supernatant. In an alternative procedure, whole blood is frozen and thawed to lyse the red cells. The sample is then diluted with two volumes of 1x SSC and the nucleated cells are pelleted by centrifugation in a microfuge for 10 minutes (Jeffreys *et al.*, 1986). Only the nucleated cells, such lymphocytes, are collected by this procedure (human erythrocytes do not have nuclei). With either procedure, the genomic DNA from the pelleted nuclei or cells is then digested by treatment with SDS and Proteinase

K. The DNA is phenol-extracted and ethanol-precipitated according to standard methods (Procedures 2.1 and 2.2). A simplified method that does not require phenol extraction and is suitable for PCR samples is described in Procedure 6.2. All of these methods yield about 10 mg of DNA per ml of blood.

EXTRACTION OF DNA FROM SERUM

Many viruses and bacteria are not cell associated, but occur free in the blood, such as hepatitis B virus. The DNA from these organisms can be recovered from blood by preparing a serum or plasma fraction and extraction with phenol. The quantity of DNA contained in these sources is extremely low, so carrier DNA must be added prior to phenol extraction and ethanol precipitation to assure quantitative recovery.

PROCEDURE 2.5

EXTRACTION OF HBV DNA FROM HUMAN SERUM
(*Keller et al.*, 1988)

Reagents:
a) Extraction Buffer

150 mM NaCl	15 ml of 1 M (or 3 ml of 5 M)
10 mM EDTA pH 8.0	1 ml of 1 M
10 mM Tris-HCl pH 7.6	1 ml of 1 M
2% SDS	20 ml of 10%
5 µg/ml salmon sperm DNA	50 µl of 10 mg/ml

dilute to 100 ml with water

b) 25 mg/ml Proteinase K (Boehringer-Mannheim)
c) Phenol:chloroform:isoamyl alcohol (25:24:1, Appendix A)
d) Chloroform:isoamyl alcohol (24:1)
e) 2 M sodium acetate
f) Cold 100% ethanol
g) Cold 70% ethanol
h) TE Buffer
    10 mM Tris-HCl, pH 7.6
    1 mM EDTA

Procedure:
1. Centrifuge heparinized whole blood or clotted blood at 10,000 xg for 10 minutes at room temperature. Remove the upper layer containing the plasma or serum.

2. Add an equal volume of extraction buffer to the serum or plasma and add Proteinase K to 250 µg/ml. Incubate at 37°C overnight.

3. Extract the sample with an equal volume of phenol:chloroform:isoamyl alcohol (25:24:1). Incubate the emulsion at 50°C for 20 minutes. Centrifuge for 10 minutes in a microfuge and transfer the aqueous layer to a new tube, leaving the interphase behind.

4. Add up to 1/2 of the original serum or plasma volume of extraction buffer to the tube containing the phenol and interphase and re-extract at room temperature. Centrifuge for 10 minutes in a microfuge.

5. Combine the aqueous layers from Steps 3 and 4 add an equal volume of chloroform:isoamyl alcohol and vortex. Centrifuge for 10 minutes in a microfuge and transfer the aqueous layer to a new tube.

6. Add 1/10 volume of 2M sodium acetate plus 2 volumes of absolute ethanol to the aqueous layer. Incubate at -20°C for 30 minutes to overnight.

7. Centrifuge for 10 minutes in a microfuge.

8. Wash the pellet with 70% ethanol, then centrifuge for 10 minutes in a microfuge.

9. Wash the pellet with 100% ethanol, then centrifuge for 10 minutes in a microfuge.

10. Aspirate off the ethanol and air-dry the pellet for 15 minutes. Resuspend the DNA in TE to 1/2 the original volume of serum used in Step 1. The final carrier DNA concentration is 10 µg/ml.

Extraction of DNA from Tissues

Tissues are often used as a source of nucleic acids for analysis. Animal and human tissues are a convenient source of genomic DNA or RNA. For example, one gram of liver tissue contains about 10^9 cells. To obtain an equivalent number of nucleated cells from blood would require about 1 liter of blood. Tissues are also collected for analysis of signs of infection (viral or bacterial) or abnormal growth (tumors). To minimize degradation of the nucleic acids, the tissues should be kept on ice or quick-frozen in liquid nitrogen and processed as soon as possible after collection. Extraction of DNA from tissues requires some preliminary processing to break up the tissue into fine pieces from which the cells can be lysed and the DNA released. The tissue can be finely minced and disrupted by homogenization (Gross-Bellard et al, 1973), or frozen tissue can be ground in a mortar and pestle or crushed with a hammer into small pieces. The pieces can then be digested with SDS and Proteinase K and phenol extracted as in Procedure 2.1.

Many tissue specimens collected by pathology departments are formalin-fixed and paraffin-embedded for subsequent analysis. The DNA in these samples is well preserved and is stable for many years. High molecular weight DNA can be extracted from these samples and examined by spot blot, Southern blot, or PCR analysis. Before the DNA can be extracted, however, the tissues must be deparaffinized by treatment with xylene. In addition, extensive Proteinase K digestion is required to reduce the high degree of cross-linking that results from formalin fixation, liberating the DNA from the proteins. Extraction of DNA is facilitated by cutting the block into thin sections (Mark *et al.*, 1987; Dyall-Smith and Dyall-Smith, 1988). The extraction of DNA from formalin-fixed, paraffin-embedded cells is described in Procedure 2.7. Alternatively sections can be mounted on microscope slides and hybridized directly to permit examination of specific sequences by *in situ* hybridization (Procedure 2.22).

The homogenization, sonication or grinding used to facilitate the break-up of large tissue fragments can shear high molecular weight DNA. If it is important to recover intact DNA, shearing forces should be minimized. The tissue should be cut as finely as possible with very sharp scissors or a scalpel and digested with 200 µg/ml of Proteinase K and 0.5% SDS in cell lysis buffer overnight. The tissue should be mixed with a fresh aliquot of 200 µg/ml Proteinase K for an additional incubation for 24 hours or until the tissue disintegrates (Procedure 2.7, steps 7 and 8). The DNA is then isolated by phenol extraction and ethanol precipitation, observing the precautions described for isolation of high molecular weight DNA (Procedures 2.1 and 2.3).

PROCEDURE 2.6

EXTRACTION OF DNA FROM FRESH OR FROZEN TISSUES

Reagents:
a) Phosphate buffered saline (PBS, Appendix A)
b) Homogenization Buffer
     0.25 M sucrose
     25 mM Tris HCl, pH 7.5
     25 mM NaCl
     25 mM $MgCl_2$

Procedure:
1. Place fresh or freshly thawed tissue into PBS in a Petri dish on ice. Mince the tissue into small pieces with scissors or a scalpel. Keep the tissue wet during processing.
2. Centrifuge the minced tissue at 1,000 xg for 10 minutes.
3. Suspend the pellet in cold homogenization buffer (about 10 ml per g).
4. Homogenize the tissue suspension in a motor-driven homogenizer at full-speed at 4oC until the tissue is completely disrupted.

5. Centrifuge at 1,000 xg for 10 minutes.
6. Resuspend the cell pellet in PBS (1-5 ml per 0.1 g of starting material). Recentrifuge at 1,000 xg for 10 minutes.
7. Resuspend the pellet in DNA lysis buffer (1 ml per 0.1 g starting material) and proceed with the phenol extractions described in Procedure 2.1.

PROCEDURE 2.7

EXTRACTION OF DNA FROM PARAFFIN-EMBEDDED TISSUES

Reagents:
a) Xylene
b) 100% ethanol
c) DNA Digestion Buffer
   50 mM Tris-HCl, pH 7.4
   10 mM NaCl
   10 mM EDTA
   1% SDS
d) 25 mg/ml Proteinase K (Boehringer-Mannheim)

Procedure:
1. Cut the tissue into 3 μm sections using a microtome and collect up to 300 mg of tissue into a 1.5 ml microcentrifuge tube.
2. Dewax the tissue by adding 1 ml of xylene and vortex. Centrifuge for 5 minutes in a microfuge. Discard the supernatant.
3. Repeat the xylene extraction two more times as in step 2.
4. Wash the pellet with 1 ml of absolute ethanol. Vortex and recentrifuge for 5 minutes in a microfuge.
5. Repeat the ethanol wash as in step 4.
6. Air-dry the pellet for about 1 hour.
7. Resuspend the pellet in an approximately equal volume of DNA-digestion buffer (1 ml per mg of starting tissue). Add Proteinase K to a final concentration of 300 μg/ml.
8. Incubate the sample at 37°C for 1-2 days until most of the tissue has disintegrated. Vortexing or brief sonication during this step will help in breaking down larger tissue fragments. If extended incubation time is required, add a fresh aliquot of Proteinase K (to 300 μg/ml) after 16 hours.
9. Pellet the debris by centrifugation in a microfuge for 10 minutes.
10. Phenol extraction of the supernatant (Procedure 2.1, starting at step 6).

Extraction of DNA from Bacteria

The purification of DNA from bacteria can be accomplished by phenol extraction and ethanol precipitation, except that additional procedures should be included to break open the cell walls (i.e., lysozyme digestion). The cell debris and polysaccharides can then be removed by the addition of 5% cetyl-trimethylammonium bromine (CTAB; Murray and Thompson, 1980). CTAB is a cationic detergent which complexes with cell walls, protein and polysaccharides and allows them to be precipitated from solution. The salt concentration must be kept above 0.5 M to ensure that the nucleic acids do not complex with the CTAB.

PROCEDURE 2.8

EXTRACTION OF DNA FROM BACTERIAL CELLS

Solutions:
a) STET Buffer
    8% sucrose
    50 mM Tris-base, pH 8.0
    50 mM EDTA
    0.1% Triton X-100
b) 50 mg/ml lysozyme
c) 10% SDS
d) 4 M NaCl
e) CTAB/NaCl
    5% (w/v) cetyl-trimethylammonium bromine
    0.5 M NaCl

Procedure:
1. Grow bacterial cells to desired density.
2. Centrifuge 1.5 ml of cells in a microfuge for 5 minutes. Drain off the supernatant.
3. Resuspend the pellet in 200 µl STET buffer.
4. Add 4 µl of the 50 mg/ml lysozyme solution to the resuspended pellet and incubate at room temperature for 5 minutes, then at 94°C for 1 minute.
5. Add SDS to a final concentration of 0.5% and Proteinase K to a final concentration of 100 µg/ml. Mix and incubate for 1 hour at 37°C.
6. Add NaCl to the reaction, to a final concentration of 0.5 M.
7. Add 1/10 volume of the CTAB/NaCl solution. Mix and incubate at 65°C for 10 minutes.
8. Perform phenol extraction and ethanol precipitation (Procedures 2.1 and 2.2)

Extraction of RNA

Many hybridization assays are performed to identify RNA sequences in biological samples. The expression of certain DNA sequences (cellular or viral) can be monitored by assaying for the presence mRNA transcripts in the cytoplasm of cells. Many viruses contain RNA genomes and even DNA viruses are often identified on the basis of their RNA transcripts because of the significant amplification of copy number. In addition, the diagnosis of several bacterial species relies on detection of the specific rRNA characteristic of that species.

The major problem in working with RNA is contamination of the sample with RNase. RNases are very stable enzymes which do not require cofactors for activity and, if appropriate precautions are not followed, will degrade the RNA before it is isolated. Many tissues and cell types contain high levels of RNase activity and RNase can also be introduced during processing. Therefore, RNase-free conditions must be maintained throughout the purification to assure the integrity of the RNA, since contamination of samples with even small quantities of RNase can lead to degradation.

PRECAUTIONS FOR WORKING WITH RNA

1. *Glassware*: All glassware used in the preparation of RNA should be baked at 250°C for 4 hours. Glassware can also be washed thoroughly and treated with 0.1% diethyl pyrocarbonate (DEPC) for 12 hours at 37°C followed by autoclaving. Autoclaving alone is generally not sufficient to inactivate RNase.

2. *Plasticware*: Sterile, disposable plasticware straight out of the package is considered RNase-free. New, non-sterile plasticware should be autoclaved before use.

3. *Solutions:* All solutions used in the preparation of RNA can be made RNase-free by treatment with DEPC. To treat solutions, add 0.2 ml DEPC per 100 ml of solution. Mix vigorously. Allow the solution to stand overnight at room temperature, then autoclave. Since DEPC is a suspected carcinogen, the procedure should be carried out in a fume hood. **Note:** RNase cannot be effectively inactivated in solutions containing Tris buffer, since Tris reacts with DEPC. To prepare solutions containing Tris, the solution should be made up with DEPC-treated water then autoclaved before use.

4. *Other precautions.* Since human hands are a major source of exogenous RNase, gloves must be worn when handling solutions, pipettes, etc., to prevent contamination. Precautions should also be taken to ensure that contaminated pipettes, glassware and solutions do not come in contact with the RNase-free materials.

RIBONUCLEOSIDE VANADYL COMPLEX-PHENOL EXTRACTION METHOD

RNA can be prepared from eukaryotic cells by phenol extraction, providing that precautions are taken to prevent RNase contamination. In this procedure the potent RNase inhibitor, ribonucleoside vanadyl complex (RVC), is added at the time the cells are lysed (Berger and Birkenmeimer, 1979). The complexes formed between ribonucleosides and the oxovanadium ion bind to many RNases and effectively inhibit their activity. The RVC can subsequently be removed by extraction with phenol containing 0.1% 8-hydroxyquinoline.

The non-ionic detergent Nonidet-P40 (NP40) is used to lyse the cell membranes while leaving the nuclear membrane intact (Favoloro *et al.*, 1980). Cytoplasmic contents, including the RNA (mRNA, rRNA and tRNA) are released into the solution, while the genomic DNA is removed centrifugation. RNA is isolated from this cytoplasmic fraction by phenol extraction and ethanol precipitation. Samples should be kept on ice and cold solutions used throughout processing. The NP40 detergent used to lyse the cell membranes should be added after the washed cells are resuspended so as to prevent the cells from clumping.

Procedure 2.9 is suitable for the extraction of RNA from tissue culture cells or washed lymphocytes. When processing tissues, it is best to start with fresh tissue. If this is not possible, use tissue that has been quick-frozen in liquid nitrogen and crush it with a hammer or pestle while still frozen. The tissue should then be homogenized in buffer containing 10 mM RVC and 10% NP40 and further processed as rapidly as possible. Excellent yields of intact RNA can be obtained by this procedure and the RNA is most stable when stored under ethanol at -20°C. The RVC solution is commercially available (BRL), but if you wish to make your own, refer to the procedure below.

PROCEDURE 2.9

PREPARATION OF RIBONUCLEOSIDE VANADYL COMPLEX (RVC)

Reagents:
a) Adenosine
b) Cytosine
c) Guanosine
d) Uridine
e) 2 M vanadyl sulfate
f) 10 N NaOH
g) 1 N NaOH
h) Nitrogen gas

Procedure:

1. To 16 ml of boiling water, add the four ribonucleosides while stirring:

   Adenosine   (MW   267.2) 267.2 mg
   Cytidine   (MW   243.2) 243.2 mg
   Guanosine   (MW   283.2) 283.2 mg
   Uridine   (MW   244.2) 244.2 mg

2. Flush the solution with nitrogen gas while adding dropwise 2 ml of 2 M vanadyl sulfate.

3. Continue to flush the solution with nitrogen gas and add 10 N NaOH dropwise to adjust the pH to approximately 6 and then with 1 N NaOH to bring the pH to 7.0. As the complex is formed the solution will turn from blue to a dark green.

4. Adjust the volume of the solution to 20 ml with water. The final concentration of RVC is 200 mM. The RVC should be diluted 1:20 (to 10 mM) for use in RNA solutions.

5. Freeze the 200 mM RVC solution (20x stock) in 1-5 ml aliquots at -20°C.

PROCEDURE 2.10

ISOLATION OF CYTOPLASMIC RNA

Reagents:

a) Phosphate buffered saline (PBS, Appendix A)

b) TKM Buffer

   10 mM Tris-HCl pH 7.0
   10 mM KCl
   1.5 mM $MgCl_2$
   3 mM dithiothreitol (DTT)

c) 200 mM ribonucleoside vanadyl complex (RVC)

d) 10% Nonidet-P40

e) 10% SDS

f) 0.5 M EDTA

Procedure:

1. Wash the cells with ice-cold PBS. Centrifuge at 1,000 xg for 10 minutes at 4°C.

2. Resuspend the washed cells at $2-10 \times 10^8$ cells/ml in ice-cold TKM buffer.

3. Add 1/20 volume of 200 mM RVC (final conc. = 10 mM) and 1/20 of volume 10% NP40 (final conc. = 0.5%) to the cells and vortex.

4. Pellet the nuclei and cell debris at 2,000 xg for 10 minutes at 4°C. Transfer the supernatant to a fresh tube.

5. Add 1/20 volume of 10% SDS (final conc. 0.5%) to the supernatant (cytoplasmic extract), mix, then add EDTA to 75 mM (0.15 volume of 0.5 M stock).
6. Perform phenol extraction and ethanol precipitation (Procedures 2.1 and 2.2).
7. Resuspend the RNA pellet in a small volume of TE buffer. Use 200 μl TE per $1-5 \times 10^8$ cells. The final volume should be kept as low as possible.

ISOLATION OF RNA USING GUANIDINIUM THIOCYANATE

Guanidinium thiocyanate, a potent chaotropic agent, can be used in combination with a strong reducing agent, 2-mercaptoethanol and a detergent to prepare intact, biologically active RNA from tissues with high RNA content. Guanidinium thiocyanate lyses and solubilizes cells while rapidly inactivating RNase activity. The DNA released by this procedure is viscous, making RNA isolation difficult. This viscosity can be reduced by homogenization or passing the solution through a narrow gauge needle. Phenol extraction is used to deproteinate the nucleic acids. The RNA can then be collected by sequential ethanol precipitation (Chirgwin *et al.*, 1979) or by pelleting the RNA through a high-density CsCl (Okayama *et al.*, 1979) or cesium trifluoroacetate (CsTFA) gradient. The centrifugation methods are more commonly used since they effectively separate RNA from DNA in a single step (Gilsin *et al*, 1974). Furthermore, the procedure is simple and the recovery of RNA is essentially quantitative.

When extracting RNA from cells growing in a monolayer, wash the cells with cold PBS, aspirate and add the guanidinium thiocyanate solution directly to the plate (2 ml of solution per 100 mm plate). Collect the lysed cells, rinse the plate of residual cells with another 1 ml of guanidinium thiocyanate solution and combine the aliquots. Extraction of RNA from tissues is somewhat more difficult, since endogenous RNase is active as the sample is being processed. The pancreas and spleen contain particularly high levels of RNase, while the liver and intestine have relatively low levels. Use tissue as fresh as possible, cut it into small pieces (less than 1 gram each) and quick-freeze it in liquid nitrogen until you are ready to process it. Once the tissue is thawed, homogenize it in the guanidinium thiocyanate solution as quickly as possible. Below are two procedures for the isolation of RNA using guanidine thiocyanate. The first method employs a cesium chloride gradient for RNA purification, while the second method uses a cesium trifluoroacetate gradient.

PROCEDURE 2.11

GUANIDINIUM THIOCYANATE METHOD FOR RNA ISOLATION I

Reagents:
a) Phosphate buffered saline (PBS, Appendix A)
b) <u>4 M Guanidinium Thiocyanate Solution</u>
    Prepare 4 M guanidinium thiocyanate (Fluka purum grade) in 0.5% sodium N-lauryl sarcosine, 25 mM sodium citrate.
    Adjust the pH to 7.0 with 1 N NaOH.
    Filter out undissolved material through a 0.2 μm filter.
    The solution is stable only for a couple of days when stored at 4°C in a dark bottle and should be prepared fresh as needed.
    Immediately before use, heat the solution to 37°C, cool to room temperature and add 2-mercaptoethanol to 2%.
c) 10% sodium lauryl sarcosine
d) Phenol:chloroform:isoamyl alcohol (25:24:1)
e) 5.7 M cesium chloride (0.96 g/ml)
f) <u>MSE Buffer</u>
    5% 2-mercaptoethanol
    0.5% sarkosyl
    5 mM EDTA, pH 7.4
g) 25 mg/ml Proteinase K (Boehringer-Mannheim)
h) 100% ethanol
i) <u>TE Buffer</u>
    10 mM Tris-HCl, pH 7.6
    1 mM EDTA.

Procedure:
1. <u>For cultured cells</u>: Wash the harvested cells with cold PBS, centrifuge at 2,000 xg for 10 minutes at 4°C and resuspend the cell pellet in guanidinium thiocyanate solution (at 1×10^7 cells/ml.). Vortex the suspended cells and proceed to step 5.
    <u>For Tissues</u>: Mince the tissue in cold PBS into fine cubes with sterile scissors or scalpel.
2. Pellet the tissue fragments at 2,000 xg for 10 minutes at 4°C.
3. Resuspend the pellet in 5 ml of guanidinium thiocyanate solution per gram of cells and homogenize the tissue rapidly (2-3 short bursts for 10-15 seconds each) of a motor-driven homogenizer. Avoid generating excess heat or foam.
4. Remove the cellular debris by centrifugation at 2,000 xg for 10 minutes at 4°C. Using a pipette, carefully transfer the supernatant to a new 15 or 50 ml polypropylene tube and vortex.

5. Incubate the solution at 65°C for 10 minutes, then draw it into a syringe fitted with a 20 gauge needle. Forcibly eject the suspension back into the tube. Repeat the procedure 8-10 times to shear the high molecular weight DNA and reduce the viscosity of the solution.

6. Extract the sample with an equal volume of phenol:chloroform:isoamyl alcohol, (25:24:1). Centrifuge at 2,000 xg for 10 minutes at 4°C.

7. Extract the aqueous layer with chloroform:isoamyl alcohol (24:1). Centrifuge at 2,000 xg for 10 minutes at 4°C.

8. Remove the aqueous layer and place it on top of 3 or 6 ml of the 5.7 M CsCl solution in a SW41 or SW27 ultracentrifuge tube (Beckman), respectively. Balance the tubes (with guanidinium thiocyanate solution) and centrifuge at 20K for 20 hours, or 25K for 16 hours at 18°C, respectively. The DNA will collect as a band at the CsCl interface, while the RNA will form a clear to opaque pellet at the bottom of the tube

9. Aspirate the CsCl solution from the top. Change to a fresh pipette after the DNA band has been removed. Aspirate the remainder of the CsCl solution, keeping the pipette tip away from the RNA pellet so as not to disturb it.

10. Resuspend the pellet in 500 μl of TE buffer. Pipette up and down to dissolve the RNA. Extract the RNA solution with phenol:chloroform:isoamyl alcohol (25:24:1). Centrifuge for 10 minutes in a microfuge to separate the phases.

11. Collect the aqueous layer and add to it 1/10 volume of 2 M sodium acetate. Precipitate the RNA by adding 2 volumes of 100% ethanol and incubate for 1 hour at -20°C.

12. Pellet the RNA by centrifuging for 10 minutes in a microfuge. Wash the pellet with 70% ethanol. Centrifuge for 10 minutes in a microfuge.

13. Wash the pellet with 100% ethanol. Centrifuge for 10 minutes in a microfuge.

14. Dissolve the pelleted RNA in TE buffer (use 200 μl per 10^9 cells). Store in aliquots at -70°C.

PROCEDURE 2.12

GUANIDINIUM THIOCYANATE METHOD FOR RNA ISOLATION II

An alternative method for purifying RNA is to separate the RNA from the guanidinium thiocyanate solution by centrifugation on a cesium trifluoroacetate (CsTFA) density gradient. CsTFA is more water-soluble than CsCl and, unlike CsCl, it promotes the hydration and solubilization of both nucleic acids and proteins. This method promotes effective dissociation of protein from the nucleic acids so that when combined with guanidinium thiocyanate extraction, phenol extraction is not necessary.

Reagents:
a) CsTFA Solution
    1.51 g/ml CsTFA (Pharmacia cat. no. 17-0847-02)
    0.1 M EDTA, pH 7.0
b) TE buffer
    10 mM Tris-HCl, pH 7.5
    1 mM EDTA

Procedure:
1. Extract the cells as in Procedure 2.11, Steps 1 -3).
2. Pellet the cell debris at 5,000 xg for 20 minutes at 15°C. Carefully transfer the supernatant to a new tube, leaving behind the pelleted debris.
3. Add 8.5 ml of CsTFA solution per SW 28.1 tube (Beckman) and carefully layer 8 ml of the supernatant from step 2 on top. Use additional guanidinium thiocyanate solution to fill the tube, if necessary. Extracts from 0.1 - 0.5 g of tissue (or 1 -5x10^8 cells) can be processed in each SW 28.1 tube.
4. Centrifuge at 25,000 rpm at 15°C in a SW 28.1 rotor (or equivalent) for 24 hours (see Procedure 2.11, Step 8). The RNA will pellet to the bottom of the tube, while the DNA will collect in a band at the interphase.
5. Aspirate the liquid from the tube, being careful not to disturb the RNA pellet. Drain the tube by inverting on a paper towel for 5 minutes.
6. Suspend the RNA in 200 µl of TE buffer by pipetting up and down and transfer the RNA to a microfuge tube. Rinse out the centrifuge tube with an additional aliquot of TE buffer, if necessary and combine the aliquots. Heat the sample at 65°C for 10 minutes and vortex to dissolve the RNA.
9. Pellet the insoluble material by centrifugation for 10 minutes and transfer the clarified RNA solution to a new microfuge tube.
10. Ethanol-precipitate and redissolve the RNA as in Procedure 2.2.

PROCEDURE 2.13

UREA-LITHIUM CHLORIDE METHOD FOR EXTRACTION OF RNA

The urea-lithium chloride method for extracting RNA is yet another technique for the isolation of RNA from mammalian cells (Birnboim, 1988). It is somewhat simpler than the guanidinium thiocyanate methods (Procedures 2.11 and 2.12) and does not require phenol extraction (Procedure 2.10). The yield of total cell RNA is high (i.e., 25 µg per 10^6 fibroblasts), it is essentially free of DNA and ribonuclease and is suitable for hybridization assays.

This method uses a chaotropic extraction solution to solubilize total cellular RNA and inhibit ribonucleases, yet still allows deproteination with Proteinase K. Proteins are effectively removed by a single extraction. The soluble nucleic acids can then be precipitated with ethanol. The sample is concentrated early in the extraction procedure so that subsequent steps can be carried out in microfuge tubes. The LiCl precipitation step (Step 12) preferentially pellets the RNA while the DNA remains in solution. This small sample volume decreases RNA losses during processing and permits the convenient processing of multiple samples.

Reagents:
a) Phosphate buffered saline (PBS, Appendix A)
b) RES Buffer
    0.5 M LiCl
    1 M urea
    0.02 M sodium citrate
    2.5 mM CDTA (cyclohexanediamine tetraacetate, Sigma), final pH is 6.8.
    Filter solution and add sodium dodecyl sulfate to 0.25%. Store solution at room temperature.
c) LiCl/Ethanol (3:1)
    3 volumes of 5 M LiCl (filtered and autoclaved)
    2 volumes of 95% ethanol.
d) 25 mg/ml Proteinase K (Boehringer-Mannheim)
e) 2 M acetic acid
f) CCS Solution
    1 mM sodium citrate
    1 mM CDTA
    0.1% SDS, pH 6.8.
    Filter and store at room temperature.
g) 2 M sodium acetate
h) 100% ethanol
i) Phenol:chloroform:isoamyl alcohol (25:24:1)
j) TE buffer
    10 mM Tris-HCl, pH 7.5
    1 mM EDTA

Procedure:

1. *Monolayer Cultures*: For processing cells growing as a monolayer on plates, the plates are washed with cold PBS and the cells solubilized with 2 ml of RES buffer per 100 mm plate. Swirl the plates to allow the solution to completely cover the cells. Use a rubber policeman to scrape the cells from the plate. Transfer the cell lysate to a centrifuge tube. Rinse the plate with an additional 1 ml RES; pool the lysates.
   Suspended Cells: For cells in suspension, wash the cells with ice-cold PBS. Centrifuge the cells at 1,000 xg for 10 minutes and aspirate off most of the supernatant. Vortex the cell pellet in the residual volume of PBS

(about 20-50 μl) to obtain a suspension. Add RES buffer to the cell suspension to obtain a final suspension of 1×10^7 cells/ml.

2. Sonicate the solution at low power for 5-10 seconds or pass repeatedly (about 8-10 times) through a 20 gauge needle to shear the DNA and reduce the viscosity of the lysate.

3. Add Proteinase K to a final concentration of 100 μg/ml and incubate the reaction at 50°C for 30 minutes.

4. Cool on ice and add 1/10 volume of 2 M sodium acetate and 2 volumes of 100% ethanol. Incubate at -20°C for 20 minutes.

5. Pellet the nucleic acid by centrifuging at 2,500 xg for 10 minutes at 4°C. Drain the ethanol, being careful not to disturb the small pellet.

6. Dissolve the pellet in 0.5 ml RES buffer (for to $1-10 \times 10^7$ cells).
    Steps 7 and 8 are optional; see comments below.

7. Add Proteinase K to the redissolved pellet to a final concentration of 100 μg/ml and incubate at 50°C for 30 minutes.

8. Extract the sample with an equal volume of phenol:chloroform:isoamyl alcohol (25:24:1). Centrifuge in a microfuge for 10 minutes.

9. Extract the aqueous layer with an equal volume of chloroform. Centrifuge in a microfuge for 10 minutes.

10. Transfer the aqueous layer to a new tube. Add 1/10 volume of 2 M acetic acid and an equal volume of LiCl/ethanol (3:1). Mix and incubate overnight at 0°C.

11. Centrifuge in a microfuge for 10 minutes. Carefully drain off the supernatant.

12. Resuspend the pellet in 0.2 ml CCS solution. Add 1/10 volume sodium acetate plus 2 volumes ethanol. Incubate at -70°C for 5 minutes or -20°C for 15 minutes. Centrifuge in a microfuge for 10 minutes.

13. Resuspend the pellet in 100% ethanol. Centrifuge in a microfuge for 10 minutes.

14. Carefully remove the ethanol. Turn the tube upside down on a paper towel for about 5 minutes. Allow the tube to air-dry for 10-15 minutes to evaporate the remaining ethanol.

15. Dissolve the pelleted RNA in 100 μl of TE buffer.

Comments:

Steps 7 and 8 are optional and need only be carried out if large amounts of nuclease are present in the original sample or if a high purity RNA preparation is desired. The RNA obtained when these steps are omitted is still suitable for slot blot and northern blot analysis. Note that LiCl-precipitated RNA dissolves slowly. The extra ethanol washes help to remove LiCl and increase the solubility of the pellet. Care should be taken during these washes not to lose any of the pelleted material. Excessive ethanol washing can lower RNA yields.

PROCEDURE 2.14

PURIFICATION OF POLY (A⁺) RNA

In studying the expression of cellular genes, it may be useful to purify the messenger RNA (mRNA) from the total cellular RNA. Because a subset of mRNAs contain poly(A) tails, they can be isolated by chromatography on oligo(dT) cellulose columns. The poly (A)⁺ mRNAs bind to the oligo(dT) sequences on the column in the presence of high salt. Nucleotides and non poly(A)-containing nucleic acids are washed through the column, while the poly (A)⁺ mRNA is eluted with low salt (Aviv and Leder, 1972). Since poly(A)⁺ RNA represents only about 1% of the total cellular RNA (the rest being rRNA, tRNA and non-polyadenylated mRNA, such as histone mRNA), a significant enrichment of mRNA sequences can be realized by this purification step.

Reagents:
a)   Oligo(dT) cellulose (Pharmacia)
b)   Column Buffer
     500 mM KCl
     10 mM Tris-HCl, pH 7.8.

c)   2 M KCl
d)   10 mM Tris-HCl, pH 7.8
e)   100% ethanol

Procedure:
1.   Prepare an oligo(dT)-cellulose column by suspending 1 g of oligo(dT)-cellulose in 5 ml of column buffer. Load into a 2 ml disposable column (or use a siliconized glass pipette plugged with glass wool) and wash with 5-10 ml of column buffer. Do not allow the column to run dry during the procedure. The column capacity is 2 mg of total RNA or the RNA extract from up to 10^9 cells (1 g).
2.   Heat the total RNA solution (dissolved in TE buffer) to 70°C for 10 minutes to denature the RNA. Add 1/3 volume of 2 M KCl (final concentration is 500 mM KCl).
3.   Apply the RNA (up to 300 µl) to the oligo(dT) column.
4.   After the sample enters the column, close off the column for about 5 minutes to allow binding of the poly (A)⁺ RNA. With larger sample volumes, it may be necessary to collect the initial eluate and reapply it to the column to assure complete binding of the poly (A)⁺ mRNA. Collect the eluate and pass it through the column two more times to assure complete binding.
5.   Wash the column with 5-10 ml of column buffer.

6.   Elute the poly(A)⁺ RNA from the column using 4 - 0.5 ml aliquots of 10 mM Tris-HCl, pH 7.8. Collect each fraction into a separate tube.

7.   To each tube add 1/10 volume of 2M sodium acetate and 2 volumes of cold ethanol. Incubate at -70°C for 30 minutes or at -20°C overnight.

8.   Centrifuge the sample at 4,000 xg at 4°C. Aspirate off the ethanol and allow the pellet to air-dry for about 15 minutes.

9.   Dissolve the pellet in 100 µl of TE buffer per gram of original cells. Typical yields are 50-150 µg of poly(A)⁺ mRNA per gram of cells.

Extraction of Nucleic Acids from other Sources

STOOL

Diarrheal diseases are among the leading causes of morbidity and mortality worldwide. Many viruses and bacteria that infect the gastrointestinal tract can be recovered from fecal specimens. Among the viral infections that can be diagnosed by an examination of stool samples are infections by picornaviruses, adenoviruses and rotaviruses. Enteric adenoviruses (adenovirus types 40 and 41 of subgenus F) have been implicated as causes of gastroenteritis in infants (Uhnoo *et al*, 1984). Numerous enteroviruses including polio, the coxsackieviruses, echoviruses and hepatitis A virus inhabit the human alimentary tract (Melnick, 1982). Specimens for virus isolation are usually stool samples or rectal swabs and virus concentrations as high as 10^6-10^9 viral particles per gram of feces can be encountered.

Rotaviruses and Norwalk viruses are important etiological agents of human gastroenteritis and account for over 50% of acute diarrhea cases presenting to hospitals in tropical and temperate areas (Kapikian, 1976). These viruses also may be shed in stools in high numbers (up to 10^{10} particles per gram). Stools collected on day 3-5 following the onset of an illness are most likely to contain virus particles; samples collected after 1 week of onset rarely contain virus (Cukor, 1984).

Many of these viruses are difficult to analyze for a number of reasons. Viral culture methods are either not available or are very expensive. Electron microscopy is effective in demonstrating the presence of virus, but usually cannot be used to identify viruses. A number of ELISA assays have been developed for these viruses, but the assays cannot always differentiate between subtypes. For these difficult cases, DNA probes are finding increased usage.

Among the most common causes of bacterial enteritis are the pathogens: *Campylobacter*, *Salmonella* and *Shigella* species and in some geographic locations: *Yersinia enterocolitica*, *Clostridium difficile* and *Vibrio parchnolyticus* and enterohemorrhagic *E. coli.* (Rosenblatt, 1985). Many of these pathogens are not efficiently recovered from stool samples by laboratory culture methods. As a result, a variety of DNA probes for the detection of these and other bacterial pathogens in stool samples are becoming available to aid in the laboratory diagnoses (Lanata *et al.*, 1985; Sethabutr *et al.*, 1985). As the number of available DNA probes for viral and bacterial pathogens in stool continues to increase and methods for their use become further refined, their use in clinical diagnosis will increase dramatically. The two procedures below (2.14 and 2.15) describe how DNA can be recovered from stool samples for use in hybridization assays.

PROCEDURE 2.15

STOOL SPECIMEN PREPARATION I - DNA EXTRACTION

Reagents:
a) Phosphate buffered saline (PBS, Appendix A)
b) 10% SDS
c) 25 mg/ml Proteinase K (Boehringer-Mannheim)

Procedure:
1. Prepare a 10% suspension of feces in phosphate buffered saline (PBS).
2. Centrifuge at 400 xg for 30 minutes to clarify the suspension. Transfer the supernatant to a new tube.
3. To the clarified supernatant, add SDS to 1% and Proteinase K to 100 µg/ml. Incubate at 50°C for 1 hour.
4. Phenol-extract and ethanol-precipitate the nucleic acid as described in Procedure 2.1 and 2.2.

PROCEDURE 2.16

STOOL SPECIMEN PREPARATION II - DIRECT SPOT BLOTTING PROCEDURE

Reagents:
a) Denaturation Buffer
   0.1 M NaOH
   1 M NaCl
b) Neutralization Buffer
   1 M Tris-HCl, pH 7.2
   1 M NaCl
c) 2x SSC

Procedure:

1. Deposit 5 μl of clarified fecal supernatant (Procedure 2.15, steps 1 and 2) directly onto nitrocellulose membranes using a manifold device (Procedure 5.4).
2. Place the nitrocellulose membrane on a piece of filter paper soaked in denaturation buffer for 20 minutes to lyse the bacteria or virus and to denature the DNA.
3. Neutralize the membrane by transferring it to a filter paper soaked with neutralization buffer.
4. Wash the filter twice with 2x SSC for 20 minutes each.
5. Bake the filter at 68°C for 1 hour.
6. Proceed with hybridization (Procedure 5.12).

URINE

Many urinary tract (kidney, urethra and bladder) infections can be diagnosed by an examination of urine specimens (Kunin, 1972). Viruses such as mumps, adenovirus and cytomegalovirus are excreted in the urine during the incubation period of infection. Human cytomegalovirus (CMV) normally causes mild or asymptomatic infections in healthy individuals, but severe infections can occur among congenitally infected infants, or in immunocompromised patients, including those with acquired immune disease (Kinney *et al.*, 1985). Diagnosis of CMV is clinically difficult and usually requires isolation of the virus by tissue culture methods. Since antiviral therapy is available for the treatment of severe CMV infections, a rapid and sensitive detection method is essential to permit therapy to be administered early in infection and to monitor the level of infection during therapy.

Excretion of CMV is somewhat sporadic, often necessitating the examination of multiple urine specimens. Spot blot hybridization is one way to rapidly monitor the levels of CMV in urine (Augustine *et al.*, 1987). Another is the amplification of CMV DNA using the polymerase chain reaction (PCR). The PCR amplification method can be used directly on urine samples without the extraction of DNA (refer to Section 6 and Olive *et al.*, 1989). For the direct detection of CMV in urine, the urine is first clarified by low speed centrifugation and the virus is pelleted using an ultracentrifuge. The nucleic acid in the pellet (which would contain the viral particles, if they are present) is then extracted with phenol and ethanol-precipitated.

PROCEDURE 2.17

EXTRACTION OF CMV FROM URINE SAMPLES
(Spector *et al.* 1984; Lurian *et al.* 1986)

Reagents:
a) Phosphate buffered saline (PBS, Appendix A)
b) <u>Lysis Buffer</u>
    0.1 M NaCl
    10 mM Tris HCl, pH 8.0
    10 mM EDTA
    200 µg/ml Proteinase K
    0.5% SDS
c) Phenol:chloroform:isoamyl alcohol (25:24:1)
d) Chloroform:isoamyl alcohol (24:1)
e) 2 M sodium acetate
f) 100% ethanol
g) <u>TE Buffer</u>
    10 mM Tris-HCl, pH 7.6
    1 mM EDTA
h) <u>Denaturation Solution</u>
    0.3 M NaCl
    1.0 M NaOH
i) <u>Neutralization Solution</u>
    0.8 M Tris HCl, pH 6.8
    0 1 M NaCl.

Procedure:
1. Use a 1-3 ml sample of urine.
2. Adjust the sample volume to 8 ml with PBS.
3. Centrifuge the sample at 2,000 xg for 5 minutes.
4. Transfer the supernatant to a new tube.
5. Centrifuge the sample at 25,000 xg for 90 minutes at 4°C in an ultracentrifuge.
6. Discard the supernatant and resuspend the pellet in 20 µl of lysis buffer.
7. Incubate 37°C 1 hour.
8. Extract with equal volume of phenol:chloroform:isoamyl alcohol (25:24:1). Centrifuge in a microfuge for 10 minutes.
9. Extract with chloroform:isoamyl alcohol (24:1). Centrifuge in a microfuge for 10 minutes.
10. Transfer the aqueous layer to a new tube and add 1/10 volume of 2 M sodium acetate and two volumes ethanol. Centrifuge and wash as in Procedure 2.2.

11. Dissolve the pellet in 20 μl of TE buffer.
12. Add 20 μl of denaturation solution. Vortex briefly and incubate the solution at room temperature for 15 minutes.
13. Neutralize the sample with 40 μl of neutralization solution.
14. Apply the sample to a membrane by slot blotting (Procedure 5.1).

OTHER SAMPLES

In the diagnosis of viral or bacterial infections, specimens can also be collected from throat and nasopharyngeal swabs or washings, sputum, dermal lesions, or cerebrospinal fluid (Smith, 1986; Lenette, 1980). The bacteria- or virus-infected cells can then be cultured or concentrated by centrifugation for direct assays. Exfoliated cells from a cervical scrape, for example, can be collected by centrifugation in a microfuge to yield a pellet of 1-5 x 10^5 cells (Henderson et al., 1987).

Buccal cells can be isolated by diluting 0.5 ml saliva with 5 ml of 1x SSC and centrifuging at 2,000 xg for 10 minutes. The cell pellet is then rinsed three times with 1x SSC and resuspended to $1x10^4$ cells/ml.. The DNA can be extracted from these cells and spotted directly on nitrocellulose (Augustin et al., 1987), or the cells may be fixed on a microscope slide (Gupta et al., 1985).

The recent use of DNA fingerprinting analysis and the polymerase chain reaction has permitted identification of individuals by analyzing DNA extracted from forensic samples such as tissue, hair or blood stains (Caskey, 1987). The most common method of DNA analysis involves the examination of restriction fragment length polymorphisms (RFLPs), a method which requires microgram amounts of relatively undegraded DNA (> 5 kb). Intact DNA has even been obtained from 2-year-old dried blood stains on cloth. A spot from 1 ml of blood (about 45 mm) can yield about 40 μg of DNA and may be of sufficient quality to give interpretable DNA fingerprint patterns (Kanter et al. 1986). The blood-stained material is cut out or dried blood is scraped directly into DNA lysis buffer and processed as in Procedure 2.3.

Hairs are one of the most frequently found forms of biological forensic evidence. The DNA in hair is located in the root end and may contain only about 0.2-0.5 μg of DNA from freshly plucked hairs and even less from shed hairs. The DNA extracted from a freshly plucked single hair root has been successfully used in DNA fingerprint analysis with single-locus probes (Wong et al., 1987). With the additional step of PCR amplification, even small or degraded DNA samples from hair can be typed by analysis of the amplified DNA fragment length, by hybridization with allele-specific oligonucleotide probes and by direct DNA sequencing (Higuchi et al., 1988).

Preparation of Cells and Tissues for *In Situ* Hybridization

The presence of viral sequences or the expression of specific genes in specific cell types can be monitored by hybridizing to cells fixed on microscope slides, to detect the nucleic acid sequences *in situ* where they normally occur (Haas *et al.*, 1984). Fixation conditions are chosen to attach the cells to the microscope slide, to preserve the cellular morphology and to immobilize the nucleic acids (Moench *et al.*, 1985). Fixation is often carried out after mounting the cells on the slide but can also be done before application to slides.

Acid-washed slides are recommended for the *in situ* detection of RNA targets, although new, ethanol-washed slides are suitable for many applications. Tissue culture cells or isolated peripheral blood lymphocytes may be deposited onto slides using a cytospin centrifuge. This flattens the cells on the slide and aids their adhesion to the slide. Alternatively, cells may simply be suspended in PBS, applied onto the slide and air-dried. During air-drying, the cells should be in a monolayer and dried quickly in an isotonic solution such as PBS or tissue culture medium. Once dried, the cells must be fixed to stabilize their morphology and immobilize the cellular structures, including the nucleic acid. Many fixation procedures use protein denaturants such as methanol or ethanol to stabilize the cells. Solutions containing formaldehyde or glutaraldehyde act by cross-linking the proteins and nucleic acids, thereby immobilizing the cellular structures.

Cells may also be fixed in suspension, before they are mounted on the slide. This helps to retain the three-dimensional structure of the cell, is consistent and is generally easier to carry out. Pre-fixed cells, however, adhere poorly to the slides, so slide pretreatments are required to prevent the cells from washing off the slides during processing.

PRETREATMENT OF SLIDES BEFORE MOUNTING CELLS OR TISSUES

Slides used for *in situ* hybridization should be thoroughly cleaned and free of dust and grease before mounting samples. When detecting RNA targets or using RNA probes, acid washing of the slides is strongly recommended.

Because of the numerous steps and harsh treatments encountered during *in situ* hybridization, problems may occur with samples sloughing off the slides, particularly when formalin-fixed, paraffin-embedded tissues are used. The pretreatment of slides with 3-aminopropyl triethoxysilane (APES) in acetone (Maddox and Jenkins, 1987), poly-L-lysine (Pardue, 1985) or gelatin: chrome alum (Rogers, 1979) helps the tissues to adhere firmly to the slide. The APES treatment is optimal for formalin-fixed tissues, since it covalently binds the tissues to glass slides. For other applications, pretreatment of the slides with Denhardt's reagent (Denhardt, 1966) may help to block non-specific binding of the labeled probe during hybridization process.

PROCEDURE 2.18

ACID WASHING OF SLIDES

Reagents:
a)   1 N HCl
b)   DEPC-treated water (see Extraction of RNA)
c)   95% ethanol

Procedure:
1.   Immerse the slides in 1 N HCl for 30 minutes at room temperature.
2.   Rinse the slides with DEPC-treated water.
3.   Wash the slides with 95% ethanol.
4.   Air-dry the slides.
5.   Repeat Steps 1-4.

PROCEDURE 2.19

PRETREATMENT OF SLIDES WITH APES

Reagents:
a)   2% (v/v) 3-aminopropyl triethoxysilane (APES, Sigma Cat. No. A-3648) in acetone.
b)   Acetone
c)   DEPC-treated water

Procedure:
1.   Immerse the slides in the APES solution for 10 seconds.
2.   Wash the slides by immersing them in acetone.
3.   Wash the slides by immersing them in DEPC-treated water.
4.   Air-dry the slides.
5.   Store them at 4°C.

PROCEDURE 2.20

PRE-TREATMENT OF SLIDES WITH POLY-L-LYSINE

Reagents:
a)   100 µg/ml poly-L-lysine (Sigma)
b)   DEPC-treated water

Procedure:
1.   Immerse the acid-washed slides in the poly-L-lysine solution for 45 minutes at room temperature.
2.   Rinse the slides two times with DEPC-treated water
3.   Air-dry the slides overnight.
4.   Store the slides at 4°C.

PREPARATION OF CELLS FOR *IN SITU* HYBRIDIZATION

A variety of cell types can be attached to microscope slides for examination by *in situ* hybridization (Haas *et al.*, 1984). Anchorage-dependent tissue culture cells can be grown on microscope slides and remain attached until fixed. Non-adherent cells, on the other hand, require special handling to keep them attached to the slide until fixation. The simplest approach is to deposit the cells on slides in a small volume of buffer and allow the buffer to air-dry. The cells may also be centrifuged onto the slides and cytocentrifuges (Cytospin I and II) have been specially designed for this purpose. The centrifuging cells against the slide aids in their attachment.

In addition to urine, sputum, cerebral spinal fluid and other sources of loose cells, slides can also be prepared from biopsied tissues. One of the simplest techniques is to make an imprint of the tissue directly on the slide. Cells are deposited by pressing or smearing a freshly-cut tissue surface onto the slide or squashing a small piece of tissue (1-2 mm) between two slides. The slides are then air-dried and immediately fixed. The imprint, squash and smear methods are particularly suitable for the examination of soft tissues such as lymph node or nerve tissue. The disadvantage of these methods is that the tissue does not retain its histological structure. If well-preserved morphology is important, the use of tissue sections is required. Sections 3-6 µm thick are cut from frozen or formalin-fixed tissues and embedded in paraffin. Frozen material, sections are allowed to adhere to the slide for 10-15 minutes before fixation. Formalin-fixed paraffin-embedded sections stick poorly to slides, so the slides must be precoated with APES (Procedure 2.19) or another coating material.

FIXATION OF CELLS FOR *IN SITU* HYBRIDIZATION

The fixation conditions used to stabilize the target cells introduce certain constraints into the hybridization assay. Conditions must be chosen that preserve the morphological features of the cell or tissue while anchoring the nucleic acid sequences in such a way that they are not prevented from hybridizing with the labeled probe. In the case of non-radioactive probes, the fixation process must also not inhibit the diffusion of other molecules (streptavidin, antibodies, or enzymes) required to detect the hybrids. Two classes of fixatives are generally used for *in situ* hybridization: precipitating fixatives and cross-linking fixatives (Moench *et al.*, 1985; Haas *et al.*, 1984). Precipitating fixatives, such as ethanol, ethanol:acetic acid (3:1) or methanol, tend to distort the cellular morphology, but can result in high signal intensities since they leave large pores in the cellular structure. However, RNA is not well immobilized by precipitating fixatives and may wash away during processing. The precipitating fixative: ethanol:acetic acid (3:1), is very effective in preserving DNA and usually results in stronger hybridization signals than the use of cross-linking reagents such as formalin.

Cross-linking reagents such as formaldehyde, paraformaldehyde or glutaraldehyde firmly anchor the RNA or DNA to cells (Moench *et al.*, 1985). These fixatives cross-link proteins and alkylate the amino groups of bases in single-stranded nucleic acids. The resulting network is very effective in retaining the cellular morphology, but tends to hinder the diffusion of probes and detection reagents. An optimum degree of cross-linking and efficient detection of RNA sequences can be achieved by fixation in 4% paraformaldehyde for 1 minute and storage of slides in 70% ethanol (Lawrence and Singer, 1985). The fixation of tissue samples can be difficult to control because of the variation in sample thickness and the resulting over- or underfixation will lead to variable results. Good results can be achieved with tissue sections by using frozen sections and performing fixation after application of the tissue to the slide.

PROCEDURE 2.21

FIXATION IN ETHANOL:ACETIC ACID

Reagents:
a) Ethanol:Acetic Acid (3:1) v/v
   3 parts ethanol
   1 part glacial acetic acid
b) 95% ethanol

Procedure:
1. Fix the cells on the slides by incubation in ethanol:acetic acid (3:1) for 15 minutes on ice.

2.   Transfer the slides to 95% ethanol and incubate for 5 minutes at room temperature.
3.   Air-dry the slides about 15 minutes. Store them desiccated at -70°C, or in 70% ethanol at -20°C.

PROCEDURE 2.22

4% PARAFORMALDEHYDE FIXATION

Note: Paraformaldehyde is a carcinogen. Wear gloves and avoid breathing vapors. Make up the paraformaldehyde solution in a fume hood. Dispose of waste appropriately.

Reagents:
a)   Phosphate buffered saline (PBS, Appendix A)
b)   Paraformaldehyde (PFA; Sigma P-6148)
c)   70% ethanol

Procedure:
1.   Dissolve 4 g of PFA in 100 mls of PBS by warming the mixture to about 50-60°C for 30 minutes in a fume hood.
2.   Let the solution cool to room temperature and filter through Whatman #1 paper before use. Store at 4°C. The PFA Solution is not stable and should be made fresh the same day it is needed.
3.   Fix the slides in the 4% PFA solution for 1-5 minutes at room temperature.
4.   Wash the slides in PBS.
5.   Store the fixed slides in 70% Ethanol at -20°C.

PROCEDURE 2.23

FORMALIN FIXATION OF SLIDES

Note: Formalin is a carcinogen. Wear gloves and avoid breathing vapors. Make up the formalin solution in a fume hood. Dispose of waste appropriately.

Reagents:
a)   Formalin Fixation Buffer
     Mix 5 ml of formaldehyde plus 0.9 g of NaCl in 90 ml of water.
     Adjust the pH to 7.4.
     Bring up to 100 ml with water.
b)   70% ethanol
c)   80% ethanol
d)   95% ethanol.
e)   Xylene

Procedure:
1. Fix the slides in formalin fixation buffer for 4 hours at 4°C.
3. Rinse the slides in water.
4. Dehydrate the slides by successive washing (1 minute each) in 70% ethanol, 80% ethanol and 95% ethanol.
5. Wash the slides in xylene for 1 minute.
6. Allow the slides to air dry for about 15 minutes.
7. Wash the slides 2 times with 70% ethanol.
8. Store the slides at -20°C in 70% ethanol.

PREPARATION OF TISSUES FOR *IN SITU* HYBRIDIZATION

Tissues from infected animals or human biopsy or autopsy samples should be quickly frozen after isolation to minimize degradation of the nucleic acids. Thin sections of frozen tissue can be cut with a cryostat and picked up on pretreated slides. The sections are air-dried and fixed immediately after drying.

Various tissues can be used for the preparation of frozen sections. Heart, liver and skeletal muscle are easily cut, while lymph node, kidney and intestine are somewhat more difficult (Lum, 1986). The tissues that are most difficult to section when frozen are brain, testis and lung. A brief outline of the procedure is described in Procedure 2.21.

Tissues can also be preserved by formalin fixation and embedding in paraffin. This method is routinely used in histology labs because of the excellent morphological retention that can be achieved (McManus and Mowry, 1963). Formalin-fixed, paraffin-embedded tissues are conveniently stored at room temperature with no deterioration of cellular morphology. For these reasons, the vast majority of tissue samples available for study are prepared in this way. Although nucleic acid sequences are preserved, the extensive cross-linking introduced by the formalin fixation can make it difficult for the probes and detection reagents to diffuse into the tissue. Good results have been reported with formalin-fixed tissue by carrying out the appropriate pretreatments and post-treatments before hybridization. A procedure for formalin fixation and paraffin embedding of tissues is given in Procedure 2.25. The pretreatments and post-treatments required for *in situ* hybridization of cut sections on microscope slides are described in Section 5, *In Situ* Hybridization.

PROCEDURE 2.24

PREPARATION OF FROZEN TISSUE SECTIONS

Reagents:
a) CryoKwik (Damon)
b) Liquid nitrogen
c) Fixative (Procedures 2.23-2.25)
d) Cryostat

Procedure:

1. Precool a beaker containing CryoKwik in a liquid nitrogen bath. The CryoKwik should remain cold, but liquid.
2. Place the tissue sample on top of a cork and insert the cork into the top of the CryoKwik such that the tissue remains just above the level of the liquid.
3. As the tissue becomes partly frozen, immerse the entire tissue into the CryoKwik. This will freeze the tissue onto the cork.
4. The tissue can be stored frozen in liquid nitrogen or at -70°C.
5. Cut sections (3-4 μm thick) from the frozen tissue using a cryostat. Several sections can be cut at one time and held temporarily in the cryostat.
6. Use a fine brush to position the section on a pretreated microscope slide (Procedures 2.18-2.20). The section will stick to the slide as soon as it makes contact and should be placed onto the slide so that it lies perfectly flat.
7. Allow the sections to air-dry for 15-30 minutes at room temperature.
8. Fix the slides immediately after drying (Procedures 2.23-2.25).

PROCEDURE 2.25

FORMALIN FIXATION AND PARAFFIN EMBEDDING OF TISSUES

Reagents:

a) 10% Neutral Buffered Formalin
   100 ml 37-40% formaldehyde solution
   900 ml water
   4.0 g mono-sodium phosphate (monohydrate)
   6.5 g disodium phosphate (anhydrous)
b) Xylene
c) Paraffin (Paraplast)
d) 0.1 - 1.0 % Elmer's white glue
e) Microtome

Procedure:

1. Incubate the tissue (0.2-1g) overnight in 10% neutral buffered formalin.
2. Dehydrate the tissue in graded ethanol solutions (70%, 80% and 95%) for 1 hour each.
3. Immerse the tissue in xylene for 1 hour.
4. Immerse the tissue in melted paraffin (follow label directions) at 58°C for 1 hour.
5. Allow the paraffin to solidify to room temperature. The formalin-fixed, paraffin-embedded tissues can be stored indefinitely at room temperature.
6. Cut sections of 3-5 μm using a histology microtome.

7. Float the sections on 45°C distilled water containing 0.1%-1% Elmer's white glue (use higher glue concentrations if sections have a small surface area).
8. Pick up sections on pretreated microscope slides and fix slides for *in situ* hybridization (Procedures 22.1-22.3).
9. Incubate the slides at 37°C overnight.
10. Slides can be stored desiccated at 4°C for several months.

IN SITU HYBRIDIZATION ON CHROMOSOMES

In situ hybridization techniques can be used to determine the location of specific sequences on chromosomes and to examine the role of chromosomal aberrations in inherited diseases. For these applications, probes are hybridized to metaphase spreads of G-banded chromosomes and the chromosomal location of hybridization detected microscopically. Probes of high specific activity and high resolution detection systems are required for the analysis of single copy genes. Successful chromosomal analysis has been reported using ^{3}H-labeled probes (Schwab *et al.*, 1984). Similar results have been obtained using biotin-labeled DNA probes and an alkaline phosphatase-conjugated streptavidin detection system (Garson *et al.*, 1987). The major requirement for this type of analysis is good metaphase spreads of G-banded chromosomes. The following example illustrates the procedure on human peripheral blood lymphocytes.

PROCEDURE 2.26

PREPARATION OF METAPHASE SPREADS

Reagents:
a) RPMI medium (Sigma) containing 10% fetal bovine serum
b) Phytohaemagglutinin-P (Difco)
c) Vinblastine sulfate (Sigma).
d) 0.075 M KCl
e) Methanol:acetic acid (3:1)

Procedure:
1. Stimulate division of human peripheral blood lymphocytes by incubating the cells with medium containing phytohaemagglutinin (PHA). Use a concentration of 1-2x10^6 cells/ml in a T175 flask and a PHA concentration of 1% in RPMI medium plus serum. Incubate the culture for 2-5 days at 37°C in this PHA medium.

2. Replace the medium with fresh RPMI-10% fetal bovine serum containing 1 mg/ml vinblastine sulfate and incubate for 1 hour at 37°C.
3. Pellet the cells at 230 xg for 5 minutes and resuspend the pellet in a hypotonic KCl solution (0.075 M). Incubate the cells for 20 minutes at room temperature.
4. Pellet the cells at 230 xg for 5 minutes. Aspirate off the supernatant and fix the cell pellet in freshly prepared methanol:acetic acid (3:1) for 40 minutes at 4°C.
5. Pellet the cells at 230 xg for 5 minutes and resuspend the pellet in fresh methanol:acetic acid.
6. Repeat step 4.
7. Spread the chromosomes on an acid-cleaned glass slide. Allow the spreads to air-dry at room temperature for 15 minutes.
8. Store the slides desiccated at 4°C and use them for hybridization experiments within 2 weeks of preparation.

PROCEDURE 2.27

GIEMSA BANDING

Reagents:
a) PBS containing 1×10^{-7}% w/v trypsin (Worthington USA).
b) Giemsa Solution
   2% Giemsa (Gurr) in pH 6.8 phosphate buffer (Gurr; BDH #33199).
c) 95% ethanol
   80% ethanol
   70% ethanol
d) 100 µg/ml DNase-free RNase (Sigma) in 2x SSC.

Procedure:
1. Incubate the slides bearing metaphase chromosomes (Procedure 2.26) in the PBS-trypsin solution for 15-20 seconds at 37°C. Transfer the slides to a prewarmed PBS solution and incubate for 1 hour at 60°C.
3. Stain slides for 8 minutes with 2% Giemsa solution.
4. Destain the slides with 95% ethanol.
5. Wash with PBS.
6. Incubate the slides for 1 hour at 37°C in the DNase-free RNase solution.
7. Dehydrate the slides through a series of ethanol washes (70%, 80% and 95%) for 1 minute each before using for *in situ* hybridization.

References

1. Augustin, S., Popow-Kraupp, T., Heinz, F. and Kunz, C. (1987): Problems in detection of cytomegalovirus in urine samples by dot blot hybridization, J. Clin. Microbiol. **25**, 1973-1977.
2. Aviv, H. and Leder, P. (1972): Purification of biologically active globin messenger RNA by chromatography on oligothymidylic acid-cellulose, Proc. Natl. Acad. Sci. USA **69**, 1408-1412.
3. Berger, S. and Birkenmeir, C. (1979): Inhibition of intractable nucleases with ribonucleoside-vanadyl complexes: Isolation of messenger ribonucleic acid from resting lymphocytes, Biochemistry **18**, 5143-5149.
4. Birnboim, H.C. (1988): Rapid extraction of high molecular weight RNA from cultured cells and granulocytes for northern analysis, Nucleic Acids Res. **16**, 1487-1497.
5. Blobel, G. and Potter, V. (1966): Nuclei from rat liver. Isolation method that combines purity with high yield, Science **154**, 1662-1665.
6. Boyum, A. (1968): Separation of leukocytes from blood and bone marrow, Scand. J. Lab Invest. **21**: (Suppl. 97).
7. Brawerman, G., Mendecki, J. and Lee, S. (1972): A procedure for the isolation of mammalian messenger ribonucleic acid, Biochemistry **11**, 637-640.
8. Buffone, G. and Darlington, G. (1985): Isolation of DNA from biological specimens without extraction with phenol, Clin. Chem. **31**, 164-165.
9. Caskey , C.T. (1987): Disease diagnosis by recombinant methods, Science **236**, 1223-1229.
10. Chirgwin, J., Przybyla, A., MacDonald, R. and Rutter, W. (1979): Isolation of biologically active ribonucleic acid from sources enriched in ribonuclease, Biochemistry **18**, 5294-5290.
11. Cukor, G. and Blacklow, N.R. (1984): Human viral gastroenteritis, Microbiol. Rev. **48**, 157-179.
12. Denhardt, D. (1966): A membrane filter technique for the detection of complementary DNA, Biochem. Biophys. Res. Commun. **23**, 641-646.
13. Dyall-Smith, M. and Dyall-Smith, D. (1988): Recovering DNA from pathology specimens. A new life for old tissues, Molecular Biology Reports (Bio-Rad Labs) **6**, 1-2.
14. Favoloro, J., Treisman, R. and Karmen, R. (1980): Translation maps of polyoma virus-specific RNA: Analysis by two-dimensional nuclease S1 gel mapping, Meth. Enzymol. **65**, 718-749.
15. Garson, J.A., van den Berghe, J.A. and Kemshead, J.T. (1987): Novel non-isotopic *in situ* hybridization technique detects small (1kb) unique sequences in routinely G-banded human chromosomes: Fine mapping of N-myc and b-NGF genes, Nucleic Acids Research **15**, 4761-4769.
16. Glisin, V., Crkvenjakov, R. and Byus, C. (1974): Ribonucleic acid isolated by cesium chloride centrifugation, Biochemistry **13**, 2633-2637.
17. Gross-Bellard, M., Oudet, P. and Chambon, P. (1973): Isolation of high molecular weight DNA form mammalian cells, Eur. J. Biochem. **36**, 32-38.
18. Gupta, J., Gendelman, H., Nughashfar, Z., Gupta, P., Rosenshein, N., Sawada, E.,

Woodruff, J. and Shah, K. (1985): Specific identification of human papillomavirusus type in cervical smears and paraffin sections by *in situ* hybridization with radioactive probes: A preliminary communication, Int. J. Gynecol. Pathol. **4**, 211-218.

19. Haas, A., Brahic, M. and Stowring, L. (1984): in *Methods in Virology*, (eds. Maramorosch, K. and Koprowski, H.) Vol. 7. Academic Press, New York.

20. Henderson, B.R., Thompson, C.H., Rose, B.R., Cossart, Y.E. and Morris, B.J. (1987): Detection of specific types of human papillomavirus in cervical scrapes, anal scrapes and anogenital biopsies by DNA hybridization, J. Med. Virol. **21**, 381-393.

21. Higuchi, R., von Beroldingen, C., Sensabaugh, G. and Erlich, H. (1988): DNA typing from single hairs, Nature **332**, 543-546.

22. Jeffreys, A. J., Wilson, V., Thein, S. L., Weatherall, D. J. and Ponder, B. A. J. (1986): DNA fingerprints and segregation analysis of multiple markers in human pedigrees, Am. J. Hum. Genet. **39**, 11-24.

23. Kanter, E., Baird, B.S., Shaler, R. and Balazs, I. (1986): Analysis of restriction fragment length polymorphisms in deoxyribonucleic acid (DNA) recovered from dried bloodstains, J. Foren. Sci. **31**, 403-407.

24. Kapikian, A.Z., Kim, H.W., Wyatt, R.G., Cline, W.L., Arrobio, J.O., Brandt, C.D., Rodriguez, W.J., Sack, S.A., Chanock, R.M. and Parrott, R.H. (1976): Human reovirus-like agent as the major pathogen associated with winter gastroenteritis in hospitalized infants and young children, N. Engl. J. Med. **294**, 965-972.

25. Keller, G.H., Cumming, C.U., Huang, D.P., Manak, M.M. and Ting, R. (1988): A chemical method for introducing haptens onto DNA probes, Anal. Biochem. **170**, 441-450.

26. Kinney, J.S., I.M. Onorato, J.A. Stewart, R.F. Pass, S. Stagno, S.H. Cheeseman, J. Chin, M.L. Kumar, A.S. Yaeger, K.L. Herrmann, E.S. Hurwitz and L.B. Schonberger. (1985): Cytomegaloviral infection and disease, J. Infect. Dis. **151**, 772-774.

27. Kunin, C. (1972): *Detection, Prevention and Management of Urinary Tract Infections: A Manual for the Physician, Nurse and Allied Health Worker.* (Lea and Febiger, Philadelphia).

28. Lanata, C., Kaper, J., Baldini, M., Black, R. and Levine, M. (1985): Sensitivity and specificity of DNA probes with the stool blot technique for detection of *E. coli* enterotoxins, J. Infect. Dis. **152**, 1087-1090.

29. Lawrence, J. and Singer, R. (1985): Quantitative analysis of *in situ* hybridization methods for the detection of actin gene expression, Nucleic Acids Res. **13**, 1777-1799.

30. Lenette, E. (1981): *A User's Guide to the Diagnostic Virology Laboratory*, (University Park Press, Baltimore, MD).

31. Lum, J. (1986): Visualization of mRNA transcription of specific genes in human cells and tissues using *in situ* hybridization, Biotechniques **4**, 32-40.

32. Lurian, N., K. Thompson and S. Farrand. (1986): Rapid detection of cytomegalovirus in clinical specimens by using biotinylated DNA probes and analysis of cross-reactivity with herpes simplex virus, J. Clin. Microbiol. **24**, 724-730.

33. Maddox, P.H. and Jenkins, D. (1987): 3-Aminopropyltriethoxysilane (APES): A

new advance in section adhesion, J. Clin. Pathol. **40**, 1256-1260.

34. Mark, A., Trowell, H., Dyall-Smith, M. and Dyall-Smith, D. (1987): Extraction of DNA from paraffin-embedded pathology specimens and its use in hybridization (histo-blot) assays. Application to the detection of human papillomavirus DNA, Nucleic Acids Res. **15**, 8565.

35. McManus, J. and Mowry, R. (1963): *Staining Methods: Histological and Histochemical.* (Harper and Row Publishers, Inc., New York, N.Y.).

36. Melnick, J.L. (1982): Enteroviruses, In *Viral Infections of Humans, Epidemiology and Control*, (A.S. Evans, ed.), (New York, Plenum Medical Books) pp. 187-251.

37. Miller, R. and Phillips R. (1969): Separation of cells by velocity sedimentation, J. Cell Physiol. **73**, 191-196.

38. Murray, M. and Thompson, W. (1980): Rapid isolation of high molecular weight plant DNA, Nucleic Acids Res. **8**, 4321-4325.

39. Moench, T., Gendelman, H., Clements, J., Narayan, O. and Griffin, D. (1985): Efficiency of *in situ* hybridization as a function of probe size and fixation technique, J. Virol. Meth. **11**, 119-130.

40. Okayama, H., Kawaichi, M., Brownstein, M., Lee, F., Yokota, T. and Arai, K. (1987): High-efficiency cloning of full-length cDNA: Construction and screening of cDNA expression libraries from mammalian cells, Methods in Enzymology **154**, 3-27.

41. Olive, D.M., M. Simsek and S. Al-Mufti. (1989): Polymerase chain reaction assay for detection of human cytomegalovirus, J. Clin. Micro. **27**, 1238-1242.

42. Pardue, M., (1985): *In Situ* Hybridization in *Nucleic Acid Hybridization* (Hames, B. and Higgins, S. eds.), (IRL Press, Oxford).

43. Rodgers, A., (1979): *Techniques for Autoradioraphy*, (Elsevier, North Holland, Amsterdam).

44. Rosenblatt, J.E., (1985): Laboratory diagnosis of infectious diarrhea: a clinician's viewpoint, in *The Role of Clinical Microbiology in Cost-Effective Health Care*, (Smith, J.W., ed.), (College of American Pathologists, Skokie, Ill.) p 105.

45. Schwab, M., Varmus, H., Bishop, J., Grzeschnik, K., Naylor, S., Sakaguchi, A. Brodeur, G. and Trent, J. (1984): Chromosome localization in normal human cells and neuroblastomas of a gene related to c-*myc*, Nature **308**, 288-291.

46. Sethabutr, O., Echeverria, P., Hanchaly, S., Taylor, D.N. and Leksomboon, U. (1985): A non-radioactive DNA probe to identify *Shigella* and enteroinvasive *Escherichia coli* in stools of children with diarrhea, Lancet **ii**, 1095-1097.

47. Smith, T. (1986): Specimen requirements: Selection, collection, transport and processing, in *Clinical Virology Manual*, (Spector, S. and Lancz, G., eds.), (Elsevier, New York, NY) pp 15-29.

48. Spector, S., T. Rua, Spector, D. and McMillan, R. (1984): Detection of human cytomegalovirus in clinical specimens by DNA-DNA hybridization, J. Infect. Dis. **150**, 121-126.

49. Uhnoo, I., Wadell, G., Svensson, L. and Johansson, M.E. (1984): Importance of enteric adenoviruses 40 and 41 in acute gastroenteritis in infants and young children, J. Clin. Microbiol. **20**, 365-372.

50. Wong, Z., Wilson, V., Patel, I., Povey, S. and Jeffreys, A. (1987): Characterization of a panel of highly variable mini-satellites cloned from human DNA, Ann. Hum. Genet. **51**, 269-288.

Section 3:
Radioactive Labeling
Procedures

Introduction

Nucleic acids labeled with radioactive isotopes are employed as probes to analyze gene structure and function in the basic research laboratory and in the clinical laboratory as diagnostic tools for the identification of disease agents, genetic disorders or familial relationships. Radioactive probes coupled with autoradiographic detection provide the highest degree of sensitivity and resolution currently available in hybridization assays. However, considerations of user safety as well as cost and disposal of radioactive waste products limit the commercial applications of radioactive probes.

All forms of nucleic acid can be labeled with radioactive isotopes: double and single-stranded DNA, RNA and synthetic oligonucleotides. Although a chemical procedure for labeling DNA and RNA with radioactive iodine was the first method available for preparing probes of high specific activity (Commerford, 1971), the majority of current radioactive labeling procedures rely upon enzymatic incorporation of the labeled moiety into the probe DNA. This usually involves the incorporation of a nucleotide labeled with ^{32}P, ^{35}S, or ^{3}H into the DNA or RNA. These labeling procedures can be divided into those that result in uniformly-labeled probes and those that result in end-labeled probes. Uniformly-labeled probes can be made to higher specific activity than end-labeled probes since they can incorporate many labeled dNTP moieties per molecule. Uniformly-labeled nucleic acids are most commonly used as probes in hybridization analysis, whereas DNA sequencing is the major application for end-labeled nucleic acids.

GENERAL CONSIDERATIONS

The possession and use of radioactive materials is regulated by law and, thus, a license issued by a government regulatory agency is necessary before radioisotopes can be used. In addition, the use, storage and disposal of radioisotopes and radiolabeled compounds may also be regulated by local and institutional agencies.

71

Special precautions must be observed by individuals using procedures that involve radioactivity to prevent contamination of themselves, their co-workers, the work area and the environment. Protective gloves should always be worn when using radioactive materials and lab coats are essential to prevent contamination of clothing. To contain and facilitate the clean-up of any possible spills, bench tops should be covered with absorbant plastic-backed paper. If spills do occur, a solution of mild detergent and warm water can be used to decontaminate equipment, work surfaces and skin. Special chemicals are available (Count-Off, DuPont; Nuclean, National Diagnostics) to assist in the removal of radioactivity. All radioactive waste must be discarded into special containers (labeled with the universal symbol for radioactivity and the name of the isotope) that are disposed of in compliance with local and institutional regulations.

Radiochemicals require special handling and storage to maintain optimum activity. Refer to the Specifications or Technical Data Sheet enclosed with each radiochemical for specific information as to optimum conditions. In general, radiochemicals should be used as soon as possible. Prolonged storage results in decomposition due to nuclear decay and free radical generation. Keep the number of times a primary source container is opened at a minimum and re-close the source container immediately after use as exposure to oxygen and water vapor will increase the rate of radiodecomposition. For the same reason, clean pipettes or syringes should always be used when removing material from the source container to prevent contamination with chemical salts. Many radiochemicals become more sensitive to temperature-induced decomposition with prolonged storage and accumulation of impurities. Therefore, radionucleotides should not be allowed to sit at room temperature for extended periods of time. ^{35}S and ^{32}P-labeled nucleotides should be thawed rapidly; ^{3}H-labeled nucleotides should be thawed in a room-temperature bath.

The choice of the radioactive isotope depends upon the application, the labeling procedures to be used and the sensitivity and resolution desired (Table 3.1). Phosphorous-32 (^{32}P) is the most commonly used isotope to label nucleic acids for several reasons. ^{32}P has the highest specific activity (9,200 Ci/mmol in pure form) and emits ß-particles of high energy (1.71 MeV); therefore, probes prepared with this radionucleotide provide maximum sensitivity in the shortest time in most autoradiographic detection procedures. Because the structure of a ^{32}P-labeled nucleoside triphosphate is essentially identical to that of its non-radioactive counterpart, the use of ^{32}P-labeled nucleotides does not inhibit the activity of DNA-modifying enzymes. Nucleoside triphosphates labeled at either the a or g position (Figure 3.1) are available commercially and can be used to label DNA with the appropriate enzymes. In addition, ^{32}P-labeled nucleotides can be obtained at various specific activities ranging from 10-3,000 Ci/mmol for a-labeled precursors and up to 5,000 Ci/mmol for g-labeled precursors, allowing the preparation of probes of very high or lesser specific activity. Because of the

TABLE 3.1 Emission properties of radioisotopes used for labeling nucleic acid probes.

Isotope	Particle Emitted	E_{max} (MeV)	Half Life	Hybridization Applications	Comments
^{14}C	ß	0.155	5568 years		low sensitivity rarely used
^{3}H	ß	0.0118	12.3 years	*In situ*	low sensitivity high resolution
^{35}S	ß	0.167	87.4 days	filter *In situ*	high sensitivity good resolution
^{125}I	λ ß	0.035 0.035	60 days	*In situ*	high sensitivity high resolution
^{131}I	λ ß	0.365 0.608	8.6 days		high radiation rarely used
^{32}P	ß	1.71	14.2 days	filter	highest sensitivity

relatively short half-life (14.3 days) of ^{32}P, ^{32}P-labeled probes cannot be stored for extended periods of time and for optimum results, should be used within a week after preparation. In addition, ^{32}P-labeled probes, especially those labeled to high specific activity, should also be used as soon as possible after preparation because the high energy beta emissions may damage the structural integrity of the probe itself and decrease its usefulness.

Special precautions should be observed when working with ^{32}P-labeled nucleotides. Shielding material, e.g. 1/2 inch thick Lucite, should be used between the investigator and source containers or reaction vials, tubes, etc., that contain high levels of ^{32}P-labeled materials. The hands and face can receive a considerable dose of radiation from an open container of ^{32}P; therefore never work over an open source container. Avoid direct eye exposure by wearing safety glasses or a face shield. Be aware that airborne contamination in the form of aerosols or dust that lead to inhalation of ^{32}P can be generated by rapid boiling, expelling solutions through syringes, or failure to clean up spills. Personal external dosimetry badges should be worn by all persons using ^{32}P. Use a Geiger-Mueller detector to monitor work surfaces, hands and clothing for the possibility of spills during the course of the labeling procedure and prior to leaving the laboratory.

The beta emissions of ^{35}S have less energy (0.167 MeV) and the specific

FIGURE 3.1   Structure of a [^{32}P]Deoxynucleoside Triphosphate.   The alpha or gamma phosphate is replaced with a radioactive ^{32}P atom.

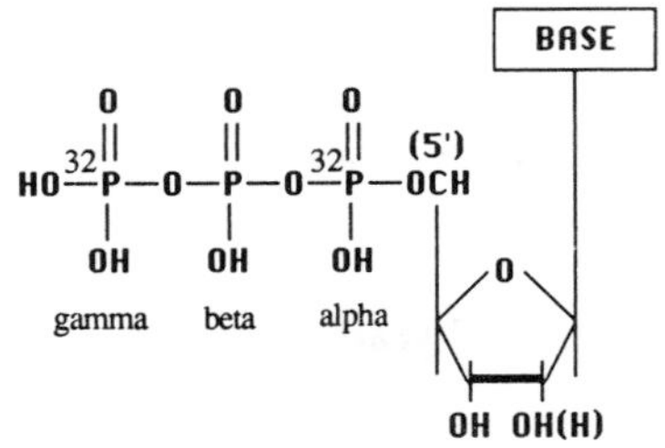

```
                                              BASE

        0       0       0
        ||      ||      ||   (5')
  HO—³²P—O—P—O—³²P—OCH
        |       |       |
        OH      OH      OH        O
      gamma    beta   alpha
                              OH OH(H)
```

activity (1,500 Ci/mmol in pure form) is approximately 6-fold lower than that of ^{32}P (Table 3.1). The lower energy of ^{35}S plus its longer half-life (87.4 days) make this radioisotope more useful than ^{32}P for the preparation of more stable, lower specific activity probes. These ^{35}S-labeled probes, although less sensitive, provide higher resolution in autoradiography and are especially suitable for *in situ* hybridization procedures. ^{35}S-labeled deoxynucleotides are commercially available at specific activities of 500-1,500 Ci/mmol; approximately one-third to one-half that of the commonly used 3,000 Ci/mmol ^{32}P-labeled deoxynucleotides. ^{35}S-labeled nucleotides contain a phosphorothioate group (P=S) in place of the phosphate group (P=O) at either the a or g position of the nucleotide (Figure 3.2). This change in nucleotide structure may inhibit the activity of certain enzymes. For example, it has been reported that DNA polymerase I incorporates a-phosphorothioate deoxynucleotide derivatives into DNA at a reduced rate (Vosberg and Eckstein, 1977). However, the nucleotide phosphorothioates (^{35}S) are suitable substrates for DNA and RNA polymerases, kinases, phosphatases as well as numerous other enzymes and can directly replace the ^{32}P-labeled analogs without procedural changes to the experimental protocols. These procedures permit the synthesis of high specific activity probes labeled with ^{35}S. Furthermore, the sixfold longer half-life of ^{35}S (relative to ^{32}P) and the inherent resistance of thiophosphodiester linkages in DNA to degradation by phosphatase significantly increase the useful life ot DNA probes labeled with ^{35}S (Vosberg and Eckstein, 1977).

^{35}S-labeled nucleotides present little external hazard to the user. The low energy beta particles barely penetrate the upper dead layer of skin and are easily contained by laboratory tubes and vials. Therefore, internal exposure from inhalation or ingestion of gaseous sulfur by-products is the major hazard. To minimize exposure, a chemical fume hood equipped with special filters should be used when opening source containers or working with large quantities of ^{35}S-labeled radiochemicals. A Geiger-Mueller survey meter can be used to monitor work surfaces and clothing for ^{35}S contamination but with significantly less sensitivity than is obtained for ^{32}P.

FIGURE 3.2 Structure of a [^{35}S]Deoxynucleoside Triphosphate. The oxygen of the alpha or gamma phosphate is replaced with a radioactive ^{35}S atom (phosphorothioate group).

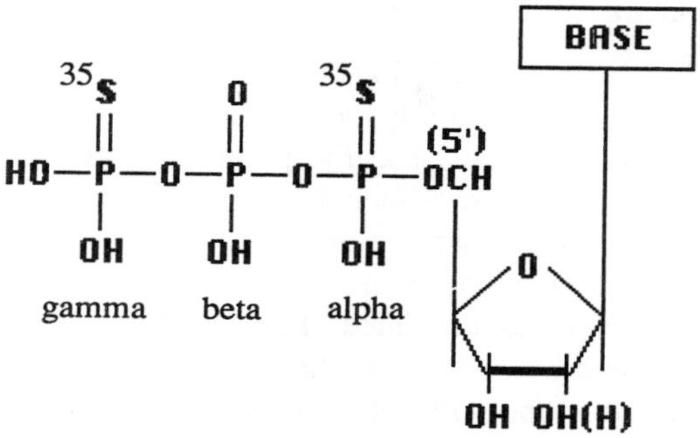

```
                                          ┌──────────┐
         35                 35            │   BASE   │
           S     O            S           └────┬─────┘
           ‖     ‖            ‖    (5')         │
     HO—P—O—P—O—P—OCH                          │
           │     │            │                 │
          OH    OH           OH           O
                                        /   \
       gamma   beta        alpha       /     \
                                      └──┬──┬──┘
                                        OH OH(H)
```

Tritium (^{3}H) has the lowest specific activity (29 Ci/mmol in pure form), the lowest energy ß-particle emissions (0.019 MeV) and the longest half-life (12.3 years) of the radioactive isotopes routinely used for probe preparation. The low specific activity of ^{3}H-labeled probes is too weak for most autoradiographic detection procedures. Although extended periods of exposure are required, ^{3}H-labeled probes have traditionally been used for *in situ* hybridization because the low energy results in maximum resolution with low background. Because the beta energy of ^{3}H is so low, it cannot penetrate the outer layer of skin. Internal exposure to ^{3}H through spills and vaporization presents the major hazard. ^{3}H cannot be detected with a Geiger-Mueller survey meter; surface wiping followed by liquid scintillation counting is the only method available to monitor this radionucleotide.

^{125}I and ^{131}I were widely used in the 1970s to label DNA and RNA by a chemical method developed by Commerford (1971). Because of the hazards associated with the use of radioactive iodine, labeling with radioiodinated nucleic acids declined with the availability of ^{125}I-labeled nucleoside triphosphates of high specific activity. ^{125}I is preferred over ^{131}I, because of its lower energies of emission and longer half-life. Both isotopes emit ß-particles and g-radiation and, thus, can provide both high sensitivity and high resolution by autoradiographic detection. The g-particles penetrate X-ray film readily, without efficient silver grain production. They can, however, be detected by the use of an intensifying screen, giving rise to strong, although somewhat diffuse, signals. Because the low energy b-particles are stopped entirely in the emulsion and give extremely high resolution, ^{125}I-labeled probes are frequently used for *in situ* hybridization. Use of plexiglass shields is recommended to provide a screen against the low energy g (and b) emissions when working with ^{125}I. The Geiger-Mueller survey meters do not efficiently monitor ^{125}I emissions and special detection equipment is required.

Labeling of DNA by enzymatic modification

NICK-TRANSLATION OF DNA

Nick-translation (Rigby *et al.*, 1977) is a rapid, easy and relatively inexpensive method for producing uniformly radiolabeled DNA of high specific activity. It is used to prepare sequence-specific probes for screening libraries, genomic DNA blots and RNA blots. Although double-stranded DNA in any form can be used for nick-translation when using recombinant plasmid probes, the probe insert is typically cut out with restriction endonucleases, purified by gel electrophoresis and nick-translated. Purified DNA fragments are essential for screening genomic DNA or cDNA libraries if there is a possibility that vector sequences in the probe will hybridize with the vector used to construct the library. In addition, more specific probes can be produced with purified DNA fragments because 100% of the DNA labeled will represent the sequences of interest. This leads to reduced background signals in the hybridization reactions. For some applications, it is unnecessary to purify the fragment from the plasmid or phage vector. The labeled DNA product of nick-translation has an average size of 600 nucleotides and should yield ^{32}P-labeled or ^{3}H-labeled DNA of up to 10^9 and 10^8 cpm/µg, respectively, under conditions where 30-60% of the deoxynucleoside triphosphate (dNTP) is incorporated.

The mechanism of nick-translation involves the combined activities of DNase I and the 5'->3' polymerase and 5'->3' exonuclease activities of *E. coli* DNA polymerase I (Rigby *et al.*, 1977). DNase I randomly introduces a single-stranded break (nick) in double-stranded DNA to create a free 3'-hydroxyl group. The 5'->3' exonuclease activity of DNA polymerase removes one or more bases at the 5' phosphoryl side of this nick. Simultaneously, DNA polymerase I catalyzes the incorporation of a nucleotide to the 3'-hydroxyl termini thus filling the gap. The nick will have been shifted along by one nucleotide in a 3' direction so that this 3' shift or translation of the nick will result in the sequential addition of new nucleotides. If radiolabeled dNTPs are incorporated in this reaction, the DNA fragment becomes labeled throughout to a uniform specific activity (Figure 3.3). Nick-translation can be used to prepare research quantities of probe quickly and efficiently and can be used for labeling both circular and linear double-stranded DNA templates. Single-stranded nucleic acids can not be labeled by this procedure.

The degree of DNase I activity is critical for optimal nick-translation; too little nicking leads to inefficient incorporation of label whereas too much nicking results in DNA fragments that are too short to be useful. However, by careful adjustment of the DNase I concentration, it is possible to obtain either probes of high specific activity and reduced length or high molecular weight probes with lower specific activity. The appropriate dilution of DNase I should be determined

FIGURE 3.3 Nick-Translation of DNA. Double-stranded DNA is subjected to limited DNase I digestion and incubated with DNA polymerase I in the presence of an [a-^{32}P]dNTP precursor. The polymerase primes DNA synthesis at the nick and incorporates the isotope into a newly synthesized chain in the 5' to 3' direction, while the 3' to 5' exonuclease digests the preexisting strand. Following denaturation, the salts, enzyme and unincorporated radionucleotides are removed from the ^{32}P-labeled probe.

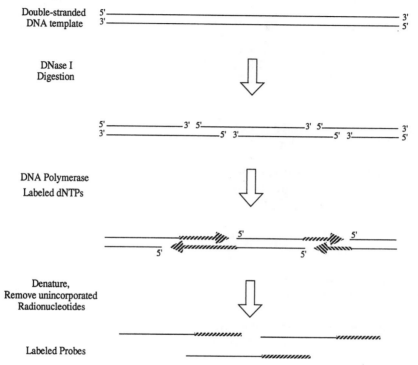

empirically for each batch of DNase I. Under optimal condition, 30-40% incorporation of the labeled nucleotides should occur within 15-45 minutes. The procedure described here makes the assumption that a 1:10,000 dilution of DNase I will yield average length (600 base pair) DNA probes of average specific activity (10^8 cpm/μg DNA) in a time period of approximately 1 hour. This assumption is adequate for preparation of radiolabeled probes for use in the majority of DNA hybridization procedures.

Nick-translation is usually carried out with one or more labeled dNTPs with the other dNTPs being unlabeled. For most applications, a single dNTP, usually [a-^{32}P]dCTP (>3,000 Ci/mmol) is used. The use of more than one labelled dNTP leads to higher specific activity of probes, but these probes are less stable and more expensive to produce. Alternatively, [a-^{35}S]dNTP can also be used for nick-translation reactions although the level of incorporation of these radiolabeled nucleotides may be decreased (Vosberg and Eckstein, 1977). Tritium-(^{3}H-) labeled dNTPs can also be incorporated into DNA probes by nick-translation but the specific activity of these probes is very low. Commercial kits for nick-translation are widely available.

PROCEDURE 3.1

LABELING OF DNA WITH RADIOACTIVE NUCLEOTIDES BY NICK-TRANSLATION

Reagents:
   (Refer to Appendix A for stock solutions)
a)   10x Nick-Translation Buffer
      200 mM Tris-HCl, pH 7.4
      50 mM MgCl$_2$
      100 mM 2-mercaptoethanol
      1 mg/ml nuclease-free bovine serum albumin, fraction V (BSA)
b)   10x dNTP Minus dCTP
      1 mM dATP
      1 mM dGTP
      1 mM TTP
c)   STOP Buffer
      200 mM NaCl
      10 mM Tris-HCl, pH 7.4
      11 mM EDTA
      0.5% sodium dodecylsulfate (SDS)
d)   DNA Polymerase I: use as obtained from supplier.
e)   DNase I
      DNase I (BRL) is available at concentrations of 2,000 to 3,000 U/mg protein in lyophilized form. A stock solution of DNase I at a concentration of 1 mg/ml should be prepared, aliquoted into 10 µl volumes and stored frozen to prevent loss of enzyme activity. For storage at -20°C in liquid form, dissolve DNase I in a solution of 20 mM Tris-HCl, pH 7.5/1 mM MgCl$_2$/50% glycerol. For storage at -70°C, dissolve DNase I in the Tris-MgCl$_2$ solution omitting the glycerol. Quick-freeze the aliquots on dry ice. DNase I stored in this manner should be thawed on wet ice and discarded after use. To minimize denaturation, DNase I should be dissolved without vortexing. In both forms, the DNase I stock solutions should be stable for one year.
f)   Yeast tRNA (Sigma) - 10 mg/ml

Procedure:
Keep all components on ice until all additions are made.
1.   Combine: 2.5 μl 10x dNTP minus dCTP

2.5 μl ₁0x nick-translation buffer

10 μl [a-³²P]dCTP (3,000 Ci/mmol) contains 100 μCi

1 μl DNase I contains 100 pg. Dilute 1 mg/ml stock 1:10,000 in 10

mM Tris, pH 7.5, 5 mM MgCl₂ immediately before use.

1 μl DNA polymerase I (5-15 U)

0.25 μg DNA template

Sufficient water to bring volume to 25 μl
2.   Mix components and incubate between 12°C to 15°C for 1.5 to 3 hours.
3.   Stop the reaction by adding 175 μl of STOP Buffer.

Comments:

   To generate probes of slightly lower specific activity, 25 μCi of 800 Ci/mmol [a-³²P]dCTP can be used. Lower specific activity probes are useful for most purposes and are less expensive to produce. This reaction can be scaled up or down depending upon the quantity of probe desired. However, it is essential to maintain the relative concentrations of DNA, [a-³²P]dATP, enzymes and unlabeled nucleotides listed above to obtain an efficient reaction.

   Poor incorporation of radiolabeled nucleotides into the probe may be caused by:

   1) Radiochemical decomposition of the labeled nucleotide.
   2) Decreased DNase I or DNA Polymerase I activity due to improper storage and/or handling.
   3) Impurities present in the substrate DNA.
   4) Too low a concentration of the labeled dNTPs.

OPTIMIZATION OF DNASE I DIGESTION

To obtain the highest specific activity probes by nick-translation, it is necessary to optimize the nick-translation reaction with regard to time and amount of DNase I for each stock of DNA polymerase. The appropriate dilution of DNase I is critical in controlling the size and specific activity of the labeled product. Parallel nick-translation reactions are set up in which various amounts (typically 50-100 pg/μl) of the DNase I stock are added. One microliter samples of the nick-translation reaction are removed prior to the addition of DNase I (0 time) and at 30-minute intervals thereafter to a maximum of 3 hours. The samples are analyzed for total counts and for counts incorporated into DNA by trichloroacetic acid precipitation as described in Procedure 3.7. Maximum incorporation of 40-50% of the total counts should occur within 60-90 minutes and plateau after this point. Having established these parameters, all subsequent nick-translation reactions using these stock solutions should be carried out with the optimized concentration of DNase I for the appropriate time.

A mixture of DNase I and DNA polymerase I in 50% glycerol is commercially available. This mixture has been titrated by the manufacturer (BRL) to provide optimum incorporation of labeled nucleotides.

LABELING DNA BY RANDOM PRIMING

This procedure for labeling DNA fragments using oligonucleotide primers and the Klenow fragment of *E. coli* DNA polymerase I was developed by Feinberg and Vogelstein (Feinberg and Vogelstein, 1983; Feinberg and Vogelstein, 1984) as an alternative to nick-translation to produce uniformly-labeled probes. Random priming offers a number of advantages over nick-translation:

1. Using [a-^{32}P]dCTP with a specific activity of 3,000 Ci/mmol, DNA probes with a specific activity greater than 1×10^9 cpm/µg can be routinely obtained in a 30 minute reaction.
2. More than 50% of the input radiolabeled nucleotide is incorporated into the DNA probe.
3. Because the input DNA is not degraded during the reaction, less than 200 ng of DNA is required for the random priming reaction and as little as 10 ng can be effectively labeled.
4. The length of the DNA fragment does not influence the reaction; therefore, small DNA fragments (100 base pairs) can be labeled as efficiently as large DNA fragments.
5. The label is incorporated equally along the entire length of the input DNA.
6. The labeled probe can be used without removal of unincorporated nucleotides.
7. Random primed probes are typically longer than those made by nick-translation when using large DNA templates, especially if the DNA template was overdigested with DNase I.
8. Both double and single-stranded DNA can be used as template for random priming.
9. Random priming can be used for smaller DNA fragments (100-500 bp), whereas nick-translation works best with longer ones (>1,000 bp).
10. Titration of DNase I activity is not necessary so that more consistent probes can be made with a variety of templates.

The major disadvantages of this procedure are that lower quantities of probe are produced than by nick-translation and circular DNA is not efficiently labeled by this method, and must first be linearized by restriction endonuclease digestion or nicked with DNase I or by alkali.

In this procedure, random sequence hexanucleotides are hybridized to the heat-denatured double-stranded or a single-stranded template at multiple sites along the DNA (Figure 3.4). The 3'-hydroxyl termini of the hexanucleotides

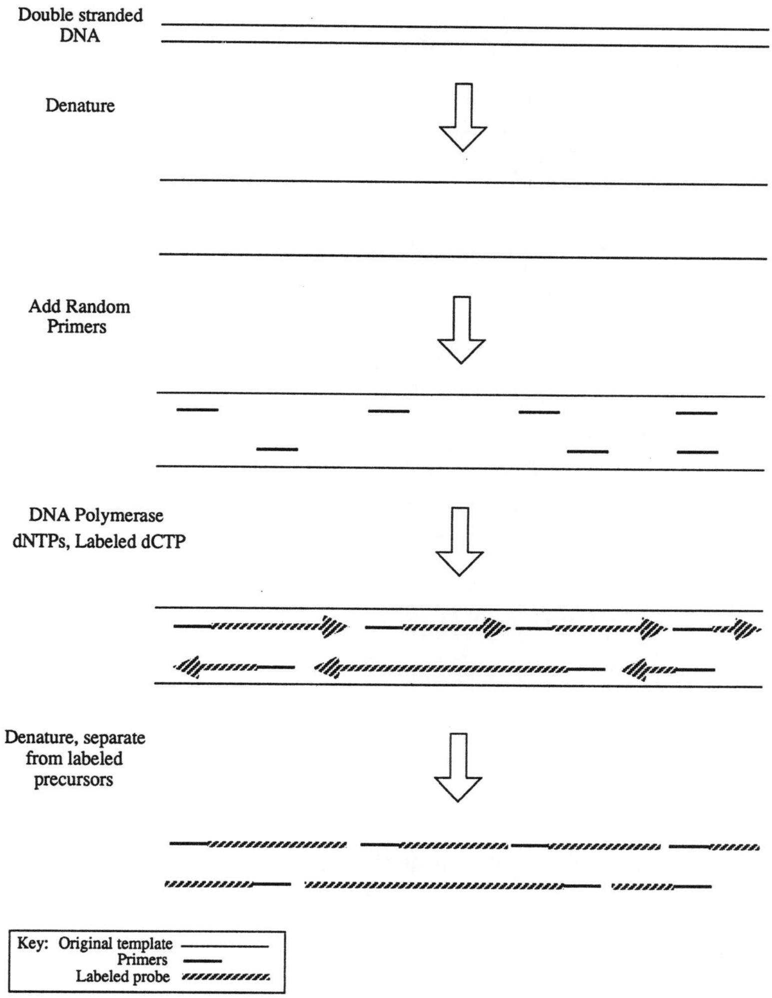

FIGURE 3.4 Random Primer Labeling of DNA. Double-stranded DNA is denatured and annealed with random oligonucleotide primers (6-mers). The oligonucleotides serve as primers for the 5' to 3' polymerase which synthesizes labeled probes in the presence of an [a-^{32}P]dNTP precursor.

serve as primers for the 5'->3' polymerase activity of the Klenow fragment of DNA polymerase I (Klenow *et al.*, 1971). When radiolabeled deoxynucleotides are present in the reaction mixture, the hexanucleotide primers are extended to generate double-stranded DNA that is uniformly radiolabeled on both strands. Because the Klenow fragment lacks the 5' to 3' exonuclease activity, its use in primer extension avoids loss of incorporated label. The 3' to 5' exonuclease activity is greatly diminished by the use of a pH 6.6 buffer, permitting synthesis of highly labeled probes. Using this method, more than 60% of the radiolabeled nucleotide can be incorporated to produce probes with specific activities greater than 10^9 cpm/μg of DNA. For random priming, [a-^{35}S], [a-^{32}P]-, [5, 5' ^{3}H]- and [5'-^{125}I]iodo-deoxynucleoside triphosphates can be used. However, [a-^{35}S]dNTPs are incorporated by DNA polymerase I at a reduced rate (Vosberg and Eckstein, 1977).

The mixture of short deoxynucleotides originally used for random priming (Feinberg and Vogelstein, 1983) was generated by pancreatic deoxyribonuclease digestion of calf thymus DNA. Recently, mixtures of synthetic hexamers in which every possible sequence combination is equally represented have become commercially available (IBI) for use as primers.

PROCEDURE 3.2

LABELING OF DNA WITH RADIOACTIVE NUCLEOTIDES BY RANDOM PRIMING

Reagents:
a) 10x DNA Polymerase I (Klenow fragment) Buffer
    500 mM Tris-HCl, pH 6.6
    100 mM MgCl$_2$
    10 mM DTT
    0.5 mg/ml nuclease-free bovine serum albumin, fraction V (BSA)
b) 10x dNTP minus dCTP
    0.5 mM dATP
    0.5 mM dGTP
    0.5 mM TTP
c) Random hexanucleotides, use as obtained from supplier
d) Large fragment of *E. coli* DNA polymerase I, use as obtained from supplier
e) 0.5 M EDTA
f) Yeast tRNA (10 mg/ml)
g) TE Buffer
    10 mM Tris-HCl, pH 7.6
    1 mM EDTA

Procedure:

1. Keep all components on ice until all additions are made.
2. Prepare DNA template: Plasmid DNA must be linearized by digestion with an appropriate restriction endonuclease prior to denaturation. Purify the DNA fragment by gel electrophoresis or ethanol precipitate the DNA to remove Mg^{++} ions that inhibit DNA denaturation.
3. Combine 30-100 μg of the DNA fragment with 1-5 μg of the random hexanucleotides. Place in a boiling water bath for 2 minutes and immediately transfer to wet ice to cool. Supercoiled plasmid DNA should be denatured in a boiling water bath for 15 minutes and immediately placed on ice to cool before addition of the hexanucleotide primers.
4. Centrifuge the reaction tube in a microfuge for a few seconds to collect the DNA solution as a single drop in the bottom of the tube. Return the tube to ice.

   Combine: 2.5 μl 10x dNTP minus dCTP
   2.5 μl 10x Klenow buffer
   5 μl [a-^{32}P]dCTP (3,000 Ci/mmol) = 50 μCi
   1 μl Klenow fragment (3-8 U)

5. Add the reaction mix to the denatured DNA. Adjust the reaction volume to 25 μl with water. Mix briefly.
6. Incubate the mixture at room temperature for 1-2 hours.
7. Stop the reaction by adding 1 μl of 0.5 M EDTA and dilute the reaction mixture to 100 μl with TE buffer.
8. Separate the labeled DNA from unincorporated radioactive precursors by standard column chromatography or chromatography through centrifuged columns as described under Purification of Radiolabeled Probes in this Section.
9. Ethanol-precipitate the labeled DNA probe fragments if desired, and determine the specific activity as described in Procedure 3.7.

SYNTHESIS OF PROBES FROM M13 TEMPLATES

Specific single-stranded radiolabeled probes can be made by first cloning the sequence of interest into an M13 bacteriophage vector (Hu and Messing, 1982). For cloning the DNA, it is convenient to use M13 vectors such as M13mp18 or M13mp19 (BRL, Promega, Pharmacia) containing the Multiple Cloning Site (MCS) sequence. DNA fragments to be cloned are first cut with restriction enzymes and ligated into the corresponding sites of the MCS in M13 using standard cloning techniques (Maniatis *et al.*, 1982). The purified single-stranded phage DNA is isolated and used as the template for generating probes. A synthetic oligonucleotide primer complementary to the region of the M13 just

FIGURE 3.5 Synthesis of Probes from M13 primers. The probe sequence is cloned
into an M13 vector at the Multiple Cloning Site (MCS). The vector is linearized with
the appropriate restriction enzyme, denatured and annealed with either an upstream
or downstream M13 primer depending on the desired polarity of the probe. In the
presence of the Klenow fragment of DNA polymerase I and an [a-^{32}P]dNTP, labeled
probes of defined size and polarity are synthesized.

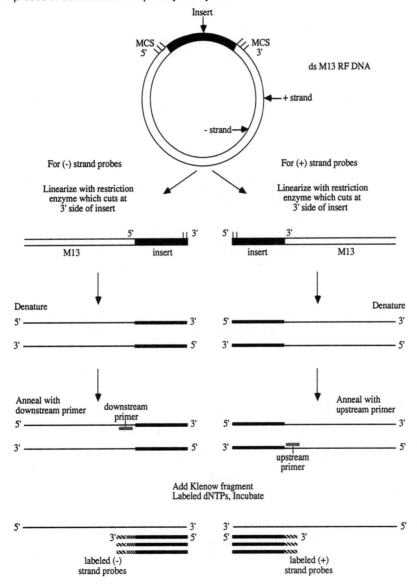

upstream of the insert (5' side) is annealed to the template and incubated in the presence of *E. coli* DNA polymerase I Klenow fragment and [a-^{32}P]dNTPs. The product of this reaction is a labeled single-stranded DNA complementary to the sequence in the phage DNA. Since this procedure generates strand specific probes, care must be taken to assure that the sequence of interest is inserted in the proper orientation. If a probe for mRNA is required, a (+) strand orientation in the clone will produce (-) strand labeled probes which will hybridize to the mRNA.

Probes of either strandedness can also be produced from the double-stranded RF form of the M13 clone containing the sequence of interest. In this case, primers complementary to the plus strand of phage DNA at the 5' side of the insert can be used to prime the synthesis of the insert strand in one orientation (Figure 3.5). For synthesis of the opposite orientation, primers complementary to the minus strand at the 3' side of the insert are used. The DNA is first linearized by digestion with restriction enzymes which will cut the double-stranded M13 DNA near the insert at the opposite end used for priming. The DNA and primers are mixed, denatured and used for synthesis of probes as described above. M13 primers are commercially available (BRL).

DNA probes generated by the nick-translation or random priming can self-anneal, limiting their available concentration for hybridizing to the target sequence. The asymmetric DNA or RNA transcripts (from M13 or pSP6 vectors, respectively, see Radiolabeled RNA Probes) do not self-anneal, so the entire labeled probe is available for hybridization, giving rise to increased sensitivity.

RADIOLABELED RNA PROBES

Radiolabeled RNA probes of high specific activity can be made from DNA sequences cloned into one of the commercially available transcription vectors. These constructs contain an RNA promoter site for the SP6, T3, or T7 RNA polymerases adjacent to a multiple cloning site into which the desired sequence can be inserted. The Riboprobe Gemini vectors, for example, pGEM-3 and pGEM-4 (Promega) provide a convenient transcription system for generating RNA probes of either (+) or (-) orientation from a single construct (Figure 3.6). These vectors contain both the SP6 and T7 RNA polymerase promoters flanking the multiple cloning site from pUC19. Following insertion of the desired sequence into the multiple cloning site, a simple color selection scheme based on inactivation of the lac Z a-peptide facilitates the screening for recombinants (Palazzolo and Meyeroivitz, 1987). The addition of the SP6 or T7 RNA polymerase in an *in vitro* transcription system in the presence of radiolabeled nucleotide triphosphate precursors allows the run-off of multiple copies of the DNA insert into labeled RNA probes from either direction (i.e. 'sense' or 'anti-

FIGURE 3.6 Synthesis of RNA Probes from Cloned DNA. The DNA sequence to be transcribed is cloned into an appropriate vector containing RNA polymerase promoters flanking a polylinker region. In the presence of RNA polymerase and a radioactive dNTP, labeled RNA transcripts are produced which are complementary to the insert DNA sequence.

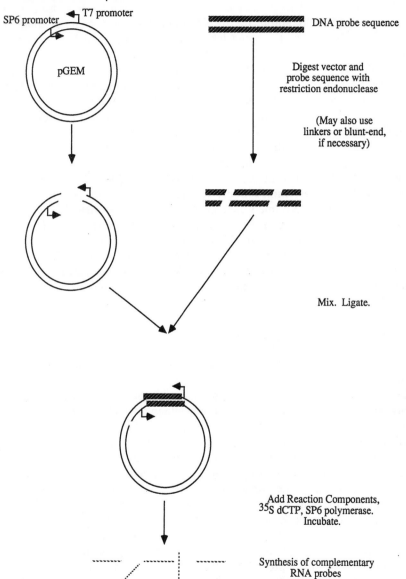

sense' probes, Johnson and Johnson, 1984). By using high concentrations (25 μM) of the ^{35}S-labeled UTP, up to 80% of the labeled UTP can be incorporated, yielding approximately 0.4 - 0.5 μg of labeled RNA probe per μg template with specific activity of 10^9 cpm/μg (Harper *et al.*, 1986). In constructing the clones to be used for probes, insert the DNA in a 5' to 3' orientation in the transcription vector pSP64 (Promega) so that the transcripts will be complementary to the RNA target. The DNA should be linearized with a restriction enzyme which cuts downstream from the sequence to be amplified. This will assure that only the insert sequences are transcribed and not those of vector. Following polymerization with the radioactive precursor, unlabeled UTP is added for a 'chase' incubation to assure that labeled probes are full length. This eliminates very short labeled sequences (5-15 nucleotides) in the probe preparation, which may lead to non-specific hybridization with other target species, increasing the background 'noise' level. The probe preparation is then digested with RNase-free DNase I to remove the DNA template and the RNA probes are purified by standard methods. Using the conditions described below, the average length of probes prepared in this manner is about 1-2,000 bases.

When performing enzymatic incubations with RNA, the addition of the RNase inhibitor, RNasin, helps to assure the integrity of the RNA. RNasin has a very high affinity for RNase ($k_i = 3 \times 10^{12}$) and is very effective in blocking its activity (Blackburn *et al.*, 1977). This inhibition is maintained over a wide range of salt and buffer conditions (0-0.5 M NaCl, pH 5-8), making it suitable in many reactions. The inclusion of RNasin in a cDNA synthesis, or *in vitro* transcription reaction, can improve the size and yield of cDNA or RNA transcripts, respectively.

Some of the advantages of using labeled RNA probes for hybridization include the following:

1. RNA:DNA and RNA:RNA hybrids are more stable than DNA:DNA hybrids, allowing the use of higher stringency conditions, increasing the signal-to-noise ratio.
2. The single-stranded RNA probes do not self-anneal so all probe molecules are available for hybridization. The original double-stranded template can be removed by digestion with DNase.
3. Only the insert is transcribed, not the vector, thus increasing the specificity of the probes.
4. Following hybridization, RNase can be used to remove unhybridized probe to reduce backgrounds.
5. Probes can be used without denaturation.
6. RNA probes are suitable for use in *in situ* hybridization.

The disadvantages include:
1. Precautions must be taken to assure RNase free conditions or the probes may become degraded prior to use.
2. The template must be linearized prior to use.

3. The size of the probe can not be easily controlled. The size of the transcripts, however, can be limited by digesting the template with restriction endonucleases at defined locations downstream from the SP6 promoter site to specify an upper limit on probe size. To prevent the accumulation of short labeled probes, a 'chase' incubation with unlabeled dNTPs can be performed after labeling with the radioactive dNTP.

PROCEDURE 3.3

TRANSCRIPTION OF ^{35}S-LABELED RNA PROBES

Note: RNase-free conditions must be maintained throughout. (Refer to Section 2 - Precautions for working with RNA, p. 44)

Reagents:
a) 5x Reaction Buffer
    200 mM Tris-HCl, pH 8.2
    30 mM MgCl$_2$
    10 mM spermidine
    50 mM dithiothreitol
    2.5 U/µl of RNasin (Boehringer-Mannheim)
    500 µg/ml of bovine serum albumin
    2.5 mM each of ATP, CTP and GTP
b) STOP Buffer
    200 mM NaCl
            10 mM Tris HCl, pH 7.4
            11 mM EDTA
            0.5% SDS

Procedure:
1. Combine the following in a microfuge tube:

    2 µl of 5x reaction buffer
    2 µl of linearized DNA template (1 µg) in DEPC-treated water
    4 µl of [a-^{35}S]UTP (DuPont; 1,000 Ci/mmol)
    2 µl of SP6 (or T7) RNA polymerase (5U; Promega)

    Incubate the reaction at 40°C for 45 minutes.

2. Add an additional 2 µl of SP6 RNA polymerase, plus 1 µl of 5 mM unlabeled UTP. Mix and incubate for an additional 15 minutes at 40°C.

Optional: Steps 3 and 4 can be included to digest the template DNA:
    3. Add RNase-free DNase I to 0.1 µg/ml and incubate an additional 15 minutes at 40°C to digest the DNA template.
    4. Dilute the sample with 100 µl of STOP Buffer.

5. Separate the labeled RNA from unincorporated radioactive precursors by column chromatography or chromatography through centrifuged columns as in described under 'Purification of Radiolabeled Probes' in this Section.
6. Determine the specific activity of the probe by precipitation with trichloroacetic acid (TCA) of 1 µl of probe, (Procedure 3.7). Calculate the probe specific activity as cpm per µg of starting DNA template.

Oligonucleotide Probes

PRODUCTION OF RNA PROBES FROM OLIGODEOXYNUCLEOTIDE TEMPLATES

The cloning vector pSP64 (Promega), which contains the SP6 RNA promoter adjacent to a multiple cloning site, can be used as the basis of generating labeled RNA probes from a DNA oligonucleotide template (Wolfl *et al.*, 1987). The oligonucleotides should be prepared to contain, in addition to the hybridization sequence, the four nucleotides (ACGA) at their 3' end, which are complementary to the 3' overhang of *Pst* I-cut DNA. The pSP64 plasmid is linearized with *Pst* I and allowed to anneal with the oligomer by virtue of their 'sticky' ends (Figure 3.7). The annealed structure, which now resembles nicked DNA, can serve as a template for *E. coli* DNA polymerase I. The 5'->3' polymerase will translate in the lower strand into the pSP64 vector and elongate the upper strand to synthesize a complementary copy of the oligonucleotide. The resulting double-stranded DNA molecule will consist of the oligonucleotide sequence attached to the pSP64 vector downstream from the SP6 promoter. This molecule can then serve as template SP6 RNA polymerase to generate labeled RNA copies of the original oligonucleotide sequence.

PROCEDURE 3.4

TRANSCRIPTION OF [³⁵S]RNA PROBES FROM SYNTHETIC SINGLE-STRANDED OLIGONUCLEOTIDES

Reagents:
a) TE Buffer
   10 mM Tris-HCl, pH 7.6
   1 mM EDTA

FIGURE 3.7   Synthesis of RNA Probes from Oligodeoxynucleotide Templates. Oligodeoxynucleotides with a 3'- *Pst* I 'sticky' end are annealed with a Pst I digested pSP64 vector.   This construct is then incubated with DNA polymerase I and unlabeled dNTPs to form a double-stranded molecule.   This molecule can then serve as a template for SP6 RNA polymerase to generate labeled RNA copies of the original oligonucleotide sequence.

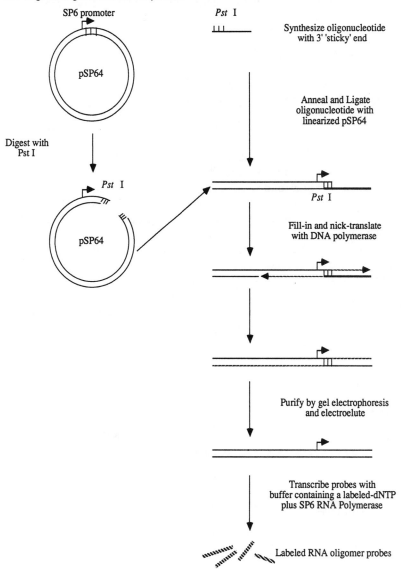

b) Transcription Mix
    2 µl   50 mM $MgCl_2$, 100 mM Tris-HCl, pH 8.5
    2 µl   0.5 mM each dATP, dCTP, dGTP, dTTP
    5 µl   4 mM dithiothreitol
    2 µl   5U/µl RNasin (Boehringer-Mannheim)
    3 µl   Water
    1 µl   DNA polymerase I (5 U/µl, holoenzyme, Boehringer-Mannheim)
c) STOP Buffer
    0.1 M EDTA,
    1% SDS

Procedure:
1. Anneal 5 µg of *Pst* I-digested pSP64 with 2 µg of oligonucleotide (50 nt) in 70 µl of TE buffer by heating to 65°C for 5 minutes and slow cooling to room temperature.
2. Centrifuge the annealed DNA for 30 seconds in a microfuge. Add 15 µl of the transcription mix to the tube.
3. Allow nick-translation and elongation to take place by incubating the tube for 2 hours at 10°C followed by a 1 hour incubation at 37°C.
4. Stop the reaction by adding 2 µl of STOP buffer. Incubate for 5 minutes at 65°C.
5. Electrophorese the reaction on a 1% agarose (low melting point) mini-gel.
6. Cut out the 3-kb band, heat at 50°C to melt the agarose and dilute the solution with 200 µl of TE buffer. Collect the DNA by ethanol precipitation or by passing it through a Nensorb column   (See 'Purification of Radiolabeled Probes' in this Section.)
7. Use the purified DNA as a template for SP6 (or T7) RNA polymerase in the presence of [a-^{35}S]dCTP (Procedure 3.3).

PREPARATION OF 'TAILED' OLIGONUCLEOTIDE PROBES

The enzyme terminal deoxynucleotidyl transferase will add deoxyribo-nucleoside triphosphates to the free 3'-hydroxyl end of a DNA molecule (Bollum, 1974). This addition of deoxynucleotides results in the formation of an elongated 'tail' at the 3' end of the probe. The large number of reporter groups that can be added in this way allows one to produce high specific activity probes. A variety of different isotopes (^{3}H, ^{32}P, ^{35}S, ^{125}I) can be used for this labeling, providing that the a-position of the phosphate or an internal residue of the base is labeled. The 'tailing' method is particularly useful for labeling synthetic oligonucleotide probes which can reach specific activities in excess of 1×10^{10} cpm/µg when using the ^{32}P-labeled precursors. Tailed probes can be prepared which have thermal dissociation properties that are indistinguishable from probes lacking tails (Collins and Hunsacker, 1985). Tailed oligonucleotide probes are suitable for the identification of cloned sequences in gene banks (Wood *et al.*, 1985), detection of point mutations in genomic DNA samples (Conner *et al.*, 1983) and for *in situ* hybridization (Lewis *et al.*, 1986).

As in the case of nick-translation and primer extension, suitable substrates which can be used for the tailing reaction include: [a-^{32}P]dCTP, [a-^{35}S]dCTP, [5, 5' ^{3}H] dCTP, or [5'-^{125}I]dCTP. Other nucleoside triphosphates (dATP, dGTP or dTTP) can also be used. Probes should not be tailed with dTTP since the tail can hybridize to the poly(A)$^{+}$ sequences in mRNA giving rise to high background signals. Similarly, probes tailed with [a-^{32}P]dATP may hybridize to poly(T) regions in genomic DNA. To minimize hybridization artifacts when using probes tailed with these precursors, the target sample should be prehybridized in the presence of excess unlabeled poly(dA) or poly(dT). Using the conditions below, the use of 200 µCi of [a-^{32}P]dCTP results in incorporation of about 60% of the precursors into the tail (about 100 residues in length) in about 30 minutes. The incorporation of [a-^{35}S]dCTP is slightly slower. The length of the tail (and the specific activity of the resultant probe) can be influenced by the relative molar concentrations of 3' ends and dNTPs. The following reaction uses a 20-mer synthetic oligonucleotide probe. Complete kits for performing tailing reactions are also available commercially (e.g. from Boehringer-Mannheim).

PROCEDURE 3.5

OLIGONUCLEOTIDE TAILING WITH TERMINAL DEOXYNUCLEOTIDYL TRANSFERASE

Reagents:
a) 5x Tailing Buffer
    5 mM CoCl$_2$
    500 mM sodium cacodylate, pH 7.0
    1 mM dithiothreitol
b) [a-^{32}P]dCTP (5,000 Ci/mmol)
c) 20 ng/µl oligonucleotide probe (20-mer)
d) 5 U/µl terminal deoxynucleotidyl transferase (Boehringer-Mannheim)

Procedure:
1. Mix the following reagents in a microfuge tube:
        10 µl 5x tailing buffer
        20 µl [a-^{32}P]dCTP = 200 µCi
         1 µl oligonucleotide probe
        18 µl water
         1 µl terminal deoxynucleotidyl transferase

2. Centrifuge briefly in a microfuge to bring the reagents to the bottom of the tube. Incubate the tube at 37°C for 45-60 minutes.
3. Stop the reaction by heating to 65°C for 5 minutes. Cool on ice.
4. Purify the probe away from unincorporated nucleotides by chromatography on Sephadex G-25, QuickSpin columns, (Procedure 3.9) or one of the alternative methods discussed under 'Purification of Radiolabeled Probes' in this Section.

LABELING OF OLIGONUCLEOTIDES AT THE 5' END

The enzyme T4 polynucleotide kinase will transfer the a-phosphorous from [g-^{32}P]ATP to a free 5' hydroxyl group (Maxam and Gilbert, 1977).   When oligodeoxyribo-nucleotides are synthesized, they are usually not phosphorylated and so contain a hydroxyl group at the 5' position. The procedure below is suitable for labeling oligomers and can also be used for dephosphorylated double or single-stranded DNA.   When labeling blunt or recessed ends of double-stranded DNA, the DNA should first be denatured by heating to 90°C for 2 minutes and quick cooling on ice. Phosphorylated DNA can be dephosphorylated with calf intestinal alkaline phosphatase or with bacterial alkaline phosphatase, then extracted with phenol and ethanol-precipitated (Maniatis *et al.*, 1982). Remaining traces of phosphatase in the subsequent labeling reaction will remove the label, leading to low specific activity probes.   It is also possible to use [g-^{35}S]ATP to label the synthetic probe at the 5' position with ^{35}S (Johnson and Johnson, 1984).   Since only one molecule of isotope is added per molecule of probe, the specific activity of the probe is a function of probe length.   Short oligonucleotide probes can be labeled to high specific activities, but for longer probes the specific activity decreases in proportion to the probe length.   The kinase labeling method is most often used in conjunction with DNA sequencing (Maxam and Gilbert, 1977).

PROCEDURE 3.6

5' END LABELING WITH T4 POLYNUCLEOTIDE KINASE

Reagents:
a) 10x Kinase Buffer
    500 mM Tris-HCl pH 7.4
    50 mM MgCl$_2$
    20 mM DTT
    1.0 mM spermidine
b) 0.1 µg/µl oligodeoxyribonucleotide probe
c) 10 U/µl T4 polynucleotide kinase
d) [g-^{32}P]ATP (3,000 Ci/mmol, DuPont)

Procedure:

1. In a 1.5 ml microfuge tube combine:

    1 0 µl oligodeoxyribonucleotide probe
    2.5 µl 10x kinase buffer
    1.5 µl T4 polynucleotide kinase
    20 µl [g-^{32}P]ATP

    Mix gently and centrifuge in a microfuge for 30 seconds to bring all of the reagents to the bottom of the tube.
2. Incubate the tube at 37°C for 45 minutes.
3. Stop the reaction by heating to 65°C for 5 minutes.
4. Purify the labeled probe away from unincorporated nucleotides by chromatography on Sephadex G-25, QuickSpin columns (Procedure 3.9), or one of the alternative methods discussed under 'Purification of Radiolabeled Probes' in this Section.

OTHER LABELING METHODS

A variety of other labeling schemes can be used for generating radiolabeled probes. These methods include enzymatic labeling protocols which are not widely used, or which have specialized applications. We make reference to them here for the sake of completion and the reader is encouraged to consult the appropriate references for further information.

DNA probes can be transcribed from RNA targets by use of the RNA-dependent DNA polymerase from avian myoblastosis virus (AMV reverse transcriptase) (Verma, 1981). This enzyme is most commonly used to transcribe mRNA into cDNA for cloning purposes (Maniatis *et al.*, 1982). Single-stranded cDNA probes can be transcribed from either single-stranded DNA or RNA templates in the presence of the reverse transcriptase, dNTPs (one or more of which can be labeled) and suitable primers. For poly(A)$^+$ mRNA, an oligo(dT) primer is most commonly used, although random primers or specific primers can also be used.

T4 DNA polymerase can be used to fill in single-stranded regions of DNA starting from a suitable primer. This polymerase possesses both a 3'->5' exonuclease activity and a 5'->3' DNA polymerase activity (O'Farrell, 1981). It is most often used to fill in 5' overhangs in DNA, such as those produced by restriction endonuclease digestion. The exonuclease activity is 200 times as active as that of DNA polymerase I and in the absence of dNTPs can be used to produce DNA molecules with recessed 3' ends. These molecules can then serve as primer templates for preparing probes by adding dNTPs (one or more of which can be labeled) and continuing the incubation to regenerate intact, double-stranded DNA molecules.

For labeling recessed 3'-ends of DNA, the large (Klenow) fragment of *E.*

coli DNA polymerase I can be used. This enzyme possesses a 5'->3' DNA polymerase activity and the 3'->5' exonuclease activity of the holoenzyme (Klenow *et al.*, 1971). By including [a-^{32}P]dNTPs in the reaction mix, these fill-in reactions will generate 3' end-labeled DNA.

When using T4 DNA polymerase and the Klenow fragment for filling in and labeling the 5' and 3' ends of restriction digested DNA, the labeled dNTPs must include residues which are complementary to the protruding end in order for labeling to take place. These procedures can also be used to generate strand-specific probes, by using restriction endonucleases which cut the labeled DNA into unequal size fragments. The fragments are separated by gel electrophoresis and each fragment will contain only a single labeled strand annealed to an unlabeled strand. The two strands can then be separated by denaturation and used in hybridization reactions.

The enzyme T4 RNA ligase can be used to label the 3'-ends of RNA molecules. This enzyme catalyzes the ATP-dependent formation of a phosphodiester bond between a 5'-terminal phosphate and a 3'-hydroxyl on adjacent RNA (or oligoribonucleotide) molecules (Unlenbeck and Gumport, 1982). A ^{32}P-labeled 3', 5'-biphosphate (labeled at the 5' position) can be used for this reaction to label the RNA (England *et al.*, 1980).

Chemical modification of DNA by the covalently coupling of ^{125}I to cytosine residues has been described by Commerford (1971). This method was further refined by Chan *et al.* (1973) and extended to RNA labeling Heiniger *et al* (1973). Although these methods are effective in labeling nucleic acids, they are no longer widely used because of the biohazards associated with radioactive iodine. The enzymatic labeling of DNA with an [^{125}I]dNTP has largely replaced these chemical labeling methods.

PROCEDURE 3.7

ESTIMATION OF SPECIFIC ACTIVITY BY TCA PRECIPITATION

Reagents:
a)   Whatman GF/C filters
b)   10% trichloroacetic acid (TCA)
c)   95% ethanol

Procedure:
1.   Add all reagents to the labeling reaction, except the enzyme. Spot duplicate 1 μl aliquots on separate Whatman GF/C filters and let them air dry. These filters will be used to determine the background TCA-precipitable cpm.
2.   After the labeling reaction is complete, again spot duplicate 1 μl aliquots on separate filters and allow them to air-dry. These filters will be used to determine the total TCA-precipitable cpm.

3. Place the filter papers in a 50 ml polypropylene tube and add 20 ml of cold 10% TCA. Gently wash the filters for about 30 seconds by inverting the tube, then discard the solution into the liquid radioactive waste.

4. Repeat the wash step two more times with 20 ml of fresh 10% TCA each and pour off the TCA. Wash the filters twice with 20 ml of cold 95% ethanol, then let them air-dry on a paper towel.

5. Measure the cpm on each filter by scintillation counting. Average the duplicate filters and calculate the background and total incorporated cpm for the entire reaction. Subtract the background from the total to obtain the net TCA-precipitable cpm. Finally, divide the net cpm by the μg of DNA in the labeling reaction to obtain the specific activity in cpm/μg.

Purification of Radio Labeled Probes

The radiolabeled probes synthesized by nick-translation, primer extension, transcription, tailing, or kinasing are purified after labeling to remove enzymes, unincorporated label and salts which may interfere with the hybridization reaction. The unincorporated labeled nucleotide can contribute significantly to non-specific background 'noise'. General approaches which work well for purification of labeled probes are ethanol precipitation, gel filtration, denaturing polyacrylamide gel electrophoresis and hydrophobic chromatography.

GEL FILTRATION METHODS

Gel filtration methods can be used to separate the labeled probe from the unincorporated nucleotides on the basis of size. Sephadex chromatography is most commonly used for this procedure. The separation depends on the different abilities of the various sample molecules to enter the pores of the Sephadex beads which are held in columns. The smaller nucleotide molecules enter the gel pores and are retained for a longer time, while the large probe molecules flow between the beads. To obtain the best separation, the sample is applied to the column in a small volume of buffer and washed into the matrix with small aliquots of buffer.

Ready to use, disposable columns are commercially available. The QuickSpin columns, available from Boehringer-Mannheim contain a pre-measured (0.8 ml) volume of swollen Sephadex G-50. These columns are designed to retain small molecules (less than 72 bp) including unincorporated nucleotides, while allowing the larger molecules (labeled probe) to flow through. The columns can be loaded with a maximum 100 μl of sample and are centrifuged to allow rapid separation and high recovery of the labeled probe.

PROCEDURE 3.8

PURIFICATION OF LABELED PROBES ON SEPHADEX COLUMNS

Reagents:
a)   Sephadex G-50 (Pharmacia)
b)   <u>TNES Buffer</u>
     10 mM Tris-HCl, pH 7.4
     1 mM EDTA
     50 mM NaCl
     0.1% SDS

Procedure:
1.   Pour 5 ml of autoclaved, pre-swollen medium grade Sephadex G-50 into disposable plastic columns (Kontes #420160 column, or equivalent). A 5 ml pipette with a glass wool plug can also be used.
2.   Equilibrate the column with TNES Buffer, then shut off the flow, leaving just enough TNES so the column will not dry out.
3.   Add 50 µl of TNES to the labeling reaction. Apply the diluted reaction to the top of the column and allow it to flow into the resin.
4.   When the sample has entered the column, add 100 µl of TNES. When this has entered the column, add additional TNES and begin collecting 0.5 ml fractions.
5.   Measure the radioactivity in 5 µl aliquots of each fraction by scintillation counting. The first peak contains the labeled probe. Pool the appropriate fractions. The second peak contains unincorporated nucleotides and should be discarded as radioactive waste. Calculate the total cpm in the probe fractions and divide by the amount of DNA used for labeling to determine the specific activity of the probe. Store frozen in aliquots.

PROCEDURE 3.9

DNA PURIFICATION ON QUICKSPIN COLUMNS

Reagent:
a)   QuickSpin columns (Boehringer-Mannheim)

Procedure:
1.   Resuspend the gel in a QuickSpin column by inverting the column several times.
2.   Remove the top and bottom caps from the column and allow the buffer to drain out.
3.   Place the column in the collection tube supplied and centrifuge for 2 minutes at 5,000 xg. Discard the collection tube containing the eluted buffer.

4.   Carefully add up to 100 µl of sample containing the labeled probe directly to the top of the gel bed.

5.   Place the column in a fresh collection tube and centrifuge for 4 minutes at 5,000 xg.

6.   The purified sample is recovered in the collection tube, while unincorporated nucleotides and salts are retained in the column.

7.   Count 1 µl of the eluted probe and calculate the specific activity (cpm/µg).

ETHANOL PRECIPITATION OF LABELED PROBES

If it is desirable to reduce the volume of the probe following separation by Sephadex chromatography, the pooled column fractions or eluate from centrifugation can be precipitated with ethanol by adding 10 µg of yeast tRNA carrier, sodium acetate to 0.3 M and 2 volumes of cold (-20°C) 100% ethanol (Procedure 2.2). Redissolve the radiolabeled DNA pellet in a small volume (i.e. 100 µl) of TE. Labeled DNA probes should be stored at -20°C in shielded containers. The probes should be thawed rapidly and boiled for 5 minutes prior to use for hybridization.

The use of ammonium acetate and ethanol for DNA precipitation have been reported to be a convenient method for separating labeled DNA from free nucleotides without the requirement of column chromatography (Maxam and Gilbert, 1980). Proteins are not precipitated in 2 M ammonium acetate and are removed in the supernatant. For very dilute solution (less than 10 µg/ml) of DNA, 10 µg of a yeast tRNA carrier can be added prior to the addition of the ethanol to improve the efficiency of the precipitation. The carrier RNA will not interfere with subsequent hybridization reactions.

PROCEDURE 3.10

PURIFICATION OF LABELED PROBES
BY ETHANOL PRECIPITATION

   Reagents:
   a)   5 M ammonium acetate
   b)   100% ethanol
        70% ethanol
   c)   TE Buffer
        10 mM Tris-HCl, pH 7.6
        1 mM EDTA

Procedure:

1. Add 0.4 volume of 5 M ammonium acetate to the DNA sample.
2. Add 2 volumes of cold 100% ethanol.
3. Precipitate the DNA in a dry ice/ethanol bath for 15 minutes or at -20°C for 1 hour
4. Centrifuge in a microfuge at 4°C for 15 minutes.
5. Wash the pellet twice with 70% ethanol and once with 100% ethanol. Centrifuge in a microfuge at 4°C for 10 minutes between washes.
6. Air-dry the pellet for about 15 minutes and dissolve the DNA in TE buffer or water.

PROCEDURE 3.11

DENATURING POLYACRYLAMIDE GELS

Oligonucleotide probes can be purified on polyacrylamide gels to obtain a product of specific size. This method is particularly useful for selecting a probe that possesses the desired number of deoxynucleotide additions after 3'-end labeling. This procedure can also be used to separate efficiently 'tailed' probes from those with short tails or untailed molecules following incubation with terminal deoxynucleotidyl transferase (Procedure 3.5).

Reagents:
a) 10x TBE Buffer (Appendix A)
b) Ultrapure urea
c) 40% acrylamide:bis-acrylamide (19:1)
d) Ammonium persulfate
e) N, N, N', N'-tetramethylethylenediamine (TEMED)
f) Denaturing Buffer
   60% deionized formamide
   0.6% bromophenol blue
   6% gel buffer

Procedure:
1. To prepare a 20% polyacrylamide-urea gel:
   Combine in a flask:

   26.25 g ultrapure urea
   31.25 ml 40% acrylamide:bisacrylamide (39:1)
   6.25 ml 10x gel buffer
   25 ml H_2O
   60 mg ammonium persulfate

   Mix well and filter through a 1µ fiter. Degas for 5 minutes.
   20 µl TEMED
   Mix by inversion.

2. Immediately after the addition of the last two reagents pour the solution into the pre-assembled forming plates.

3. Add the well-forming combs ¿ ɪd allow the gel to polymerize at room temperature for 1-2 hours.

4. Add 5 µl of denaturing buffer to the probe. Heat the samples to 90°C for 2 minutes and apply to individual wells.

5. Electrophorese at 100 V until the bromophenol blue has traversed approximately 75% of the gel. The dye will migrate at the same rate as a 12-mer.

6. Remove the gel, cover with plastic wrap and overlay a sheet of X-ray film in the dark to autoradiographically localize the position of the probe.

7. Align the film with the gel to localize the probe. Cut out the gel piece containing the labeled probe and elute the probe from the gel by crushing it in a 1.5 ml microfuge tube. Dilute the crushed gel fragment with with 500 µl TNES and shake the solution overnight on a rotary shaker at room temperature.

8. Pass the solution through a 0.2 µ syringe filter to remove the gel fragments.

HYDROPHOBIC CHROMATOGRAPHY - NENSORB COLUMNS

Reverse-phase (hydrophobic) chromatography can be used to remove both protein and salts from DNA preparations. Thus it is an easy way to remove enzymes from DNA after digestion or unincorporated nucleotides after labeling. A convenient format for reverse-phase chromatography is a prepacked column from DuPont called Nensorb.

PROCEDURE 3.12

PURIFICATION OF CLONED DNA ON NENSORB COLUMNS

The column capacity is 20 µg of DNA plus protein. Pass all solutions through the column using a syringe attached to the top. At each step, stop before the last of the buffer enters the column. After the activation step, do not allow air to enter the column or the yield will be affected.

Reagents:
a) Nensorb columns (DuPont)
b) Methanol
c) 0.1 M Tris-HCl, pH 8.0
d)   50% ethanol
    100% ethanol
e) 4 M sodium acetate

Procedure:

1. Pre-wash the Nensorb cartridge with 1 ml of methanol to activate the resin.
2. Wash the cartridge with 2 ml of 0.1M Tris-HCl, pH 8.0 to equilibrate the resin.
3. Apply up to 20 μg of DNA in 1 ml of 0.1M Tris, pH 8.0, per column. Collect the eluate and reapply it to the column two more times.
4. Wash the cartridge with 2 ml of 0.1M Tris-HCl, pH 8.0.
5. Wash the cartridge with 2 ml of water to remove the Tris buffer.
6. Add 1 ml of 50% ethanol to elute the labeled probe. Collect 0.5 ml fractions into microfuge tubes and allow the column to run dry.
7. To precipitate the eluted DNA add 50 μl of 4M sodium acetate and 500 μl of isopropanol to each tube, incubate at -20°C for 1 hour and collect the pellet by centrifugation for 10 minutes in a microfuge.
8. Wash the pellet with 70% ethanol and recentrifuge.
9. Dissolve the pellet in water or TE buffer and store frozen.

Reverse-phase chromatography can also be used for the purification of synthetic oligonucleotides after synthesis. The hydrophobic dimethoxy trityl moiety, which protects the 5' hydroxyl group, can be used as a 'handle' to purify oligonucleotides by reverse-phase chromatography. The chromatography matrix (C_{18}-silica) is available in prepacked columns from DuPont (Nensorb prep) or Applied Biosystems (OPC). We prefer the Nensorb column because it has a larger capacity (50 OD units or 1 mg). Although the columns are essentially the same, the instructions supplied with each differ. Our modified protocol for oligonucleotide purification on Nensorb prep columns is outlined in Procedure 3.13.

PROCEDURE 3.13

PURIFICATION OF TRITYLATED OLIGONUCLEOTIDE PROBES

Reagents:
a) Concentrated ammonium hydroxide (Applied Biosystems)
b) 0.3M sodium acetate
c) 100% ethanol
d) 0.1 M triethylammonium acetate, pH 7.0 (TEAA)
    Add 14 ml of reagent grade triethylamine to 900 ml of water. Adjust the pH to 7.0 with glacial acetic acid. Adjust to a final volume of one liter with water.
e) Methanol (HPLC grade)
f) 12% acetonitrile/88% TEAA
g) 10% acetonitrile/90% TEAA
h) 0.5% trifluoroacetic acid (TFA), reagent grade
i) Methanol:water (35:65)

Procedure:

1. Set the program on your DNA synthesizer for 'trityl group on'. After synthesis, store the column, containing the completed oligomer, dry at 4°C until it can be eluted.

2. Elute the finished 5'-amino oligonucleotide from the column. The following volumes are for a 0.2 μmole column. Attach a 1 ml syringe to the column. Using another 1 ml syringe, attached to an 18-gauge needle, remove 0.5 ml of concentrated ammonium hydroxide (Applied Biosystems) from the stock bottle. Remove the needle and attach the syringe to the other end of the column. Pass the ammonium hydroxide back and forth through the column several times by pushing with one plunger and pulling with the other. Leave the column immersed in ammonium hydroxide for 15-30 minutes.

   Remove the solution from the column by pulling it into one of the syringes and eject it into a screw-top 1.5 ml microfuge tube. Repeat the entire process with another 0.5 ml aliquot of ammonium hydroxide.

3. The base-protecting groups are removed from the eluted DNA by adding 10 μl of 0.5 N NaOH (for stability of the oligomer) and heating the solution at 55°C overnight (16 hours). Cool the tube on ice and centrifuge before opening. Transfer the solution to a 15-ml polypropylene tube, cover with Parafilm and poke small holes in the Parafilm with a needle. Freeze the solution in a dry ice bath and lyophilize until dry (usually about 18 hours). Redissolve the dried oligomer in 200 μl of water and re-lyophilize until dry. This double lyophilization assures efficient removal of ammonium ions. Resuspend the residue in 300 μl of 0.3 M sodium acetate and precipitate the DNA by adding 900 μl of 100% ethanol. Chill to -20°C and centrifuge to collect the pellet. Repeat the precipitation, wash the pellet with 70% ethanol and dry under vacuum. Redissolve the pellet in 4 ml of 0.1 M TEAA (for a 0.2 μmole column) immediately before purification. Measure the A_{260} of an aliquot and calculate the concentration using an extinction coefficient of 35 $\mu g/OD_{260}$ (Procedure 2.3).

4. Prepare a Nensorb prep column by placing it in a ring stand and attaching a 20 ml syringe to the bottom as directed by the manufacturer. Pass 10 ml of methanol through the column to activate the resin. For all steps, use a flow rate of about 10 ml/minute. *Avoid pulling any air through the resin after activation*; this will greatly affect the recovery.

5. Equilibrate the column with 10 ml of 0.1 M TEAA.

6. Pass the 4 ml of sample through the column twice.

7. Wash the column with 25 ml of acetonitrile/TEAA. Use 12%/88% for 19-mers and smaller; use 10%/90% for 20-40-mers. This step removes failure sequences, salts and other contaminants.

8.   Pass 25 ml of 0.5% TFA through the column to hydrolyze the trityl group from the oligonucleotide.
9.   Wash the column with 10 ml of 0.1 M TEAA.
10. Replace the 20 ml syringe with a 3 ml syringe. Pull 5 ml of 35% methanol/65% water through the column 1 ml at a time. Place each into a separate microcentrifuge tube. For the sixth fraction, pull all remaining liquid from the column, leaving it dry.
11. Measure the UV absorbance of a 1/10 dilution of each fraction. The DNA is usually in fractions 3-5.
12. Pool, aliquot and lyophilize the oligomer. The oligomer can be stored dry at -70°C until use.
13. To use the oligomer, redissolve the pellet in 200-500 µl of water and measure the A_{260} to calculate the concentration.

References

1.   Blackburn, P., Wilson, G. and Moore, J. (1977): Ribonuclease inhibitor from human placenta, J. Biol. Chem. **252**, 5904-5910.
2.   Bollum, F. J. (1974): Terminal deoxynucleotidyl transferase, in *The Enzymes*, (Boyer, P. D., ed), Vol. 10, chapter 5.
3.   Chan. H-C., Ruyechan, W. T. and Wetmur, J. G. (1976): *In vitro* iodination of low complexity nucleic acids without chain scission, Biochemistry **15**, 5487-5490.
4.   Collins, M. and Hunsaker, W. (1985): Improved hybridization assays employing tailed oligonucleotide probes: A direct comparison with 5' end-labeled oligonucleotide probes and nick-translated plasmid probes, Anal. Biochem. **151**, 211-224.
5.   Commerford, S. (1971): Iodination of nucleic acids in vitro, Biochemistry **10**, 1993-1999.
6.   Conner, B. Reyes, A., Morin, C., Itakura, K.,Teplitz, R. and Wallace, R., (1983): Detection of sickle cell b^s-globin allele by hybridization with synthetic oligonucleotides, Proc. Natl. Acad. Sci.USA **80**, 278-282.
7.   England, T. E., Bruce, A. G. and Uhlenbeck, O. C. (1980): Specific labeling of 3'-termini of RNA with T4 RNA ligase, Methods in Enzymology **65**, 65-74.
8.   Feinberg, A.P. and Vogelstein, B. (1983): A technique for radiolabeling DNA restriction endonuclease fragments to high specific activity, Anal. Biochem. **132**, 6-13.
9.   Feinberg, A.P. and Vogelstein, B. (1984): A technique for radiolabeling DNA restriction endonuclease fragments to high specific activity, Addendum Anal. Biochem. **137**, 266-267
10. Harper, M. E., Marselle, L. M., Gallo, R. C. and Wong-Staal, F. (1986): Detection of lymphocytes expressing human T-lymphotropic virus type III in lymph nodes and peripheral blood from infected individuals by *in situ* hybridization, Proc. Natl. Acad. Sci. USA **83**, 772-776.

11. Heiniger, H. J., Chen, H. W. and Commerford, S. L. (1973): Iodination of ribosomal RNA *in vitro*., Int. J. Appl. Radiat. Isotop. **24**, 425-427.
12. Hu, N. and Messing, J. (1982): The making of strand-specific M13 probes, Gene **17**, 271-277.
13. Johnson, M. and Johnson, B. (1984): Efficient synthesis of high specific activity ^{35}S-labeled human b-globin pre-mRNA, Biotechniques **2**, 156-162.
14. Klenow, H., Overgard-Hanson, K. and Patkar, S. (1971): Proteolytic cleavage of native DNA polymerase into two different catalytic fragments, Eur. J. Biochem. **22**, 371-381.
15. Lewis, M., Arentzen, R. and Baldino, F. (1986): Rapid, high-resolution *in situ* hybridization histochemistry with radioiodinated synthetic oligonucleotides, J. Neurosci. Res. **16**, 117-124.
16. Maniatis, T., Fritsch, E. and Sambrook, J. (1982): in *Molecular Cloning: a Laboratory Manual*, Cold Spring Harbor Laboratory, Cold Spring Harbor, New York.
17. Maxam, A. and Gilbert, W. (1977): A new method for sequencing DNA, Proc. Natl. Acad. Sci. USA, **74**, 560-564.
18. Maxam, A. and Gilbert, W. (1980): Sequencing end-labelled DNA with base-specific chemical cleavages, Methods in Enzymology **65**, 499-560.
19. O'Farrell, P. (1981): Replacement synthesis method of labelling DNA fragments, *FOCUS (Bethesda Research Laboratories/Life Technologies Inc.)* **3**, 1.
20. Palazzolo, M. and Meyeroivitz, E. (1987): A family of lambda phage cDNA cloning vectors, lSWAJ, allowing the amplification of RNA sequences, Gene **52**, 197-206.
21. Rigby, P.W.S., Dieckman, M., Rhodes, C. and Berg, P. (1977): Labeling deoxyribonucleic acid to high specific activity in vitro by nick-translation with DNA polymerase I, J. Mol. Biol. **113**, 237-251.
22. Uhlenbeck, O. C. and Gumport, R. I. (1982): T4 RNA ligase, in *The Enzymes*, (Boyer, P. D., ed), Vol. 15, chapter 2.
23. Verma, I. M. (1981): Reverse transcriptase, in *The Enzymes*, (Boyer, P. D., ed), Vol. 14, chapter 6.
24. Vosberg, H. and Eckstein, F. (1977): Incorporation of phosphothioate groups into fd and fx174 DNA, Biochemistry **16**, 3633-3640.
25. Wood, W., Gitshier, J., Lasky, L. and Lawn, R. (1985): Base composition-independent hybridization in tetramethylammonium chloride: A method for oligonucleotide screening of highly complex gene libraries, Proc. Natl Acad. Sci. USA **82**, 1585-1588.
26. Wolfl, S., Quaas, R., Hahn, U. and Wittig, B. (1987): Synthesis of highly radioactively labelled RNA hybridization probes from synthetic single-stranded DNA oligonucleotides, Nucleic Acids Res. **15**, 858.

Section 4:
Non-Radioactive
Labeling Procedures

Introduction

Just as the radioimmunoassay (RIA) has been steadily replaced by its non-radioactive counterpart, the enzyme-linked immunosorbent assay (ELISA), so too are radioactively-labeled DNA probes being replaced by non-radioactive versions. Modification of DNA with non-radioactive detectable groups is more difficult than antibody or antigen modification because DNA contains none of the conveniently reactive groups common to proteins, such as primary amines, sulfhydryl groups or carboxylic acid groups. Therefore, many innovative labeling procedures have been developed in order to prepare sensitive DNA probes. The non-radioactive labeling procedures can be divided into two major groups.

The first group includes enzymatic labeling procedures, the second group, the non-enzymatic or chemical labeling procedures. The enzymatic labeling techniques usually result in a greater degree of modification with a resulting increase in sensitivity over the non-enzymatic procedures. The disadvantages of enzymatic labeling procedures are their complexity, poor reproducibility, expense and difficulty in scaling up. Chemical labeling methods, on the other hand, are usually inexpensive and simple. Some chemical systems are quite versatile in that different detectable groups may be attached to the DNA probe using the same basic chemistry. Non-radioactive RNA probes are rarely used because most of the labeling procedures work either exclusively or best with DNA. In addition, while RNA probes offer few advantages over DNA probes, extra care is required to avoid degradation during labeling, hybridization and detection. For more information, refer to 'biotinylated RNA probes' in this section.

Non-radioactive probes are about as sensitive as ^{32}P-labeled probes, when the specific activity of the radioactive probe is $1\text{-}5\times10^8$ cpm/µg, but are usually less sensitive when compared with probes of 10^9 cpm/µg of greater. In general, the enzymatic non-radioactive techniques (nick-translation, random priming) yield the most sensitive probes, but these techniques are not as suitable as the chemical methods for labeling large quantities (>50 µg) of probe. The information in Table 4.1 can be used to compare detection sensitivities of some of the reported labeling schemes.

TABLE 4.1 Comparison of Non-Radioactive Nucleic Acid Labeling Methods. NR, Not reported.

LABELING METHOD	DETECTION	REFERENCE	AFFILIATION	SENSITIVITY
ENZYMATIC MODIFICATION				
cloned DNA				
biotin-dUTP nick translation	AP-streptavidin	Langer et al. 1981 Leary et al. 1983	Enzo Biochem	NR 1.4x10^6 copies
biotin-dUTP tailing	AP-streptavidin	Brakel and Engelhardt 1985	Enzo Biochem	1x10^6 copies
biotin-dATP nick translation	AP-streptavidin	Gebeychu et al. 1987	BRL/LifeTechnologies	5x10^4 copies
digoxigenin-dUTP	AP-anti digoxigenin	Heiles et al.1988	BoehringerMannheim	2x10^4 copies
oligonucleotides				
3' tailing with biotin-dUTP	AP -streptavidin	Kumar et al. 1988	INSERM	1x10^7 copies
CHEMICAL MODIFICATION				
cloned DNA				
AAIF	AP-double antibody Eu-double antibody	Tchen et al. 1984 Syvanen et al. 1986	INSERM Orion	4x10^6 copies 2x10^5 copies
sulfonation	double antibody	Poverenny et al. 1979	Orgenics	2x10^5 copies
enzymes	direct	Renz and Kurz 1984	EMBO	2x10^6 copies
biotin-angelicin	double antibody	Albarella et al. 1989	Miles	NR
photobiotin	AP-streptavidin Eu-streptavidin Gold-antibody	Forster et al. 1985 Dahlen et al. 1987 Tomlinson et al. 1988	BRESA Orion Miles	4x10^6 copies 1x10^6 copies 6x10^5 copies
photo-DNP	double antibody	Keller et al. 1989	Biotech Research	1.5x10^5 copies
transamination	AP-streptavidin Europium	Viscidi et al. 1986 Dahlen et al. 1988	Johns Hopkins Wallac	4x10^4 copies 3x10^6 copies
activated linker arm (BSPSE)	various	Landes 1986 Fink et al. 1980	Integrated Genetics	NR NR
mercury	HS-hapten double antibody	Hopman et al. 1986	U. Leiden	7x10^6 copies
Br-linker-hapten	double antibody	Keller et al. 1988	Biotech Research	8x10^5 copies
biotin hydrazide	AP-streptavidin	Reisfeld et al. 1987	Weizmann Inst	2x10^5 copies
biotin hydrazide	AP-streptavidin	Takahashi et al. 1989	Showa U.	1x10^6 copies
diazo biotin	AP-streptavidin	Rothenberg et al. 1988	Weizmann Ins	NR
DNA binding protein/biotin	acid phosphatase-streptavidin	Syvanen et al. 1985	Orion	1x10^6 copies
Biotin-psoralen	perox-streptavidin	Sheldon et al. 1986	Cetus	6x10^4 copies
Eu-psoralen	fluorescence	Oser et al. 1988	Max Planck Inst.	6x10^5 copies

Table 4.1 cont.

LABELING METHOD	DETECTION	REFERENCE	AFFILIATION	SENSITIVITY
CHEMICAL MODIFICATION				
oligonucleotides				
5'-amino	fluorescent primer	Smith *et al.* 1985	Cal Tech	NR
amino-cytosine	various groups	Ruth 1984	Molecular Biosystems	NR
amino-cytosine+ enzyme	direct	Jablonski *et al.* 1986	Molecular Biosystems	3×10^6 copies
5'-amino + enzyme	direct	Li *et al.* 1987	U. Adelaide	3.5×10^6 copies
		Sproat *et al.* 1987	EMBO	NR
SH-oligo + enzyme	direct	Chu and Orgel 1988	Salk Inst.	NR
Biotin-UMP	perox-Streptavidin	Cook *et al.* 1988	Enzo Biochem	3×10^8 copies
amino-cytosine+ enzyme	direct	Urdea *et al.* 1988	Chiron	1.2×10^7 copies

ENZYMATIC MODIFICATION

The first non-radioactive DNA probes, of a practical design, were described in the scientific literature by Langer *et al.* (1981). This early probe labeling scheme employed biotin-labeled deoxyribonucleotide triphosphates, incorporated into the probe DNA by enzymatic polymerization. The modified nucleotides, in turn, were developed as the result of years of experimentation with mercurated nucleotides and polynucleotides (Dale and Ward, 1975; Dale *et al.*, 1973; Dale *et al.*, 1975). The most widely used modified nucleotide is biotin-11-dUTP, as shown in Figure 4.1.

The molecule incorporates the following features: modification at the C-5 position where it will not interfere with hydrogen bonding, a double bond to minimize flexing of the linker arm and a linker arm long enough to ensure access of detection reagents to the biotin. This and other modified nucleotides can be incorporated into DNA by nick-translation (Leary *et al.*, 1983) or onto the ends of DNA by tailing (Riley *et al.*, 1986). After hybridization, these biotin-labeled probes are detected using avidin or streptavidin-enzyme conjugates. Streptavidin is superior to avidin for DNA detection because it exhibits far less nonspecific binding. Unlike avidin it contains no carbohydrate and has a neutral isoelectric point (Chaiet and Wolf, 1964). When combined with a precipitating substrate, the probe:immobilized target hybrid is visualized as a colored band or spot on nitrocellulose, (Leary *et al.*, 1983) or as cellular staining following *in situ* hybridization (Brigati *et al.*, 1983). These labeling and detection methods result in probes with a lower detection limit of 0.5-2 picograms, or about 5×10^4 copies of target nucleic acid.

FIGURE 4.1 Structure of Biotin-11-dUTP. This is the biotin-modified nucleotide most frequently incorporated into DNA by enzymatic labeling procedures.

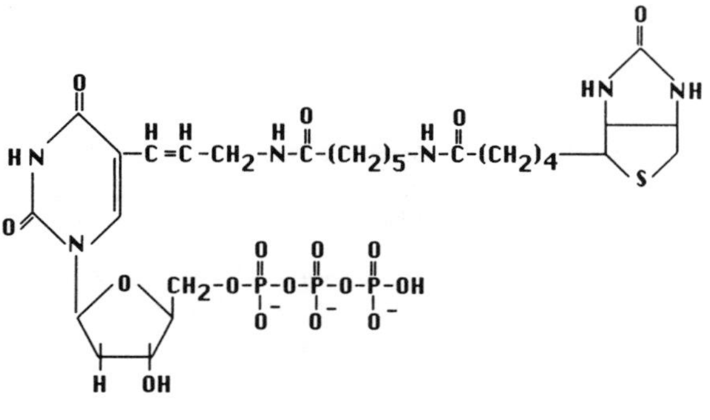

FIGURE 4.2 Structure of Biotin-14-dATP. This compound is an alternative to biotin-11-dUTP and can be incorporated into DNA by most enzymatic labeling procedures.

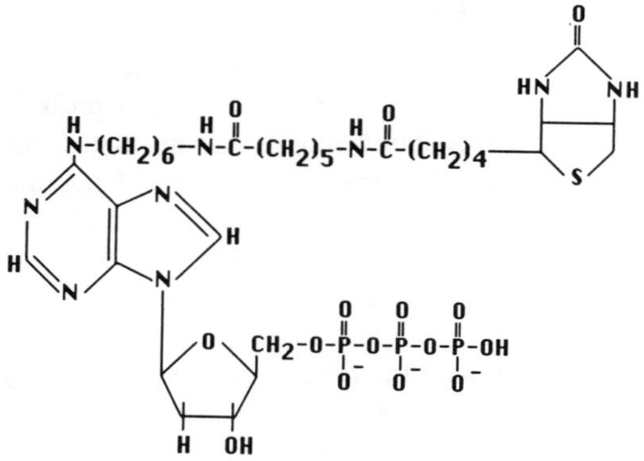

FIGURE 4.3 Structure of 8-Aminohexyl-dATP. AH-dATP is an amino-modified nucleotide which can be tailed onto DNA using terminal transferase. The free amino group can subsequently be modified with various detectable groups.

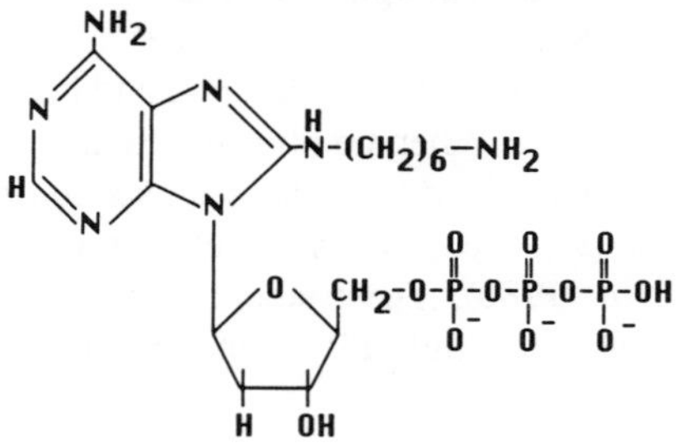

Of the various possible nucleoside triphosphate modifications, only a few result in a product which can be incorporated into DNA. The pyrimidines dUTP or dCTP modified at the C-5 position, with a linker arm ending in a detectable group, remain excellent substrates for DNA polymerase and terminal transferase. Likewise, dATP modified at the N-6 position (Gebeychu *et al.*, 1987), illustrated in Figure 4.2, can be incorporated into DNA by either enzyme. Purines modified at the C-8 position (dATP, dGTP) are not efficient substrates for DNA polymerase. However, they are excellent substrates for terminal transferase if modified only with a linker arm. One such compound is 8-aminohexyl-dATP, illustrated in Figure 4.3. The detectable group is easily added to the free amino group on the linker arm after tailing (in the form of N-hydroxysuccinimide-biotin, for instance).

Enzymatic incorporation of a biotinylated nucleotide is the 'standard' non-radioactive DNA-labeling procedure with which all others are compared and biotin remains a convenient label because it can be efficiently detected in one 10-minute streptavidin binding step. In order to detect a hapten with equal sensitivity it usually requires the use of two high-affinity antibodies and at least two hours of incubation time. One exception to this rule is a commercial labeling kit which incorporates digoxigenin-dUTP into DNA by random priming (Table 4.2). Sensitivities equivalent to biotin-dUTP-labeled probes are achieved using a single enzyme-conjugated antibody in a 30-minute incubation. Biotin is potentially a poor choice as a detectable group when working with food or bacterial samples which may contain biotin-binding proteins or interfering amounts of endogenous biotin.

PROCEDURE 4.1

LABELING OF DNA WITH MODIFIED NUCLEOTIDES BY NICK-TRANSLATION

There are four modified dNTPs which are commercially available: biotin-dUTP, biotin-dATP and digoxigenin-dUTP. The digoxigenin-dUTP is sold as part of a labeling kit and is sold separately (Table 4.2). Nick-translation kits may be purchased from BRL or Boehringer-Mannheim and used according to their instructions, substituting the modified dNTP for the radioactive dNTP. A nick-translation kit especially for biotinylation of DNA is available from BRL (Table 4.2).

Reagents:
a)   10x Nick-Translation Buffer
                500 mM Tris, pH 7.5
                100 mM $MgCl_2$
                80 mM ß-mercaptoethanol
                500 µg/ml BSA (Sigma A-8022 or BRL nuclease-free)

Table 4.2 Commercial Availability of Reagents for the Preparation and Detection of Non-Radioactive Nucleic Acid Probes.

Type Cat. No.	Description	Supplied	Company
LABELING REAGENTS			
enzymatic			
1093088	digox-11-dUTP	25 uM soln.	Boehringer Mannheim
9509S	biotin-7-dATP	0.4 mM soln	BRL
NU-806	biotin-11-dUTP	0.3 mM soln.	Enzo Biochem
NU-811	biotin-16-dUTP	0.3 mM soln.	Enzo Biochem
NU-815	biotin-11-UTP	20 mM soln.	Enzo Biochem
NU-816	AA-UTP (NH$_2$)	10 mM soln.	Enzo Biochem
B7645	biotin-11-dUTP	powder	Sigma
B5770	biotin-17-ATP (N^6)	powder	Sigma
B6020	biotin-11-UTP	powder	Sigma
5021-1	biotin-21-dUTP	0.5 mM soln.	Clontech
203104	biotin-21-dUTP	500 uM soln.	Calbiochem
chemical			
SP1000	photoprobe biotin	powder	Vector
8186SA	photobiotin	powder	BRL
5000-1	photoactivatable biotin	powder	Clontech
LABELING KITS			
8247SA	Bionick (nick-translation)	bio-14-dATP nick translation reagents	BRL
K1021-1	nick-translation	biotin-21-dUTP nick translation reagents	Clontech
K1017-1	3' end labeling	biotin-21-dUTP end labeling reagents	Clontech
K1019-1	mixed primer labeling ˙eagents	biotin-21-dUTP mixed primer labeling	Clontech
203215	nick-translation	biotin-21-dUTP nick translation reagents	Calbiochem
DETECTION KITS			
8279SA	Blugene System	AP-streptavidin NBT & BCIP	BRL
8239SA	DNA Detection System	biotin-AP streptavidin	BRL
K1035-1	Gene-Tect	AP-streptavidin NBT & BCIP	Clontech
LABELING & DETECTION KITS			
enzymatic			
1093 657	Genius Kit	digox-dUTP AP-anti-digox	Boehringer Mannheim
chemical			
51800	Chemiprobe Kit	sulfonation reagents mouse anti-sulfocytosine AP-RAM	FMC Bioproducts
76-001-1	MercuProbe Kit	mercuration reagents biotinylation reagents detection reagents	ICN Biomedicals

b)   1 mg/ml DNaseI (Sigma). Dissolve in the buffer given in Procedure 3.1.
c)   5 mM dNTPs (Boehringer-Mannheim, Appendix A)
d)   10 mg/ml yeast tRNA in water (Boehringer-Mannheim)
e)   Biotin-dUTP (Enzo), biotin-dATP (BRL), digoxygenin-dUTP (Boehringer-Mannheim)
f)   *E coli.* DNA polymerase I, Klenow fragment (Boehringer-Mannheim)

Procedure:

1.   Use closed circular or linear double-stranded plasmid DNA or an isolated double-stranded fragment. Labeling of the entire plasmid will provide the best sensitivity, since label can be incorporated into the vector as well as the insert DNA. In some situations, however, labeling of the isolated insert fragment will result in better specificity. Linearized DNA and isolated fragments can be purified by hydrophobic chromatography (Procedure 3.12) or organic exraction (Procedure 2.2).

2.   Combine on ice:

0.5 µg probe DNA
5 µl 10x nick translation buffer
1 µl of a 1/10,000 dilution of DNase I in water   (2 ng/ml final)
1 µl each of 3 dNTPs (- modified dNTP)   (100 µM final)
Modified dNTP   (to 200-500 µM final)
Dilute to 40 µl with water
1 µl DNA polymerase   (5-10 U)

Incubate for 1 hour at 15°C. Stop the reaction by adding 4 µl of 0.25 M EDTA, 2 µl of 10 mg/ml tRNA and 150 µl of 10 mM Tris, pH 7.5. The labeled probe may be separated from unincorporated nucleotides by alcohol precipitation or molecular sieve chromatography.

3.   Alcohol precipitation: Add 20 µl of 4 M LiCl, 500 µl of -20°C ethanol and mix well. (Better separation of DNA from soluble nucleotides is obtained using LiCl during ethanol precipitation, because the lithium salts of dNTPs are more soluble in aqueous ethanol than their corresponding sodium salts.) Store at -20°C for 30 minutes, centrifuge at 12,000 xg, wash the pellet with 70% and 100% ethanol and drain the pellet by inverting for a few minutes. Redissolve the pellet in 20 µl of water (50 µg/ml) and store at -20°C.

4.   Molecular sieve chromatography: Probe purification may also be performed on small Sephadex G-50 columns as described in Procedure 3.8.

PROBE TESTING

The success of radioactive probe labeling is determined by direct measurement of the probe's specific radioactivity. It is usually not practical to measure directly the incorporation of modified nucleotides or non-radioactive detectable groups into DNA, but they can be measured indirectly by hybridization. Test strips containing dilutions of homologous target are prepared (below) and an aliquot of the newly labeled probe is hybridized overnight at a concentration of 200 ng/ml. Hybridization and detection are performed as described in Procedures 5.15 and 5.17.

PROCEDURE 4.2

PREPARATION OF TARGET TEST STRIPS

Prepare a solution of 10x SSC containing 10 µg/ml of sheared salmon sperm DNA.
Nick the target plasmid as follows:

100 µg plasmid DNA	x µl
10 N NaOH	2 µl
Water to	200 µl

Incubate at 65°C for 15 minutes. Add 10 µl of 4 M sodium acetate and 500 µl of ethanol, chill 15 minutes to precipitate and centrifuge. Wash the pellet with cold 70% and 100% ethanol and dry. Redissolve the pellet in 150 µl of water. Determine the recovery by measuring the UV absorbance and electrophorese an aliquot on an agarose gel to assess the size distribution.

Starting with 1 µg of nicked plasmid in 100 µl of water:

DNA	10x SSC/DNA	ng/µl	pg/µl
4 µl	36 µl	1	1,000

Prepare 1:5 serial dilutions in the 10x SSC/DNA buffer:

0.2	200
0.04	40
0.008	8
0.0016	1.6

Boil and chill to denature, then spot 1 µl of each dilution on dry nitrocellulose strips (1x4 cm), on Saran Wrap. Spot 1 µl of the SSC/DNA buffer as a negative control. Let the spots dry at room temperature, then bake the filter at 80°C in a vacuum oven for one hour. To label the strips, write carefully with a soft pencil. Many strips can be prepared simultaneously and stored in heat-seal bags at room temperature for at least one year.

As discussed in Procedure 3.2, the incorporation of nucleotides by random priming is an alternative to nick-translation with a number of advantages. The procedure works well with single-stranded DNA, with small quantities of DNA template as well as with short templates. The incorporation of labeled nucleotides by random priming is generally more efficient than by nick-translation. Random primer labeling kits may be purchased from BRL or Boehringer-Mannheim and used according to their instructions, substituting the modified dNTP for the radioactive dNTP. A non-radioactive random priming labeling and detection kit is available from Boehringer-Mannheim (Table 4.2).

PROCEDURE 4.3

LABELING OF CLONED DNA WITH MODIFIED NUCLEOTIDES BY RANDOM PRIMING

Reagents:
a) 10x Random-priming Buffer
    500 mM Tris, pH 6.6
    100 mM $MgCl_2$
    10 mM B-mercaptoethanol
    500 µg/ml BSA (Sigma or BRL)
b) 5 mM each of dATP, dCTP, dTTP and dGTP (Boehringer-Mannheim)
c) 10 mg/ml yeast tRNA in water (Boehringer-Mannheim)
d) *E coli.* DNA polymerase I, Klenow fragment (Boehringer-Mannheim)
e) Modified dNTP
    Biotin-dUTP (Enzo)
    Biotin-dATP (BRL)
    Digoxigenin-dUTP (Boehringer-Mannheim)
f) Random hexanucleotides (Pharmacia)
g) 1 M Tris, pH 7.5
h) 0.5 M EDTA

Procedure:
1. Use linearized plasmid DNA, an isolated fragment, or single-stranded M13 DNA.
2. Combine 1 µg of probe DNA and 5 µg of hexanucleotide primers. Denature by boiling for 5 minutes, then quickly transfer the tube to ice and incubate for 10 minutes to allow for primer annealing.

3. Combine on ice:

    5 µl of 10x random-priming buffer
    1 µl of each of three dNTPs
    x µl of modified-dNTP   (100 µM final)
    make up to 48 µl with water
    2 µl DNA polymerase   (5-10 U)

    _____

                    50 µl total

Add the above reaction mixture to the denatured primers and probe DNA. Incubate 2 hours at 37°C. Longer incubation times may result in the synthesis of template-independent material and a loss of hybridization specificity. Stop the reaction by adding 2 µl of 0.5 M EDTA, 2 µl of 10 mg/ml tRNA and 150 µl of 10 mM Tris, pH 7.5. The labeled probe may be separated from unincorporated nucleotides by alcohol precipitation or molecular sieve chromatography as described in Procedure 4.1.

TAILING OF CLONED DNA FRAGMENTS

Deoxynucleotide triphosphates can be 'tailed' onto DNA fragments using the enzyme terminal transferase. As discussed in Section 1, terminal transferase can incorporate the widest variety of modified nucleotides onto the 3' terminus of DNA. Steps 1-4 below contain the procedure for tailing with biotin-dUTP or dCTP, biotin-dATP, digoxigenin-dUTP or aminohexyl-dATP (AH-dATP, Procedure 4.4). The biotinylated nucleotides are the easiest to use and are all about equivalent in labeling efficiency (for sources see Table 4.2). AH-dATP is used to incorporate an unusual detectable group, such as a hapten and steps 5-8 describe the further modification of AH-dATP-labeled DNA with detectable groups. When tailing a 3' overhang, the use of a modified nucleotide alone results in tails of 10-50 residues, depending on the modified nucleotide. However, the addition of dCTP at a dCTP:biotinylated nucleotide molar ratio of 2:1, results in tails of about 200 residues and optimum sensitivity. This sensitivity is a result of more incorporation of the modified nucleotide as well as the spacing between modified residues provided by the dCMP residues.

PROCEDURE 4.4

TAILING OF CLONED DNA FRAGMENTS WITH MODIFIED NUCLEOTIDES

Reagents:
a) Terminal transferase (BRL)
b) <u>5x Tailing Buffer</u>
    Concentrated reaction buffer is usually supplied with the terminal

transferase. When diluted to 1x concentration, it contains: 100 mM potassium cacodylate, pH 7.0, 1 mM $CoCl_2$ and 0.2 mM dithiothreitol. Appendix A contains a protocol if you wish to prepare your own).

c) 5 mM dCTP
d) Modified dNTP
   Biotin-dUTP (Enzo)
   Biotin-dATP (BRL)
   Digoxigenin-dUTP (Boehringer-Mannheim)
   AH-dATP (Procedure 4.5)
e) 5 M ammonium acetate
f) Isopropanol
g) Cold 100% ethanol
   Cold 70% ethanol

Procedure:

1. DNA restriction fragments are purified by gel electrophoresis, electroeluted without carrier RNA, purified by DEAE-cellulose chromatography, extracted with phenol:chloroform and ethanol-precipitated. Phenol:chloroform extraction must be performed to remove any residual restriction enzyme. Alternatively, the electroeluted DNA may be purified on a Nensorb column (Procedure 3.12). Probes of 0.5 kb to 3 kb in length will give the best signal when labeled by tailing. Also note that 3' protruding ends tail most efficiently (i.e., after *Pst* I digestion).

2. The purified fragment may be 'nicked' with DNase I (Sigma D4763) to generate more ends for tailing by terminal transferase. DNase I is stored in aliquots at 1 mg/ml in water. It is diluted to 0.05 µg/ml in 0°C water just before use. Aliquots are thawed only once. Typically 1 µg of DNA in 50 µl is adjusted to 2 mM $MgCl_2$ and 2.4 µl of a 0.05 µg/ml DNase I solution is added. After incubation at 16°C for 1-5 minutes, the reaction is then heated at 60°C for 10 minutes to inactivate the enzyme.

3. The following reagents are added directly to the 1 µg of nicked DNA:

5x tailing buffer	20 µl
Modified dNTP	x µl (to 100 µM final)
5.0 mM dCTP	4 µl (200 µM final)
Water to	100 µl
Mix and add:	
Terminal transferase 50 units	

4. After incubating the reaction at 37°C for 45 minutes, the tailed DNA is precipitated by adding 40 µl of 5 M ammonium acetate and 300 µl of isopropanol. Incubate for 15 minutes on ice. After centrifugation, the pellet is washed in 70% ethanol, 100% ethanol, dried and redissolved in

150 µl of water. If a biotin or digoxigenin-labeled dNTP is used in the reaction, the probe is ready to use. If an AH-dATP is used in the labeling, the pellet should be dissolved in 150 µl of 0.1M NaHCO$_3$, pH 9.0 and a detectable group attached as described below.

Labeling of AH-dATP-Modified DNA

Additional reagents:

a)   1 M sodium bicarbonate, pH 9.0
b)   Dimethylsulfoxide (DMSO)
c)   Reactive Detectable Groups
      N-hydroxysuccinimide-biotin (NHS-biotin, Pierce)
      N-hydroxysuccinimide-aminocaproic acid-dinitrophenyl (NHS-DNP, Appendix A)
      Dinitrofluorobenzene (Sigma)

5.   Any detectable group which reacts with a primary amine can be used. Three examples are: NHS-biotin, NHS-aminocaproic acid-dinitrophenyl and dinitrofluorobenzene. Dissolve 1 mg of the compound in 100 µl of DMSO, depending on the detectable group desired. The NHS moiety is light sensitive; avoid strong light. This will yield a 10 mg/ml solution of the activated detectable group. Centrifuge briefly in a microfuge to pellet any insoluble material. After using, discard any left-over solution; it must be made up just before use for best results.

6.   To 10 µg of AH-dATP-tailed DNA add 100 µl of DMSO and 50 µl of the 10 mg/ml solution of the activated detectable group. Incubate at room temperature for 60 minutes in the dark. Precipitate by adding 100 µg of tRNA, 140 µl of 5 M ammonium acetate and 980 µl of isopropanol. Incubate on ice for 15 minutes and centrifuge for 10 minutes.

7.   After centrifugation, wash the pellet in 100% ethanol, dry the pellet and redissolve it in 100 µl of water. Reprecipitate, using 10 µl of 4 M sodium acetate and 250 µl of ethanol, wash the pellet with 70% ethanol, 100% ethanol and dry. Redissolve the DNA in 200 µl of water (50 µg/ml). The labeled fragment may be used immediately in a hybridization reaction or it may be further purified over a column of Sephadex G-50 (Procedure 3.8).

8.   The labeling efficiency may be checked by hybridizing the probe to target dilutions as described in Procedure 4.2.

The modified nucleotide AH-dATP is not commercially available, so it must be synthesized starting with dATP (Lee *et al.*, 1977). It is useful for the enzymatic incorporation of non-standard detectable groups (groups other than biotin or digoxigenin) onto cloned DNA probes and oligonucleotide probes. The structure of the compound is illustrated in Figure 4.3.

PROCEDURE 4.5

SYNTHESIS OF 8-AMINOHEXYL-DATP (AH-DATP)

Reagents:
a) 2 M Ammonium Bicarbonate
    316 g in 2 liters of water
    Adjust to pH 8.0 with NH_4OH.
b) 1 M Sodium Acetate
    13.6 g per 100 ml
    Adjust to pH 4.5 with glacial acetic acid.
c) Isobutyric acid/Ammonium hydroxide/Water
       82.0 ml water
       2.5 ml concentrated NH_4OH
    165.0 ml isobutyric acid
d) DEAE-Sephacel (Pharmacia)
    De-fine about 200 ml in water before pouring column. Column volume is
    160 ml.   It is equilibrated with about 1.5 liters of 2 M ammonium
    bicarbonate, then equilibrated with about 2 liters of water.
e) Bromine
f) Chloroform
g) dATP (disodium salt, Boehringer-Mannheim)
h) 1 M sodium acetate, pH 4.5
i) 1,6-diaminohexane (Aldrich)
j) Isobutyric acid/NH_4OH/water (66:1:33)
k) Ninhydrin reagent (Sigma)

Procedure:
1. Dissolve 250 mg of disodium dATP in 2 ml of water and add 8 ml of 1 M
    sodium acetate, pH 4.5. In a fume hood, add 270 µl of bromine with
    vigorous stirring. Caution: bromine is extremely toxic if inhaled; contact
    with skin causes burns. After 15 minutes with constant stirring, transfer
    the solution to a disposable 50 ml polypropylene tube and extract 3 times
    with an equal volume of chloroform (also in the fume hood). Dispose of
    excess bromine properly.
2. In order to bleach the solution, add about 0.2 g of solid sodium thiosulfate
    (Sigma) in small portions until a pale yellow color is obtained.
3. To precipitate the product (8-Br dATP), add 3 volumes of cold ethanol (-
    20°C), adding one volume at a time with stirring. Incubate at -20°C for 1
    hour. This should be done in 50 ml Oak Ridge tubes, which can be
    centrifuged in the Sorvall SS-34 rotor. Centrifuge the tubes at 10,000 rpm
    at -20°C for 10 minutes and decant the supernatant from the oily pellet.

4.   Dry the pellet briefly on a lyophilizer (or in a fume hood) and redissolve it in a total of 10 ml of water. Two ml of 1,6-diaminohexane (melt at 60°C, then centrifuge and use the clear top layer) are added and the solution incubated at 60°C for 3 hours. During the three hours, the progress of the reaction is monitored by measuring the absorbance at 260 and 280 nm. The A_{280}/A_{260} ratio should increase from 0.74 to more than 1.2 by the end of the reaction.

5.   Dilute the reaction by adding 600 ml of water and adjust the pH to 8.0 with dilute HCl. Bind the sample to a pre-equilibrated DEAE-Sephacel (Pharmacia) column, then wash the column with 5 column volumes of water (900 ml). This washing step removes any unreacted diaminohexane. All of the above steps, up to the start of the column washing, should be completed in one day. The column may be washed overnight.

6.   The product is eluted from the column with a linear 0-0.5 M ammonium bicarbonate gradient. The total volume of the gradient is 700 ml; the fraction size is 5 ml. The fractions having an A_{280}/A_{260} ratio greater than 1.15 are pooled and lyophilized. They should be lyophilized for at least 48 hours to remove all trace of ammonium bicarbonate. After redissolving the material in 10 ml of water, it is checked for 8-Br dATP contamination by thin layer chromatography (TLC).

7.   Use ascending chromatography on fluorescent silica gel plates to detect any 8-Br dATP contamination. One µl per spot is adequate. Include at least one lane with some known AH-dATP. The solvent system is isobutyric acid/ammonium hydroxide/water (66:1:33). The nucleotides appear as dark spots under short-wave UV light. The final material is also checked for a positive ninhydrin reaction (which indicates a free amino group) on a thin layer chromatogram. Allow the chromatogram to dry overnight in a fume hood, then spray with ninhydrin reagent and heat at 70°C until the control spots appear. The 8-AH-dATP will appear as a purple spot. The relative migration of the various compounds upon TLC is: dATP, Rf = 0.22; 8-Br dATP, Rf = 0.29 and 8-AH-dATP, Rf = 0.64.

8.   The modified nucleotide is then adjusted to pH 7.0. If it is cloudy, it is filtered through a 0.22 µ filter on a syringe and the UV absorbance is again measured. It is stored in solution at -70°C.

Physical Properties of AH-dATP:
   A_{280} units/mg = 24.7
   Molecular weight = 765
   A_{280}/A_{260} ratio of pure material = 1.60-1.70

BIOTINYLATED RNA PROBES

RNA transcript probes have a some advantages over DNA probes. They are single-stranded, so there is no denaturation required and no interference from a complementary strand, if the vector DNA is digested after the RNA synthesis. RNA probes form more stable hybrids with their targets than DNA probes. In some *in situ* hybridization protocols, the excess RNA probe can be enzymatically digested to reduce background. Biotin-11-UTP (Enzo, Sigma) can be incorporated into RNA transcripts synthesized by SP6, T3 and T7 RNA polymerases (McCracken, 1985). Biotin-17-ATP (Sigma) may also be incorporated into RNA transcripts, but the efficiency of its incorporation, relative to biotin-11-UTP, has not been documented. The amount of RNA polymerase used in each reaction must be increased compared with reactions containing non-biotinylated nucleotides, because the incorporation is not as efficient. Even when using increased enzyme, the yield of RNA will be about half of that obtained from radioactive labeling reactions but, the length of the transcripts is unaffected. The amino-allyl analog of UTP (AA-UTP, Enzo), which contains a linker arm without the biotin attached, is incorporated more efficiently than biotin-UTP, but an additional step is required: amino-allyl modified DNA is subsequently reacted with an NHS-ester of biotin to obtain a biotin-labeled probe (Procedure 4.3).

PROCEDURE 4.6

INCORPORATION OF BIOTINYLATED
NUCLEOTIDES INTO RNA TRANSCRIPTS

Labeling kits (without modified nucleotides) are available from BRL and Boehringer-Mannheim.

Reagents:
a) Biotin-11-UTP (Sigma, Enzo)
b) SP6 or T3 RNA polymerase (BRL, Boehringer-Mannheim)
c) <u>Template DNA</u>
    Cloning vectors are available from BRL and Promega. The DNA must be linearized with a restriction enzyme before RNA synthesis. Refer to the manufacturer's instructions.
d) 1 M Tris, pH 8.0
e) 1 M $MgCl_2$
f) 10 mM spermidine
g) 50 mM dithiothreitol
h) 5 mM each of ATP, CTP and GTP

Procedure:
1. The following amounts of template and enzyme are for a 50 µl reaction:

SP6	T3
40 mM Tris, pH 8.0	40 mM Tris, pH 8.0
6 mM MgCl$_2$	8 mM MgCl$_2$
2 mM spermidine	2 mM spermidine
1 mM DTT	25 mM NaCl
400 µM each of ATP, CTP, GTP	1 mM each of ATP, CTP, GTP
1 mM biotin-11-UTP	1 mM biotin-11-UTP
1 µg template	500 ng template
50 units SP6 RNA polymerase	45 units T3 RNA polymerase

2. Incubate the reaction at 37°C for 1 hour.
3. The DNA template may be digested with RNase-free DNase (Boehringer-Mannheim) as described in Procedure 3.3. This enzyme is included in the labeling kits.
4. Stop the reaction by adjusting to a final concentration of 1% SDS.
5. Separate the RNA transcripts from unincorporated nucleotides by gel filtration (see Procedure 3.8).

CHEMICAL MODIFICATION

The first practical chemical labeling scheme employed the carcinogen, AAIF (7-iodo-N-acetoxy-N-2-acetylaminofluorene), which covalently binds to guanosine residues in DNA (Tchen *et al.*, 1984). The structure of AAIF and its guanosine conjugate are shown in Figure 4.4. Detection was by means of a rabbit anti-AAIF first antibody, followed by an alkaline phosphatase conjugated goat anti-rabbit IgG second antibody. This pioneering work established that a DNA probe, labeled with a hapten, was essentially as useful as a biotin-labeled probe. That is, 4x10^6 copies of target nucleic acid could be detected after hybridization. Although the biotin-avidin affinity constant is 10^{15} and antibody-hapten affinity constants (for high affinity antibodies) are usually about 10^{12}, the amplification provided by the enzyme-conjugated second antibody makes up for this difference. Disadvantages of the AAIF system are the toxicity of AAIF and the long developing procedure following hybridization. This developing procedure typically involves blocking the blot for 1 hour, incubating with each antibody for 1 hour followed by washing steps and color development with alkaline phosphatase substrates for at least 2 hours.

Another early hapten-based labeling system was based on the sulfonation of cytosine residues by bisulfite (Poverenny *et al.*, 1979) as depicted in Figure

FIGURE 4.4 Structure of the Guanine:AAIF Reaction Product. When AAIF reacts with DNA, it modifies the C-8 position of guanine. The structure of the resulting conjugate is shown above.

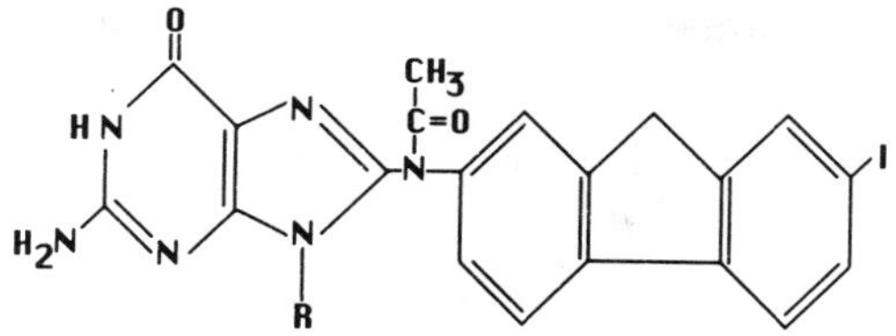

FIGURE 4.5 Sulfonation of Cytosine Residues. The reaction of cytosine (1) with bisulfite results in 6-sulfo-cytosine (2). Further reaction with o-methylhydroxylamine yields the 4-methoxy, 6-sulfonate derivative (3).

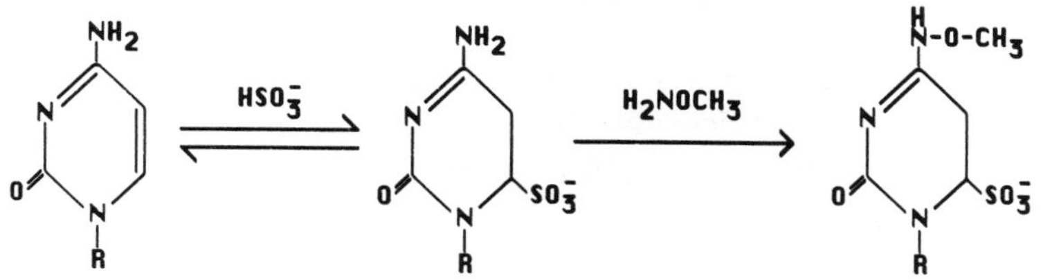

(1)   (2)   (3)

4.5. Labeling of the probe is extremely easy and inexpensive because it relies on simple, inorganic reagents. Contaminating protein and RNA do not seem to interfere with the labeling chemistry. After hybridization, the probe is detected using a monoclonal anti-sulfonate first antibody, followed by an alkaline phosphatase conjugated anti mouse IgG second antibody. Polyclonal antibodies raised against sulfonated DNA or sulfonated cytosine are not acceptable for detection because they exhibit anti-DNA activity which results in a non-specific background signal. Even immunopurification does not completely remove this background. As with AAIF-labeled probes, a long developing procedure is associated with sulfonated probes. A kit for performing the modification and detecting the modified DNA is available from FMC bioproducts (Table 4.2).

CHEMICAL LABELING WITH BIOTIN

One of the simplest and most popular chemical labeling procedures uses a light-sensitive compound developed by Forster *et al.* (1985) to chemically modify DNA with biotin. Photobiotin is a linker arm with biotin coupled to one end and an aryl azide group coupled to the other end (Figure 4.6). In the presence of visible light, the aryl azide is converted into a reactive aryl nitrene moiety which

FIGURE 4.6 Structure of Photobiotin. The aryl azide moiety is converted by light to a reactive aryl nitrene which couples to DNA, resulting in biotinylation.

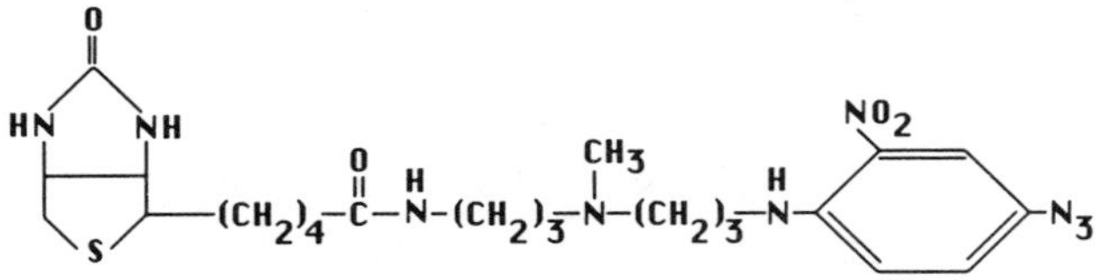

BIOTIN───────────── LINKER ARM ──────── ARYL AZIDE

reacts readily with DNA or RNA. The reaction is relatively specific for adenines, presumably at the N-7 position (Keller *et al.*, 1989). Double or single-stranded DNA is combined with a 2-fold weight excess of photobiotin, irradiated with a sunlamp and the labeled DNA is recovered by butanol extraction and ethanol precipitation. Approximately 1/50 bases is modified under these conditions. Only fragments greater than 200 nucleotides should be labeled with photobiotin; shorter probes label inefficiently. This compound is perhaps the only practical *chemical* method for labeling RNA with biotin.

PROCEDURE 4.7

PHOTO-BIOTIN LABELING OF DNA

Reagents:
a)   Photobiotin (Vector #SP-1000)
     In subdued light, add 500 μl of autoclaved water to a 500 μg vial and dissolve completely. Aliquot 100 μl per tube and store at -20°C for up to 4 months.
b)   1 M Tris, pH 8.0
c)   *sec*-Butanol
d)   4 M sodium acetate
e)   Cold 100% ethanol
     Cold 70% ethanol

Procedure:
1.   Plasmid DNA must be enzymatically linearized or nicked with NaOH (Procedure 4.2). M13 DNA and isolated fragments need no pretreatment before labeling. All DNA samples must be dissolved in water for efficient labeling. Tris buffer and proteins will interfere with the labeling, because they are a source of primary amines.
2.   If the probe is to be used for *in situ* hybridization, the DNA should not be nicked, but digested with *Hae* III. This will result in a reproducible

preparation of small fragments which are necessary for good sample penetration. Use 10 units of *Hae* III per µg and incubate at 37°C for 2 hours. Run 0.5 µg of the digest on a minigel to ensure complete digestion. Remove the restriction enzyme and any other impurities by chromatographing the reaction on a Nensorb column (Procedure 3.12). Redissolve in water to a concentration of about 500 µg/ml. Accurately determine the concentration of the redissolved DNA using UV absorbance.

3. Perform all steps, prior to irradiation, in very dim light or under a photographic safelight. Dissolve photobiotin (Vector Laboratories, BRL) to 1 mg/ml in water. Store at -20°C in a light-proof box.

4. To label DNA, combine in a 1.5 ml microcentrifuge tube:

nicked DNA (up to 30 µl)	10 µg
1 mg/ml photo-biotin	20 µl
water to	50 µl

50 µl total

6. Vortex, open cap of tube and irradiate for 10 minutes on ice under a GE sunlamp (#RSM, 275 W) placed 10 cm above the tube. The lights may now be turned on. Add 100 µl of 0.1 M Tris, pH 8.0 and extract 2x with 100 µl of sec-butanol (discard upper phase). Add 75 µl of water, 10 µl of 4 M sodium acetate and 250 µl of ethanol. Incubate 15 minutes on ice. Centrifuge and wash the pellet with 500 µl of 70% and 100% ethanol and dry. Redissolve to 50 µg/ml with 200 µl of water.

7. The reaction may be scaled up or down, using 2 µg of photobiotin per µg of DNA.

CHEMICAL LABELING WITH A HAPTEN

The hapten counterpart of photobiotin is photo-DNP, a photoactivatable 2,4-DNP labeling reagent described by Keller *et al.* (1989). Photo-DNP consists of a linker arm with a 2,4-dinitrophenyl moiety on one end and an aryl azide moiety on the other end. The synthesis and structure of photo-DNP are diagrammed in Figure 4.7. Since photo-DNP is not commercially available, its synthesis is described in Procedure 4.8. This general scheme can be adapted to any detectable group which contains a primary amine or to which a primary amine can be attached. The detection sensitivity of photo-DNP-labeled probes is essentially the same as for photobiotin-labeled probes, provided a high-affinity anti-DNP antibody is available. These probes may result in lower *in situ* hybridization backgrounds than biotin-labeled probes, owing to the use of antibodies during detection in place of streptavidin. The disadvantage of using photo-DNP is the long detection time required with most antibody detection schemes.

FIGURE 4.7 Synthesis of Photo-DNP. 2,4-dinitrobenzene sulfonic acid (1) and 1,6-diaminohexane (2) are reacted to form 6-(2,4-dinitrophenylamino)-1-aminohexane, compound (3). Compound 3 is reacted with the bifunctional linker arm sulfo-SANPAH, compound (4) to generate compound (5): 6-(2,4-dinitrophenylamino)-1-aminohexyl-6-(4'-azido-2'-nitrophenylamino) hexanoate (photo-DNP).

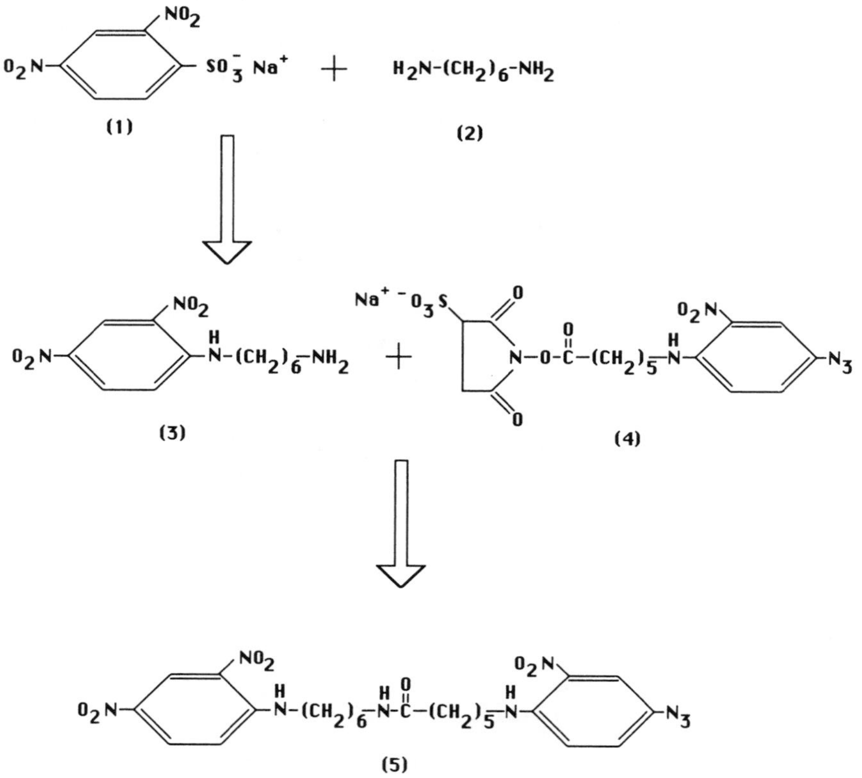

HAPTEN----------------LINKER ARM---------------ARYL AZIDE

PROCEDURE 4.8

PHOTO-DNP LABELING OF DNA

Reagents:
a)   Photo-DNP, about 5 mg/ml in DMSO (Procedure 4.9)
b)   1 M Tris, pH 8.0
c)   Isopropanol
d)   4 M sodium acetate
e)   Cold 100% ethanol
       Cold 70% ethanol
f)   Dimethylsulfoxide (DMSO)

Procedure:

1. Plasmid DNA must be enzymatically linearized or nicked with NaOH (Procedure 4.2). M13 DNA and isolated fragments need no pretreatment before labeling. Before labeling, all DNA samples must be dissolved in water. Tris buffer and proteins will interfere with the labeling, because they are a source of primary amines.

2. If the probe is to be used for *in situ* hybridization, the DNA should not be nicked, but digested with *Hae* III (Procedure 4.7).

3. Perform all steps, prior to irradiation, in very dim light or under a photographic safelight. The DNA does not need to be denatured before labeling.

To label DNA, combine:

nicked DNA (2-10 µg)	10 µl
DMSO	25 µl (final concentration must be >70%)
photo-DNB/ µg DNA	2 µg

40-50 µl total

Vortex, open the tube and irradiate 10 minutes on ice under a sunlamp (GE #RSM, 275 W) positioned 10 cm above the reaction tube. Add 165 µl of water, 20 µl of 4 M sodium acetate and 500 µl of isopropanol. Wash pellet with 70% & 100% ethanol and dry. Redissolve to 50 µg/ml in 200 µl of water.

5. If the probe is difficult to dissolve, heat probe at 60°C for 10 minutes to solubilize, then spin in the microfuge for 5 minutes to remove remaining insoluble debris. Labeled DNA can be stored at -20°C for 1-2 years.

PROCEDURE 4.9A

SYNTHESIS OF PHOTO-DNP

[6-(2,4-dinitrophenylamino)-1-aminohexyl-6-(4'-azido-2'-nitrophenylamino) hexanoate]
(Keller *et al.*, 1989)

Reagents:

a) Sulfo-SANPAH (Pierce)
b) DNP-diaminohexane (Procedure 4.9b)
c) 1 M sodium bicarbonate, pH 9.0
d) Chloroform
e) Dimethylsulfoxide (DMSO)
f) Chlorofrom:methanol (85:15)

Procedure:

1. Perform all steps in very dim light or under a photographic safelight. Dissolve 8 mg of sulfo-SANPAH (1×10^{-5} moles) in 4.5 ml of water in a 10 ml polypropylene tube. Add 0.5 ml of 0.1 M $NaHCO_3$, pH 9.0. SANPAH is a heterobifunctional linker arm; use SANPAH within 4 months of opening.

2. Add 2 ml of 10 mM DNP-diaminohexane (2.6×10^{-5} moles). Incubate at room temperature for 2 hours in the dark.

3. Centrifuge 10 minutes at 2,000 xg to precipitate the oily, orange product. Pour off and discard the supernatant.

4. Dissolve the pellet in 3 ml of $CHCl_3$ and transfer to a 50 ml polypropylene tube. Extract the $CHCl_3$ layer 5 times with 25 ml of water. For each extraction, vortex at top speed for 15 seconds, centrifuge 2 minutes at about 1,000 xg and remove the aqueous supernatant with a glass pipette. Chloroform will melt plastic pipettes. Spot 1 μl aliquots on a TLC plate as described below. Divide the material into 3 microfuge tubes, dry off $CHCl_3$ in a Speed Vac and redissolve the pellets in a total of 1 ml of DMSO. Store at -20°C in 200 μl aliquots (no-defrost freezer) shielded from light. Storage life is about 6 months.

5. Analyze the purity by TLC on fluorescent silica gel plates (Kodak, #13181) using chloroform methanol (85:15) as the solvent (lights may be on). A square glass Coplin jar works well as a mini developing tank. Photo-DNP migrates with the solvent front ($R_f = 1.0$) as an orange-brown spot. There may be a trace of yellow (DNP-diaminohexane) at $R_f = 0.31$. Any SANPAH appears as a brownish-red spot at the origin. The presence of any SANPAH or more than a trace of DNP-diaminohexane indicates the reaction should be extracted three more times with water.

6. Determine the concentration by measuring the UV absorbance: dilute 1/200 in 70% DMSO. Typical readings:

A_{260}	A_{280}	A_{320}	A_{363}	A_{363}/A_{320}	A_{363}/A_{260}
1.120	0.820	0.222	0.715	3.20	0.64

Calculate the yield from the A_{363} reading. A 1 M solution of 2,4-DNP has an A_{360} reading of 1.74×10^4 and photo-DNP has a molecular weight of 560. Thus using the A_{363} reading from above:

0.715(200) = 143 OD/ml

$143/1.74 \times 10^4 = 8.2 \times 10^{-3}$ M (.001 liters) = 8.2×10^{-6} moles DNP

8.2×10^{-6} (560) = 4.60 mg/ml

PROCEDURE 4.9B

SYNTHESIS OF DNP-DIAMINOHEXANE

[6-(2,4-dinitrophenylamino)-1-aminohexane] (Keller *et al.*, 1988)

Reagents:
a) DNP-sulfonic acid (Kodak)
b) 1,6-diaminohexane (Aldrich)
c) Methylene chloride (Aldrich)
d) 100% methanol
e) Chloroform:methanol (85:15)
f) Ninhydrin reagent (Sigma)

Procedure:
1. Dissolve 1g of DNP-sulfonic acid in 40 ml of water in a 50 ml tube. Set up two reactions. Add 2.33 ml of 1,6-diaminohexane to each tube. React overnight at room temperature in the dark.
2. Centrifuge to pellet the precipitates and pour off the supernatant. Dry pellets briefly in a fume hood. Wash pellets 3 times with 40 ml of water to remove the excess diaminohexane. Centrifuge after each wash and pour off supernatant.
3. Extract each pellet 3 times with 40 ml of methylene chloride, centrifuge to separate phases and filter through Whatman #1 paper. Dry the filtrate in a glass tray under a fume hood.
4. Dissolve the residue in 3 aliquots of 100 ml of methanol and filter through Whatman #1 paper. Check the concentration as described below and concentrate to 10 mM if necessary. To concentrate, pour into a glass tray and allow to dry inside a fume hood. Store at 4°C in screw-cap polypropylene tubes.
5. Analyze the purity by TLC on fluorescent silica gel plates (Kodak, #13181) using chloroform methanol (85:15) as the solvent . A square glass Coplin jar works well as a mini developing tank. DNP-diaminohexane should migrate as a single yellow spot and will turn purple when sprayed with ninhydrin reagent and heated to indicate a free amino group. Be certain that no purple spot appears at the origin (1,6-diaminohexane).
6. Dilute 5 µl into 1 ml of water and measure the UV absorbance. Typical readings:

Dilution	A363	A363/ml	Concentration
201	1.026	206	12 mM

Rf = 0.26
Yield is about 70 ml of a 10 mM solution.

FIGURE 4.8 Modification of DNA with Bisulfite and Ethylenediamine. The reaction of cytosine (1) with bisulfite results in 6-sulfo-cytosine (2). Further reaction with ethylenediamine yields the N4-aminoethylene derivative (3). The free amine can be modified with various detectable groups to obtain a hybridization probe.

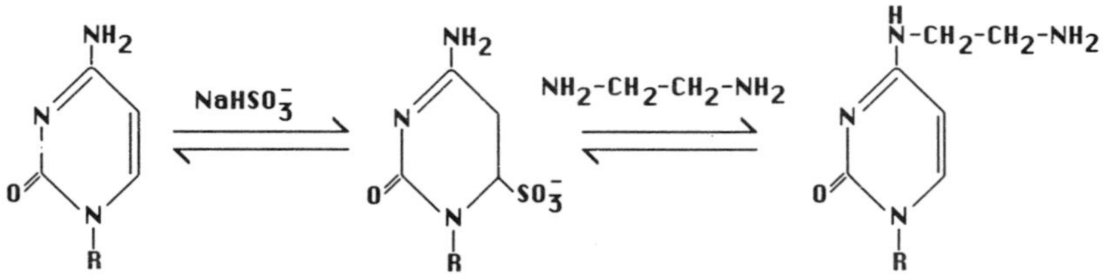

NH$_2$ NH$_2$ $\overset{H}{N}$-CH$_2$-CH$_2$-NH$_2$

NaHSO$_3^-$ NH$_2$-CH$_2$-CH$_2$-NH$_2$

O   O   SO$_3^-$ O

R   R   R

(1)   (2)   (3)

LINKER ARM MODIFICATION OF DNA

The two chemical techniques described below allow the attachment of linker arms to cloned DNA. These are versatile techniques because the linker arm modified DNA can then be labeled with a variety of detectable groups or it can be covalently attached to solid supports (i.e., styrene beads or wells) which would not covalently bind unmodified DNA.

Viscidi *et al.* (1986) described a method in which the cytosines of DNA or RNA are modified at the N-4 position with a linker arm of ethylenediamine in the presence of bisulfite (Figure 4.8). This process also introduces a sulfone moiety at the C-6 position. Their work was based on the earlier findings of Poverenny *et al.* (1979) and Budowsky *et al.* (1972). Under optimum conditions about 30-40 bases are modified per 1,000 bases. Following attachment of the ethylenediamine linker arm, detectable groups, such as NHS-biotin, can be added by reaction with the primary amine. Advantages of this procedure are the use of common reagents, versatility and sensitivity. Disadvantages include, modification of an H-bonding site, and a long preparation time (2 days). The procedure below has been modified by using a longer linker arm (C$_6$ versus C$_4$).

PROCEDURE 4.10

MODIFICATION OF DNA WITH BISULFITE AND DIAMINOHEXANE

Reagents:
The following solutions should be prepared just before use:
a)   9 mM Hydroquinone
       Dissolve 0.5 g of hydroquinone (Sigma) in 5 ml of 95% ethanol (optional).

b)   Modification Solution
     Water   1 ml
     conc. HCl   1 ml
     1,6-diaminohexane* 1 ml   (3 M)
     Sodium bisulfite   0.475 g   (1 M)
     Water to: 5 ml

The pH should be about 6.0, adjust if necessary. Add 50 μl of the hydroquinone solution, if desired. It is included as a free radical scavenger, but in our experience it is not necessary.

*Add a few grams of 1,6-diaminohexane (Aldrich) to a polypropylene tube and incubate at 60°C to melt the solid. Allow it to cool slightly, but not solidify. Quickly transfer 1 ml of the solution to avoid solidification inside the pipette.

c)   4 M sodium acetate
d)   Cold 100% ethanol
     Cold 70% ethanol
e)   N-hydroxysuccinimide-long chain-biotin (Pierce)
f)   Dimethylsulfoxide (DMSO)
g)   1 M sodium bicarbonate

Procedure:

Preparation of Aminohexyl-DNA

1.   Plasmid DNA must first be linearized with a restriction enzyme or chemically nicked with NaOH (Procedure 4.2). The following labeling reaction uses 20 μg of denatured DNA. It may be scaled up or down as desired, but keep the DNA stock concentration at about 1 mg/ml and use 9 volumes of modification solution.

     Denatured DNA, 1.0 mg/ml 20 μl (20 μg)
     Modification solution   180 μl
     _____
                       200 μl total

2.   Incubate the reaction at 42°C for 3 hours.
3.   Dialyze the reaction against water (3 changes of 500 ml) overnight at 4°C.
4.   Transfer to a microfuge tube, measure the volume and add 1/10 volume of 4 M sodium acetate and 2.5 volumes of 100% ethanol. Chill for 30 minutes at -20°C and centrifuge at full speed for 10 minutes. Wash the pellet with 70% ethanol, followed by 100% ethanol and dry briefly.
5.   Dissolve the pellet in 400 μl of water to a final concentration of 50 μg/ml. The linker arm modified DNA may be stored indefinitely at -20°C or it may immediately be modified with a detectable group, such as biotin.

Modification of Aminohexyl-DNA with Biotin

6. The NHS moiety is light sensitive - avoid strong light. Immediately before use, dissolve about 2 mg of N-hydroxysuccinimide-long chain-biotin (Pierce) in DMSO to a concentration of 10 mg/ml.

7. Combine:

AH-DNA	185 µl (10 µg)
1 M NaHCO3, pH 9.0	22.5 µl
10 mg/ml NHS-biotin	17.5 µl (175 µg)

225 µl total

Incubate in the dark at room temperature for 1 hour.

8. Recover the biotin-labeled DNA by adding 25 µl of 4 M sodium acetate and 625 µl of 100% ethanol. Chill 30 minutes at -20°C and centrifuge at full speed for 10 minutes. Wash the pellet with 70% ethanol, followed by 100% ethanol and dry briefly.

9. Dissolve the pellet in 200 µl of water (50 µg/ml final) and store at -20°C. This modified DNA should be stable for 1-2 years. Test the labeled DNA by hybridizing it to dilutions of unlabeled complementary DNA as discussed in Procedure 4.2.

BROMINE-MEDIATED DNA MODIFICATION

DNA may be reacted with N-bromosuccinimide at alkaline pH, resulting in bromination of a fraction of the thymine, guanine and cytosine residues. The bromine is subsequently displaced by a primary amino group of the linker arm. The other end of the linker arm may be a free amine or it may have a detectable group pre-attached to it (Keller *et al.*, 1988). Optimum labeling is achieved at a bromine:base molar ratio of 0.5, yielding 30-35 modified bases per 1,000 bases. Two advantages of this method are modification of sites not involved in hydrogen bonding and rapid labeling. In addition, interstrand crosslinking is avoided when the detectable group is preattached to the linker arm. Figures 4.9 and 4.10 illustrate the two variations of this method. In the three-step procedure illustrated in Figure 4.9, the DNA is brominated, the linker arm displaces the bromine and the detectable group is later added to the free end of the linker arm. In the two-step version in Figure 4.10, the DNA is brominated and the bromine is displaced by a detectable group-linker arm conjugate. Bromine-mediated labeling is not compatible with RNA because of the alkaline reaction conditions.

PROCEDURE 4.11

MODIFICATION OF DNA WITH BROMINE AND DIAMINOHEXANE

Reagents:

a) 8 mM N-Br-Succinimide
    Dissolve 14.2 mg of N-Br-succinimide (Sigma) in 10 ml of water. Store in 1 ml aliquots at -20°C for up to 6 months. Thaw only once, then discard.

b) 80 mM Diaminohexane
    CORROSIVE-WEAR GLOVES   Scrape solid 1,6-diaminohexane (Aldrich) into a 50 ml plastic tube and melt at 60°C. Add 100 µl to 9.9 ml of water. Store at 20°C for up to 6 months in 500 µl aliquots.

c) 4 M sodium acetate

d) Cold 100% ethanol
    Cold 70% ethanol

e) Reactive Detectable Groups
    N-hydroxysuccinimide long chain biotin (NHS-biotin, Pierce)
    N-hydroxysuccinimide-aminocaproic acid-dinitrophenyl (NHS-DNP, Appendix A)
    Dinitrofluorobenzene (Sigma)

f) Dimethylsulfoxide (DMSO)

g) 1 M sodium bicarbonate

Procedure:

1. Use single-stranded M13 DNA or linear, nicked (Procedure 4.2) or enzyme cut and purified (Procedure 3.12) denatured double-stranded DNA for the following reactions.

2. Combine in a microfuge tube:

M13 DNA	20 µg
1 M NaHCO$_3$, pH 9.6	20 µl
Water to	196 µl

    Mix and chill tube on ice for 5 minutes:
8 mM N-Br-succinimide	4 µl

    ---

    200 µl total

    Incubate for 10 minutes on ice.

Three-Step Labeling

3. Add 25 µl of an 80 mM 1,6-diaminohexane solution to the 20 µg of brominated DNA and incubate the reaction at 50°C for 1 hour.

FIGURE 4.9   Modification of DNA with Bromine and Diaminohexane. Single-stranded DNA is incubated with bromine under alkaline conditions to yield bromine at the C-8 position of guanine (shown), the C-5 position of cytosine and possibly the C-6 position of thymidine. The bromine is subsequently displaced by an excess of 1,6-diaminohexane to yield the aminohexyl derivative of the base. The free amino group can be further modified with a detectable group or attached to an insoluble matrix.

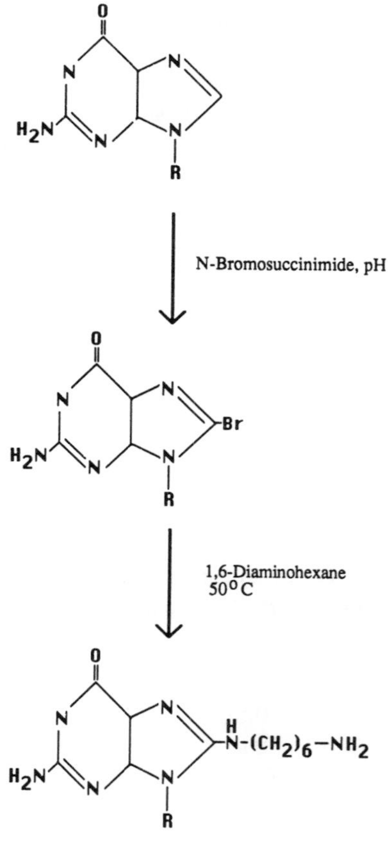

(guanine)

N-Bromosuccinimide, pH 9.6

(8-bromo guanine)

1,6-Diaminohexane
50°C

(8-aminohexyl guanine)

4.   Place tube on ice and add 25 μl of 4 M sodium acetate and 500 μl of ethanol. Incubate at -20°C for 30 minutes. After centrifugation, the pellet is washed in 70% and 100% ethanol and dried. Dissolve pellet in 200 μl of water and repeat precipitation. Wash and dry pellet.

5.   Dissolve the pellet in 100 μl of water, then add 100 μl of DMSO. Add 35 μl of water, 15 μl of 1 M NaHCO$_3$, pH 9.0 and 50 μl of a 10 mg/ml solution of NHS-aminocaproic acid-DNP, dinitrofluorobenzene or NHS-biotin in DMSO. Incubate at room temperature for 1 hour in the dark, then chill on ice.

FIGURE 4.10 Modification of DNA with Bromine and a Linker-Arm Hapten. Single-stranded DNA is incubated with bromine under alkaline conditions to yield bromine at the C-8 position of guanine (shown), the C-5 position of cytosine and possibly the C-6 position of thymidine. The bromine is subsequently displaced by an excess of DNP-diaminohexane resulting in covalent attachment of the free amino group to the base.

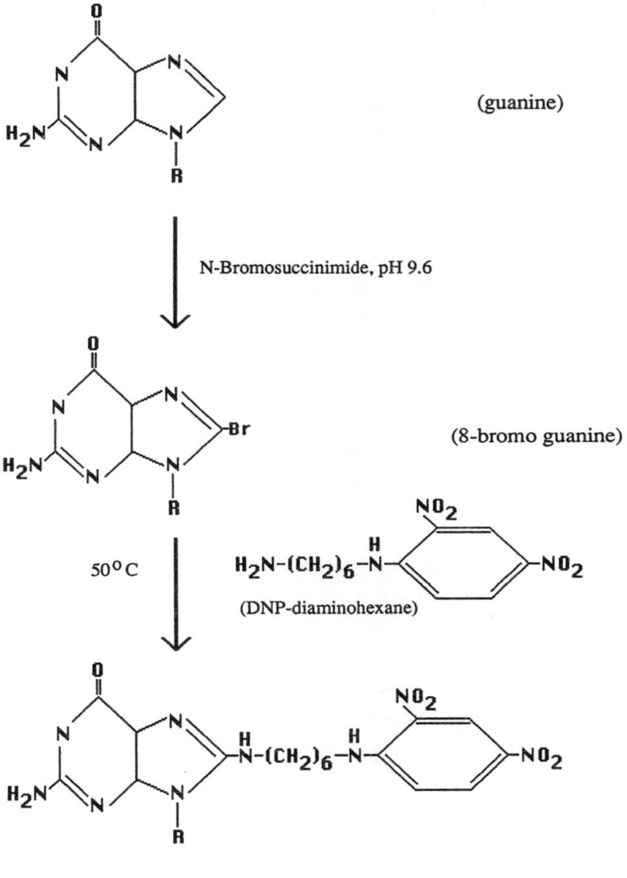

(guanine)

N-Bromosuccinimide, pH 9.6

(8-bromo guanine)

50° C

$H_2N-(CH_2)_6-N-$

(DNP-diaminohexane)

(DNP-8-aminohexyl guanine)

6.   Precipitate by adding 140 µl of 5 M ammonium acetate and 980 µl of isopropanol. Incubate for 10 minutes on ice and centrifuge. Wash pellet with 70% and 100% ethanol and dry. Redissolve pellet in 400 µl of water (50 µg/ml). The labeling efficiency of the DNA can be checked by hybridization to a test strip as described in Procedure 4.2.

Two-Step Labeling
(When a detectable group conjugated to a linker arm is available)
3.   Add 25 μl of 10 mM DNB-diaminohexane (in methanol, Procedure 4.9) to the 20 μg of brominated DNA and incubate the reaction at 50°C for 1 hour in the dark.
4.   Place tube on ice and add 25 μl of 4 M sodium acetate and 500 μl of ethanol. Incubate at -20°C for 30 minutes. After centrifugation, the pellet is washed in 70% and 100% ethanol and dried.
5.   Redissolve the pellet in 200 μl of water (50 μg/ml). Test the labeled probe as described in Procedure 4.2.

OLIGONUCLEOTIDE PROBES

Tailing with a modified dNTP is the most efficient *enzymatic* method for labeling oligonucleotide probes with non-radioactive moieties. The modified nucleotides are added onto the 3' end of the probe in the presence of terminal transferase. Using a modified nucleotide alone, about 10-20 residues are added to the probe. The resulting hybridization signal is not as strong as expected, because only a portion of the detectable groups will be available for detection because of steric hindrance. Longer "tails" containing dCMP residues, which serve as spacers and increase tailing efficiency, will result in stronger signals. However, these tails may cause some non-specific binding depending on probe length and sequence.

Probes which will be labeled by enzymatic tailing should not be detritylated on the synthesizer. The presence of this hydrophobic group will simplify purification of the DNA. Tritylated oligo probes can ꭎe cleaned up by C$_{18}$ (Nensorb) chromatography as described in Procedure 3.13. More complete purification can be accomplished by gel electrophoresis as described in Procedure 4.14. HPLC purification may also be employed, but owing to the vast number of HPLC systems, column resins and buffer systems, such a discussion is outside the scope of this book.

The conditions below are similar to those in Procedure 4.3 for tailing cloned DNA. However, for labeling oligomers, the concentration of 3' ends, rather than the weight of DNA, must be relatively constant. Detectable group-modified dNTPs such as bio-dUTP or digoxigenin-dUTP may be used or AH-dATP may be used and modified later with a detectable group. The use of dCTP is optional since long tails containing cytosine may hybridize non-specifically to target DNA. Note that a single linker-arm ribonucleotide triphosphate can also be added to the 3' ends of oligonucleotide probes using terminal transferase (Kumar *et al.*, 1988) and can be modified later with a detectable group. Examples are C8-aminohexyl-ATP and N6-aminohexyl-ATP, both available from Sigma. Do not use dCTP with ribo-NTPs because it will act as a strong competitive inhibitor.

PROCEDURE 4.12

ENZYMATIC TAILING OF OLIGONUCLEOTIDE PROBES

Reagents:
a) Terminal transferase (BRL)
b) 5x Tailing Buffer
    Concentrated reaction buffer is usually supplied with the terminal transferase. When diluted to 1x concentration, it contains: 100 mM potassium cacodylate, pH 7.0, 1 mM $CoCl_2$ and 0.2 mM dithiothreitol. (Appendix A contains a protocol if you wish to prepare your own.)
c) 5 mM dCTP
d) Modified dNTP
    Biotin-dUTP (Enzo)
    Biotin-dATP (BRL)
    Digoxigenin-dUTP (Boehringer-Mannheim)
    AH-dATP (Procedure 4.5)
e) 4 M sodium acetate
f) Cold 100% ethanol
    Cold 70% ethanol
g) 10 mg/ml yeast tRNA in water (Boehringer-Mannheim)

Procedure:
1. Combine on ice:

Oligonucleotide (3pmol)	x μl (i.e., 20ng of a 20'mer)
5x tailing buffer	20 μl
5.0 mM dCTP	4 μl (200 μM final)
Modified nucleotide	x μl (to 100 μM final)
Add water to	100 μl
Mix and add:	
Terminal transferase	50 units

    Incubate the reaction at 37°C for one hour. The probe may be recovered rapidly by alcohol precipitation or in more purified form by gel electrophoresis.

2. Alcohol precipitation: Recover the tailed probe by adding 50 μg of tRNA, 15 μl of 4 M sodium acetate and 375 μl of 100% ethanol. Incubate for 1 hour at -20°C then pellet the DNA in a microfuge at full speed for 10 minutes. After removing the supernatant, the pellet is washed with 70% ethanol, then 100% ethanol, dried briefly and redissolved in water to a concentration of about 500 ng/ml.
3. Gel purification: Alternatively, the tailed probe may be purified by gel electrophoresis on polyacrylamide gels (Procedure 4.14).

4.   Test the labeled probe as described in Procedure 4.14. If the probe was tailed with AH-dATP, refer to Procedure 4.4, 'Labeling of AH-dATP-Modified DNA.'

The *chemical* attachment of non-radioactive labels to synthetic oligonucleotide probes requires procedures somewhat different from those used for cloned probes. The most efficient procedures chemically modify the probe with a reactive primary amine during synthesis, so that it can easily be modified with a detectable group after synthesis. Table 4.1 lists a number of methods which depend on incorporation into the probe of a 5' linker arm ending in an amino group. Other methods incorporate a linker arm-modified base or a biotin-modified base into the probe. Reagents for introducing a 5'-amino group onto an oligonucleotide probe are commercially available. One example is Aminolink II, from Applied Biosystems, the manufacturer of the most popular DNA synthesizers. Aminolink II is added as the last step in the synthesis program, since oligomers are synthesized in the 3' to 5' direction. Once the amino-modified oligonucleotide is purified, the amino group is typically modified with biotin, peroxidase or alkaline phosphatase.

The addition of a single biotin group to the end of an oligonucleotide probe has been shown to provide a sensitive signal (Cook *et al.*, 1988). An internal biotin-labeled nucleotide will provide less sensitivity than an end-labeled one, presumably because the internal label is less accessible. Multiple biotins on the end of such a probe will provide a stronger signal than a single biotin. Generic reagents are available (Cruachem, Clontech) for the addition of single or multiple 5'-amino groups.

PROCEDURE 4.13

SYNTHESIS AND PURIFICATION OF AMINO-OLIGONUCLEOTIDE PROBES

Reagents:
a)   Aminolink II (Applied Biosystems)
b)   Concentrated ammonium hydroxide (Applied Biosystems)
c)   4 M sodium acetate
d)   Cold 100% ethanol
      Cold 70% ethanol

Procedure:
1.   Set up your DNA synthesizer with all four bases and Aminolink II. To use Aminolink II on synthesizers other than those from Applied Biosystems, check with the manufacturer and Applied Biosystems. Program Aminolink II addition as the last step in the synthesis. Set the program for trityl group on, since the finished DNA will not contain a trityl group because

Aminolink II contains none. After synthesis, store the column, containing the completed oligomer, dry at 4°C until it can be eluted.

2.   Elute the finished 5'-amino oligonucleotide from the column. The following volumes are for a 0.2 μmole or 1 μmole column. Attach a 1 ml syringe to the column. Using another 1 ml syringe, attached to an 18 gauge needle, remove 0.5 ml of concentrated ammonium hydroxide (Applied Biosystems) from the stock bottle. Remove the needle and attach the syringe to the other end of the column. Pass the ammonium hydroxide back and forth through the column several times by pushing with one plunger and pulling with the other. Leave the column immersed in ammonium hydroxide for 15-30 minutes.

Remove the solution from the column by pulling it into one of the syringes and eject it into a screw-top 1.5 ml microfuge tube. Repeat the entire process with another 0.5 ml aliquot of ammonium hydroxide.

3.   Deblock the eluted DNA by heating the oligomer in its 1 ml of solution at 55°C overnight (16 hours). Cool the tube on ice and centrifuge before opening. Transfer the solution to a 15 ml polypropylene tube, cover with Parafilm and poke small holes in the Parafilm with a needle. Freeze the solution in a dry ice bath and lyophilize until dry (usually about 18 hours). Redissolve the dried oligomer in 200 μl of water and re-lyophilize until dry. This double lyophilization assures efficient removal of ammonium ions which can interfere with subsequent labeling. Resuspend the residue in 300 μl of 0.3 M sodium acetate and precipitate the DNA by adding 900 μl of 100% ethanol. Chill to -20°C and centrifuge to collect the pellet. Repeat the precipitation, wash the pellet with 70% ethanol and dry under vacuum. Redissolve the pellet in water, 300 μl for a 0.2 μmol column and 3 ml for a 1 μmol column. Measure the A_{260} and calculate the concentration using an extinction coefficient of 35 $\mu g/OD_{260}$. Store in aliquots at -70°C.

4.   The DNA may be purified by electrophoresis on a polyacrylamide gel (Procedure 4.13), but recovery will be greater if gel purification follows the final labeling step (biotin or enzyme attachment).

5.   Recover the DNA by ethanol precipitation and redissolve in water to a final concentration of 1 mg/ml. The DNA is now ready to label with the detectable group of your choice.

ADDING DETECTABLE GROUPS TO AMINO-OLIGONUCLEOTIDES

The choice of detectable group depends upon the hybridization conditions, hybridization format and personal preference. Biotin is an excellent label for general use, because it is easy to incorporate and it provides a strong hybridization signal. Direct enzyme labeling, on the other hand, shortens the detection process and sometimes results in lower backgrounds than obtained with biotin-labeled probes.

Alkaline phosphatase-labeled probes can be incubated at 50°-60°C for 1–2 hours without significant loss of enzyme activity. This property makes alkaline phosphatase-labeled probes the best choice for filter hybridization and for many *in situ* hybridization applications. The only disadvantage of this label is in hybridization formats where a soluble signal is required, such as in microtiter plates. No sensitive and soluble colorimetric substrate for alkaline phosphatase is readily available. The only choice is the old standard: p-nitrophenyl phosphate. There are sensitive chemiluminescent substrates for alkaline phosphatase, but they require a luminometer or exposure to film for detection (Procedure 5.19).

On the other hand, horseradish peroxidase-labeled oligonucleotides can be detected with tetramethyl benzidine, which is sensitive and gives rise to a soluble, colored product. Such probes have the disadvantage of being limited to hybridization temperatures of 37°-50°C to preserve enzyme activity. Hybridization at these temperatures may not be very stringent and so may compromise specificity. In order to combine 60°C hybridization conditions and peroxidase detection, oligonucleotide probes should be labeled with biotin and detected after hybridization with a peroxidase-streptavidin conjugate. Certain other labels, such as aromatic haptens and fluorescent groups, may result in probes exhibiting high non-specific background signals, because of their hydrophobic character (Urdea *et al.*, 1988).

PROCEDURE 4.14

BIOTIN LABELING OF OLIGONUCLEOTIDE PROBES

Reagents:
a) Oligomer Hybridization Buffer
     0.25g PVP (40,000 MW)   (0.5% final)
     0.25g BSA   (0.5% final)
     0.25g SDS   (0.5% final)
     12.5 ml of 20x SSC   (5x final)
     Water to 50 ml
     Store buffer at -20°C.
b) N-hydroxysuccinimide-long chain-biotin (NHS-LC-biotin, Pierce)
c) 1 M NaHCO$_3$, pH 9.0
d) 10 mg/ml tRNA (Boehringer-Mannheim)
e) 4 M sodium acetate
f) Oligomer hybridization buffer (Procedure 4.2)
g) 20x SSC
h) 10% SDS
i) 3% BSA/1x Wash Buffer (Procedure 5.17)
j) Streptavidin-alkaline phosphatase (BRL)
k) NBT/BCIP substrate solution (Appendix A)

FIGURE 4.11 Preparation of a Biotin-Labeled Oligonucleotide Probe. A 5'-amino derivatized oligonucleotide probe and N-hydroxysuccinimide long chain biotin are reacted at alkaline pH to form the biotinyl-linker arm-oligonucleotide product.

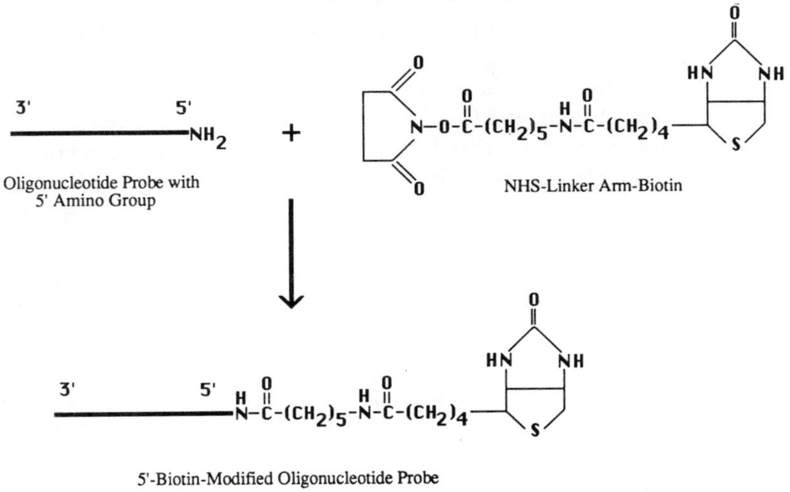

Oligonucleotide Probe with
5' Amino Group

NHS-Linker Arm-Biotin

5'-Biotin-Modified Oligonucleotide Probe

Procedure:

The reaction scheme is outlined in Figure 4.11.

1. Combine in a microfuge tube:

Amino-oligo	200 μl (20 μg)
1 M NaHCO$_3$, pH 9.0	20 μl
NHS-LC-biotin	50 μl (10 mg/ml in DMSO)

    270 μl total

2. Incubate the reaction for 2 hours at room temperature in the dark. To recover, add 5 μl of 10 mg/ml tRNA, 25 μl of 4 M sodium acetate and 500 μl of ethanol. Redissolve in 100 μl of water (200 μg/ml final). Test the labeled probe as described below.

3. Test hybridization of biotin-labeled oligonucleotides:
    a) Prehybridize a nitrocellulose strip, containing dilutions of target plasmid DNA complementary to the probe, in 2.5 ml of oligomer hybridization buffer at 50-65°C for 15 minutes (Procedure 4.2).
    b) Add 1 μl of labeled oligo (200 ng) to 2 ml of hybridization buffer.
    c) Discard prehybridization solution and add probe solution to bag. Hybridize 30 minutes at 50-65°C.
    d) Wash strip twice in 2x SSC/0.1% SDS at 50-65°C for 5 minutes each.

e) Wash strip twice in 2x SSC at room temperature for 5 minutes each.

f) Block strip in 3% BSA/1x wash buffer for 10 min.

g) Incubate strip with 1 µg/ml streptavidin-alkaline phosphatase in 3% BSA/1x wash buffer for 10 minutes.

h) Wash strip 3 times in wash buffer.

i) Develop strip in NBT/BCIP substrate solution for 2 hours.

4. The biotinylated probe may be further purified by gel electrophoresis as described by Urdea (1987). Prepare a 20% (for oligos up to 35 bases) or a 10% (for oligos over 35 bases) denaturing polyacrylamide gel using a 19:1 ratio of acrylamide:bisacrylamide. The gel should be 0.15 cm thick and contain TBE buffer with urea: 90 mM Tris, 90 mM boric acid, 2.7 mM EDTA, pH 8.3, with 8.3 M urea. Pre-electrophorese the gel at 30 mA for 15 minutes in TBE running buffer, pH 8.3. Flush the wells with running buffer.

5. Samples up to 50 µg are dissolved in 20 µl of 90% formamide containing 1% Ficoll (Pharmacia) and 0.01% bromophenol blue and heated at boiled for 2 minutes. After loading about 7 µl per lane, the gel is run at 30 mA for 2.5-4 hours or at 7-10 mA overnight.

6. To visualize the bands, the gel is removed from the glass plates and overlayed on fluorescent silica TLC plates, covered in plastic wrap. The gel is illuminated from above using a short wavelength UV lamp and the bands appear as shadows on the fluorescent background. A photographic record may be made using a Polaroid camera with a green filter (Kodak #50). Cut out the desired bands with a razor blade.

7. Place the gel slice into a 10 ml polypropylene column (Econo column, Bio-Rad) along with 5 ml of 0.1 m Tris, pH 8.0, 0.5 M NaCl and 5 mM EDTA and incubate at room temperature overnight. Drain the buffer from the column and recover the DNA from the buffer by ethanol precipitation or by chromatography on a Nensorb column (Procedure 3.13).

ENZYME CONJUGATION I

One of the simplest and most elegant procedures for conjugating amino-oligonucleotides with enzymes was reported by Urdea et al., (1988). They employed a highly hydrophobic linker (p-phenylene diisothiocyanate, DITC), the excess of which can easily be extracted from the oligonucleotide after the reaction. After coupling the enzyme to the DITC-oligomer, the conjugate is easily and efficiently purified by polyacrylamide gel electrophoresis. The reaction scheme is illustrated in Figure 4.12.

PROCEDURE 4.15

ENZYME LABELING OF OLIGONUCLEOTIDE PROBES USING A HOMOBIFUNCTIONAL LINKER ARM

Reagents:
a)   p-Phenylene diisothiocyanate (DITC, Aldrich)
b)   Horseradish peroxidase (Boehringer-Mannheim #814407)
c)   Alkaline phosphatase (Boehringer-Mannheim, #567752)
     Supplied at 10 mg/ml in 3 M NaCl
d)   0.1 M sodium borate, pH 9.3
e)   Dimethylformamide
f)   7% Polyacrylamide gel in TBE (Procedure 4.14)
g)   1 M sodium phosphate, pH 7.5
h)   Phosphate buffered saline (Appendix A)

Procedure:
All steps are performed at room temperature.
1.   Preparation of DITC-oligomer

NH_2-oligomer	70 µg (dry in a 1.5 ml microfuge tube)
0.1 M Na borate, pH 9.3	25 µl
10 mg DITC in dimethylformamide	500 µl

525 µl total

Incubate in the dark for 2 hours. Transfer the solution to a 10 ml polypropylene tube and add 3 ml of n-butanol. Mix, add 3 ml of water and mix again. Centrifuge and discard the yellow upper layer. Repeat extractions with n-butanol until the volume is about 50 µl, then dry completely on a lyophilizer or Speed-Vac.

2.   Coupling of enzyme to the DITC-oligomer: Dissolve 2 mg of horseradish peroxidase in 200 µl of 0.1 M Na borate, pH 9.3. If peroxidase from another source is used, the enzyme must be free of ammonium ions; dialyze against borate buffer if necessary. Add the enzyme to the dried DITC-oligomer and incubate in the dark overnight.

3.   Purification of the conjugate: To purify the peroxidase-oligomer away from the free DNA and free enzyme, the conjugate is run on a 7% polyacrylamide gel under non-denaturing conditions (TBE buffer). The gel is run until the bromophenol blue tracking dye is about 2/3 of the way down the gel. The peroxidase-oligomer conjugate can be visualized as a brown band about midway down the gel.

FIGURE 4.12 Preparation of an Enzyme-Labeled Oligonucleotide Probe using a Homobifunctional Linker Arm. A 5'-amino derivatized oligonucleotide probe is first activated with the linker arm DITC to introduce an isothiocyanate moiety. This activated group can then react with the free amino groups on an enzyme to produce an enzyme-conjugated probe.

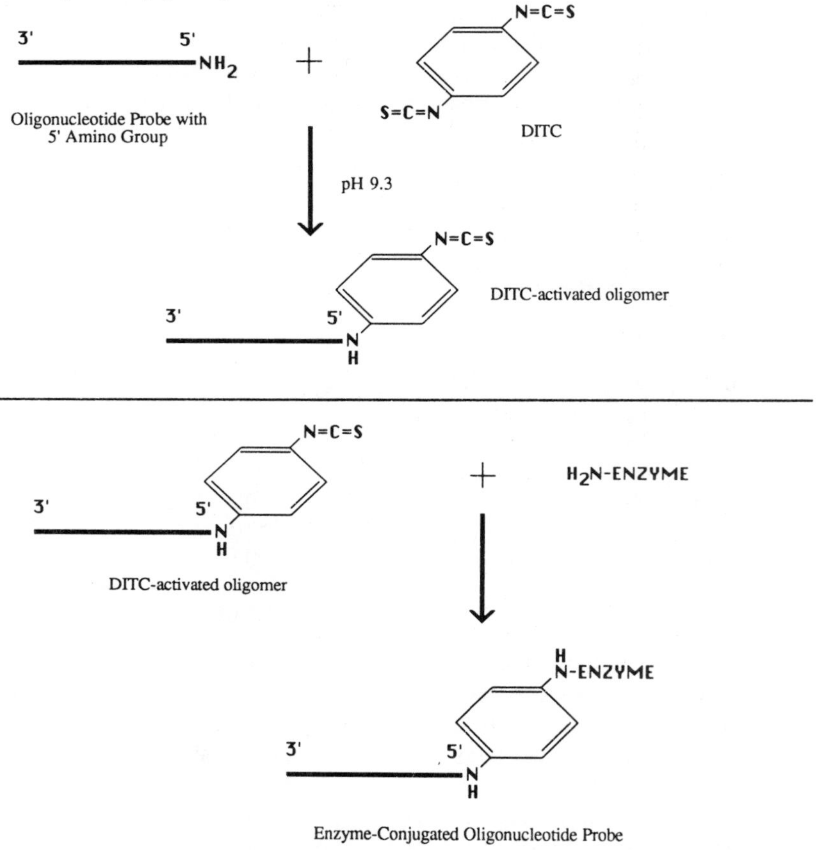

Enzyme-Conjugated Oligonucleotide Probe

4.   Recover the conjugate by cutting out the band and place it in a stoppered 10 ml Econo-column (Bio-Rad) with 3 ml of 0.1 M sodium phosphate, pH 7.5. Incubate the gel slice in the column overnight in the dark. Collect the buffer from the bottom of the column. Prewash a Centricon 10 (Amicon) micro-concentrator twice with water. Add the conjugate to the concentrator and centrifuge at about 2,000 xg to concentrate. Wash the concentrator twice with 1 ml aliquots of PBS.

5. Storage of the conjugate: The purified conjugate may be stored frozen in aliquots at -20°C, in 50% glycerol at -20°C, or it may be lyophilized and stored at 4° or -20°C.

6. Alkaline phosphatase conjugation: For alkaline phosphatase-conjugated probes, the above procedure is followed with minor modifications. Two miligrams (200 µl) of alkaline phosphatase is added to a Centricon 30 micro-concentrator (Amicon) with 2 ml of 0.1 M sodium borate, pH 9.3 and centrifuged at 2,000 xg until the volume decreases to about 50 µl. The equilibrated, concentrated enzyme is then reacted with the DITC-oligomer as above. The purification procedure is the same except that the band is visualized by UV shadowing and the gel slice is eluted with 0.1 M Tris, pH 7.5 containing 0.1 M NaCl, 10 mM $MgCl_2$ and 0.1 mM $ZnCl_2$. The final product may be stored as described above or at 4°C with 0.05% sodium azide.

7. Testing of labeled probes:

    a) Prehybridize a nitrocellulose strip, containing dilutions of target plasmid DNA complementary to the probe (Procedure 4.2), in 2.5 ml of oligo hybridization   buffer (Procedure 4.13) at 50-65°C (depending on enzyme label and base composition) for 15 minutes .

    b) Add 100 ng of labeled oligo to 2 ml of oligo hybridization buffer.

    c) Discard prehybridization solution and add probe solution to bag. Hybridize 30 minutes at 50-65°C.

    d) Wash strip twice in 2x SSC/0.1% SDS at 50°C for 5 minutes each.

    e) Wash strip twice in 2x SSC at room temperature for 5 minutes each.

    f) For alkaline phosphatase-labeled probes, develop the strip in NB / BCIP substrate solution (Appendix A) for 2 hours.

    g) For peroxidase-labeled probes, develop the strip in precipitable TMB substrate solution (Kirkegaard & Perry) for 30-60 minutes.

ENZYME CONJUGATION II

In contrast to the homobifunctional linker arm used in Procedure 4.14, the following procedure employs a longer, heterobifunctional linker arm to couple enzymes to the 5'-amino group of the oligonucleotide probe. The use of different reactive groups on the ends of the linker arm prevents cross-linking of probe or enzyme. The general reaction scheme for coupling an enzyme to an amino-oligonucleotide using the heterobifunctional linker arm sulfo-SANPAH is outlined in Figure 4.12. Sulfo-SANPAH is light-sensitive, so steps 1-3 must be performed in very dim light or under a photographic safelight.

FIGURE 4.13 Preparation of an Enzyme-Labeled Oligonucleotide Probe using a Heterobifunctional Linker Arm. An enzyme is activated to bind an amino-oligonucleotide probe by first reacting in the dark with the NHS end of the heterobifunctional linker arm SANPAH. In the presence of light, the aryl azide end of SANPAH reacts with the 5'-amino derivatized oligonucleotide to produce an enzyme-conjugated probe.

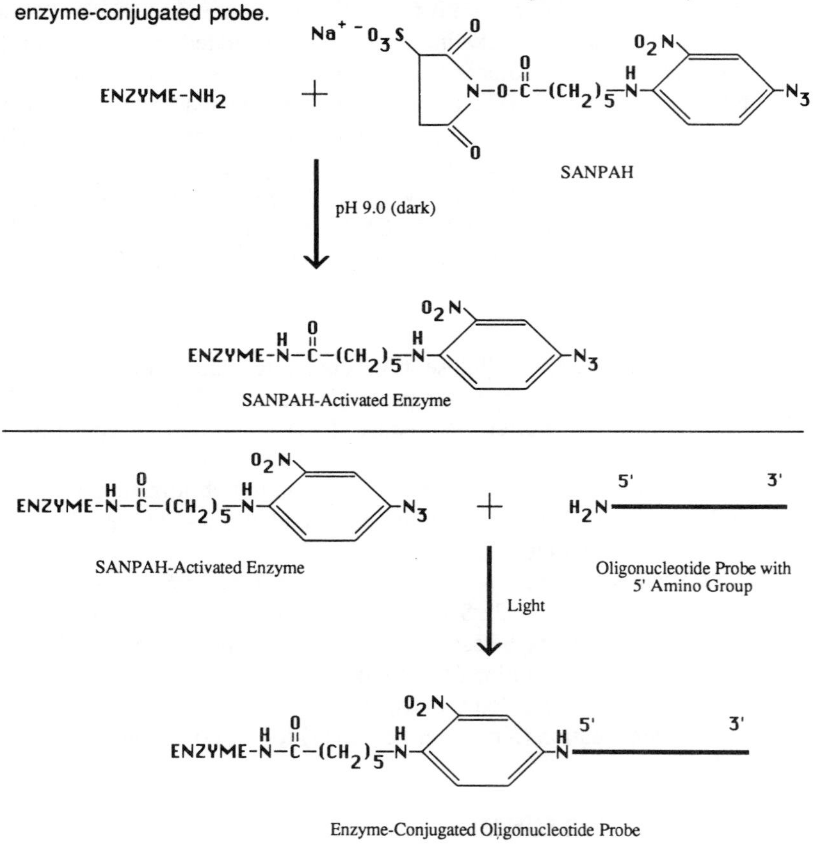

SANPAH

pH 9.0 (dark)

SANPAH-Activated Enzyme

SANPAH-Activated Enzyme   +   Oligonucleotide Probe with 5' Amino Group

Light

Enzyme-Conjugated Oligonucleotide Probe

PROCEDURE 4.16

ENZYME LABELING OF OLIGONUCLEOTIDE PROBES USING A HETEROBIFUNCTIONAL LINKER ARM

Reagents:
a)   Sulfo-SANPAH (Pierce)
b)   Horseradish peroxidase (Boehringer-Mannheim #814407)
c)   Alkaline phosphatase (Boehringer-Mannheim, #567752)
       Supplied at 10 mg/ml in 3 M NaCl
d)   1 M NaHCO$_3$, pH 9.0
e)   0.1 M NaCl
f)   0.1 M Tris, pH 8.0

Procedure:

1. Preparation of SANPAH-alkaline phosphatase:

10 mg/ml alkaline phosphatase	170 µl (1.7 mg)
1 M NaHCO$_3$ pH 9.0	20 µl (0.1 M)
10 mg/ml sulfo-SANPAH in H$_2$O	10 µl (100 µg, 12-fold molar excess)

    200 µl total

2. Incubate for 2 hours at room temperature in the dark. Dialyze against 4 changes of 250 ml of 0.1 M NaCl at room temperature in the dark. Measure the final volume to determine the concentration. It should be about 8.5 mg/ml. Store at -20°C.

3. Labeling of a 5'-amino oligonucleotide with SANPAH-alkaline phosphatase:

Amino-oligo (100 µg/ml in water)	250 µl (25 µg)
SANPAH-Alkaline phosphatase 75 µl (127 µg AP)	(3.3-fold molar excess)

    325 µl total

    Irradiate the reaction on ice for 10 minutes under a sun lamp (GE #RSM, 275W). Add 175 µl of 0.1 M Tris, pH 8.0 to bring the volume to 500 µl (50 µg/ml). Store at -20°C.

4. Test the probe as described in Procedure 4.15.

5. The conjugate may be purified by gel electrophoresis as described in Procedure 4.15. Peroxidase-conjugated probes may be synthesized by using similar molar ratios of SANPAH and enzyme.

References

1. Albarella, J.P., Minegar, R.L. Patterson, W.L., Dattagupta, N. and Carlson, E. (1989): Monoadduct forming photochemical reagents for labeling nucleic acids for hybridization, Nucleic Acids Res. **17**, 4293-4308.

2. Brakel, C.L. and Engelhardt, D.L. (1985): in Kingsbury, D.T. and Falcow, S. (eds.), Rapid detection and identification of infectious agents, Academic Press, New York, pp. 235-243.

3. Brigati, D.J., Myerson, D., Leary, J.J., Spalholz, B., Travis, S.Z., Fong, C.K.Y., Hsiung, G.D. and Ward D.C. (1983): Detection of viral genomes in cultured cells and paraffin-embedded tissue sections using biotin-labeled hybridization probes, Virology, **126** 32-50.

4. Budowsky, E.I., Sverdlov, E.D. and Monastyrakaya, G.S. (1972): New method of selective and rapid modification of the cytidine residues, FEBS Lett. **25**, 201-204.

5. Chaiet, L. and Wolf, F.J. (1964): The properties of streptavidin, a biotin-binding protein produced by *Streptomycetes*, Arch. Biochem. Biophys. **106**, 1-5.

6. Chu, E.C.F. and Orgel, L.E. (1988): Ligation of oligonucleotides to nucleic acids or proteins via disulfide bonds, Nucleic Acids Res. **16**, 3671-3691.

7. Cook, A.F., Vuocolo, E. and Brakel, C. (1988): Synthesis of a series of biotinylated oligonucleotides, Nucleic Acids Res. **16**, 4077-4095.

8. Dahlen, P., Hurskainen, P., Lovgren, T. and Hyypia, T. (1988): Time-resolved fluorometry for the identification of viral DNA in clinical specimens, J. Clin. Microbiol. **26**, 2434-2436.

9. Dahlen, P., Syvanen, A.C., Hurskainen, P., Kwiatkowski, M., Sund, C., Ylikoski, J., Soderlund, H. and Lovgren, T. (1987): Sensitive detection of genes by sandwich hybridization and time-resolved fluorometry, Molecular and Cellular Probes **1**, 159-168.

10. Dale, R.M.K. and Ward, D.C. (1975): Mercurated polynucleotides: New probes for hybridization and selective polymer fractionation, Biochemistry **14**, 2458-2469.

11. Dale, R.M.K., Martin, E., Livingston, D.C. and Ward, D.C. (1973): The Synthesis and enzymatic polymerization of nucleotides containing mercury: Potential tools for nucleic acid sequencing and structural analysis, Proc. Natl. Acad. Sci. USA **70**, 2238-2242.

12. Dale, R.M.K., Martin, E., Livingston, D.C. and Ward, D.C. (1975): Direct covalent mercuration of nucleotides and polynucleotides, Biochemistry **14**, 2447-2457.

13. Fink, G., Fasold, H., Rommel, W. and Brimacombe, R. (1980): Reagents suitable for the crosslinking of nucleic acids to proteins, Anal. Biochem. **108**, 394-401.

14. Forster, A.C., McInnes, J.L., Skingle, D.C. and Symons, R.H. (1985): Non-Radioactive hybridization probes prepared by the chemical labeling of DNA and RNA with a novel reagent, photobiotin, Nucleic Acids Res. **13**, 745-761.

15. Gebeychu, G., Rao, P.Y., SooChan, P., Simms, D.A. and Klevan, L. (1987): Novel biotinylated nucleotide analogs for labeling and colorimetric detection of DNA, Nucleic Acids Res. **15**, 4513-4534.

16. Heiles, B.J., Genersch, E., Kessler, C., Neumann, R. and Eggers, H.J. (1988): *In situ* hybridization with digoxigenin-labeled DNA of human papillomaviruses (HPV 16/18) on HeLa and SiHa cells, Biotechniques **6**, 978-981.

17. Hopman, A.H.N., Wiegant, J., Tesser, G.I. and Van Dujin, P. (1986): A Non-Radioactive *in situ* Hybridization Method Based on Mercurated Nucleic Acid Probes and Sulfhydryl-Hapten Ligands, Nucleic Acids Res. **14**, 6471-6488.

18. Jablonski, E., Moomaw, E.W., Tullis, R. and Ruth, J.L. (1986): Preparation of oligodeoxynucleotide-alkaline phosphatase conjugates and their use as hybridization probes, Nucleic Acids Res. **14**, 6115-6128.

19. Keller, G.H., Cumming, C.U., Huang, D.P., Manak, M.M. and Ting, R. (1988): A Chemical method for introducing haptens onto DNA probes, Anal. Biochem. **170**, 441-450.

20. Keller, G.H., Huang, D.P. and Manak, M.M. (1989): Labeling of DNA probes with a photoactivatable hapten, Anal Biochem. **177**, 392-395.

21. Kumar, A., Tchen, P., Roullet, F. and Cohen, J. (1988): Nonradioactive labeling of synthetic oligonucleotide probes with terminal deoxynucleotidyl transferase, Anal. Biochem. **169**, 376-382.

22. Landes, G.M. (1986): Labeled DNA, U.S. Patent #4,626,501.

23. Langer, P.R., Waldrop, A.A. and Ward, D.C. (1981): Enzymatic synthesis of biotin-labeled polynucleotides: Novel nucleic acid affinity probes, Proc. Natl. Acad. Sci. USA **78**, 6633-6637.

24. Leary, J.J., Brigati, D.J. and Ward, D.C. (1983): Colorimetric method for visualizing biotin-labeled DNA probes hybridized to DNA or RNA immobilized on nitrocellulose: Bio-blots, Proc. Natl. Acad. Sci. USA **80**, 4045-4049.

25. Lee, C.Y., Lazarus, L.H., Kabakoff, D.S., Russell, P.J., Laver, M. and Kaplan, N.O. (1977): Purification of kinases by general ligand affinity chromatography, Arch. Biochem. Biophys. **178**, 8-18.

26. Li, P., Medon, P., Skingle, D.C., Lanser, J.A. and Symons, R.H. (1987): Enzyme-linked synthetic oligonucleotide probes: non-radioactive detection of *Esherichia coli* im faecal specimens, Nucleic Acids Res. **15**, 5275-5287.

27. McCracken, S. (1985): Preparation of RNA transcripts using SP6 RNA polymerase, Focus **7** (2), 5-8; Focus **9** (4), 10.

28. Oser, A., Roth, W.K. and Valet, G. (1988): Sensitive non-radioactive dot-blot hybridization using DNA probes labeled with chelate group substituted psoralen and quantitative detection by europium ion fluorescence, Nucleic Acids Res. **16**, 1181-1196.

29. Poverenny, A.M., Podgorodnichenko, V.K., Bryksina, L.E., Monastyrskaya, G.S. and Sverdlov, E.D. (1979): Immunochemical approaches to DNA structure investigation-I, Molecular Immunology **16**, 313-316.

30. Reisfeld, A., Rothenberg, J.M., Bayer, E.A. and Wilchek, M. (1987): Non-radioactive hybridization probes prepared by the reaction of biotin-hydrazide with DNA, Biochem. Biophys. Res. Commun. **142**, 519-526.

31. Renz, M. and Kurz, C. (1984): A colorimetric method for DNA hybridization, Nucleic Acids Res. **12**, 3435-3444.

32. Riley, L.K., Marshall, M.E. and Coleman, M.S. (1986): Method for biotinylating oligonucleotide probes for use in molecular hybridizations, DNA **5**, 333-337.

33. Rothenberg, J.M. and Wilchek, M. (1988): p-Diazobenzoyl-biocytin: a new biotinylating reagent for DNA, Nucleic Acids Res. **16**, 7197.

34. Ruth, J.L. (1984): Chemical synthesis of non-radioactively-labeled DNA hybridization probes, DNA **3**, 123.

35. Sheldon, E.L., Kellogg, D.E., Watson, R.E., Levinson, C.H. and Erlich, H.A. (1986): Use of nonisotopic M13 probes for genetic analysis: application to class II loci, Proc. Natl. Acad. Sci. USA **83**, 9085-9089.

36. Smith, L.M., Fung, S., Hunkapiller, M.W., Hunkapiller, T.J. and Hood, L.E. (1985): The synthesis of oligonucleotides containing an aliphatic amino group at the 5' terminus: Synthesis of fluorescent DNA primers for use in DNA sequence analysis, Nucleic Acids Res. **13**, 2399-2412.

37. Sproat, B.S., Beijer, B. and Rider, P. (1987): The synthesis of protected 5'-amino-2',5'-dideoxyribonucleoside-3'-O phosphoramidites; applications of 5'-amino oligodeoxyribonucleotides, Nucleic Acids Res. **15**, 6181-6196.

38. Syvanen, A.C., Alanen, M. and Soderlund, H. (1985): A complex of single-strand binding protein and M13 DNA as hybridization probe, Nucleic Acids Res. **13**, 2789-2802.

39. Syvanen, A.C., Laaksonen, M. and Soderlund, H. (1986): Fast quantification of nucleic acid hybrids by affinity-based hybrid collection, Nucleic Acids Res. **14**, 5037-5048.

40. Takahashi, Y., Arakawa, H., Maeda, M. and Tsuiji, A. (1989): A new biotinylating system for DNA using biotin aminocaproyl hydrazide and glutaraldehyde, Nucleic Acids Res. **17**, 4899-4900.

41. Tchen, P., Fuchs, R.P.P., Sage, E. and Leng, M. (1984): Chemically modified nucleic acids as immuno-detectable probes in hybridization experiments, Proc. Natl. Acad. Sci. USA **81**, 3466-3470.

42. Tomlinson, S., Lyga, A., Huguenel, E. and Dattagupta, N. (1988): Detection of biotinylated nucleic acid hybrids by antibody-coated gold colloid, Anal. Biochem. **171**, 217-222.

43. Urdea, M.S. (1987): Design, chemical synthesis and molecular cloning of a gene for human epidermal growth factor, Methods in Enzymol. **146**, 22-41.

44. Urdea, M.S., Warner, B.D., Running, J.A., Stempien, M., Clyne, J. and Horn, T. (1988): A comparison of non-radioisotopic hybridization assay methods using fluorescent, chemiluminescent and enzyme-labeled synthetic oligodeoxyribonucleotide probes, Nucleic Acids Res. **16**, 4937-4956.

45. Viscidi, R.P., Connelly, C.J. and Yolken, R.H. (1986): Novel chemical method for the preparation of nucleic acids for nonisotopic hybridization, J. Clin. Microbiol. **23**, 311-317.

Section 5:
Hybrization Formats and Detection Procedures

Introduction

Various formats can be used for the detection of specific hybridization. Solution hybridization formats offer the fastest hybridization rates of the commonly used hybridization formats (Britten *et al.*, 1974). However, the difficulties in separating the free and hybridized probe have limited routine use of this format in the laboratory. Far more common are methods which involve the immobilization of one of the reacting nucleic acids on a solid support, while the other is free in solution. Such mixed phase hybridization methods offer convenient formats for the detection of nucleic acid hybrids since unreacted molecules can be easily washed away after hybridization, leaving only those which are specifically bound. The solid support can be a nitrocellulose or nylon filter, latex or magnetic beads, or microtiter plates. Immobilization has an additional advantage, it prevents self-annealing of the target molecule.

The principles governing probe-excess immobilized target hybridization are basically similar to those governing solution hybridization (Meinkoth and Wahl, 1984). However, relative to solution hybridization,the rate of hybridization with one strand immobilized on on a membrane is slower by a factor of 7-10 due to the requirement for diffusion of the soluble nucleic acid into the filter (Flavell *et al.*, 1974; also see discussion in Section 1). Nitrocellulose membranes have been traditionally used in many filter hybridization applications because of their convenience and low background signals. More recently, however, nylon based membranes which are more durable and exhibit higher binding capacities have provided a valuable alternative to nitrocellulose in many applications.

Several filter based hybridization systems are in common use. The 'spot' or 'dot blot' hybridization method uses target nucleic acid immobilized as spots on a filter and can be used for semi-quantitative detection of specific nucleic acid sequences (Kafatos *et al.*, 1979). The size of a specific nucleic acid can be analyzed by separating the DNA fragments (Southern blot) or RNA species (northern blot) by gel electrophoresis and transferring them to a filter for

149

hybridization with specific labeled probes (Alwine *et al.*, 1977; Southern, 1975). Membrane hybridizations are also useful for screening bacterial colonies such in the selection of recombinant molecules (Grunstein and Hogness, 1975).

Sandwich hybridization is a composite format utilizing two probes, one for capture and another for detection. While the detection probe is soluble, the capture probe may or may not be immobilized during hybridization, but is always immobilized during detection. The use of capture DNA sequences immobilized in microtiter wells potentially allows the simultaneous analysis of a large number of biological samples (Keller *et al.*, 1989). Sandwich hybridization and other interesting formats are discussed in detail at the end of this section.

In situ hybridization methods allow the examination of specific sequences directly in fixed cells or tissues. Intact cells or tissues are fixed on microscope slides using conditions which retain their morphology and cellular structures. After hybridization, the location of the probe molecules in the cells can be examined microscopically (Gall and Pardue, 1969) The concentration of hybridization signal within a very small area (inside the cell) gives this format greater sensitivity than other unamplified formats.

In this section, hybridization formats using filters, slides and microtiter wells will be discussed and detailed.

FILTER HYBRIDIZATION

Hybridization membranes are highly porous, solid-phase supports which provide a large surface area to bind nucleic acids. Once immobilized on membranes, nucleic acids can be identified by hybridization.

Nitrocellulose membranes are often used for immobilizing nucleic acid in hybridization assays. These membranes are convenient to use and give low background signals with both radioactive and nonradioactive probes. The chemical nature of the binding of the nucleic acids to nitrocellulose has not been well characterized, but is assumed to be non-covalent (Meinkoth and Wahl, 1984). However, after baking at 80°C for two hours the nucleic acids are firmly retained and will not detach even during stringent treatments. The low, non-specific binding of proteins to nitrocellulose makes these membranes particularly useful for use with non-isotopic probes where antibodies or enzymes must be used to develop the hybridization signal.

The use of nitrocellulose does have certain drawbacks. Nucleic acid binding is dependent on transfer conditions and high salt concentrations (>10x SSC) are required (Bresser and Gillespie, 1983). Small nucleic acid fragments (<200 bp) bind inefficiently (Meinkoth and Wahl, 1984). Furthermore, the fragility of these membranes makes them difficult to manipulate or use in transfers involving large gels. Thus, they do not stand up well to multiple rehybridization cycles.

Nylon based membranes are an attractive alternative to nitrocellulose because they offer greater strength and durability and can covalently bind nucleic acid fragments as small as 10 base pairs (Cannon *et al.*, 1985; Reed and Mann, 1985). Cationic nylon membranes such as Zeta-Probe (Bio-Rad), MagnaGraph (MSI), Biodyne B (Pall) or Gene-Screen Plus (DuPont) tightly bind single-stranded DNA and RNA under a wide range of conditions, even in low ionic strength buffers. Baking is not required for the binding of single-stranded nucleic acids to most nylon membranes, although ultraviolet crosslinking appears to be helpful in retaining small DNA fragments (Gross *et al.*, 1985). Extensive UV cross-linking, however, can interfere with hybridization efficiency, particularly when short A-T rich probes are used. Following hybridization and detection with the first probe, the probe can be stripped from the membrane without removing the target DNA. The flexibility and durability of nylon membranes permit them to be stripped and rehybridized many times. The binding of nucleic acids to charged nylon membranes is dependent upon both hydrophobic and ionic interactions, giving much tighter binding than with nitrocellulose. Thus, the nucleic acid binding capacity of these membranes ($350-500$ $\mu g/cm^2$) is much higher than of nitrocellulose ($80-100$ $\mu g/cm^2$). Nylon based membranes also have a high affinity for proteins and this presents particular problems when using non-isotopic probes. Even when preblocked with various protein solutions (BSA, milk or casein) the background signals on nylon membranes are generally higher than with nitrocellulose (Johnson *et al.*, 1984). This seems to be a result of non-specific binding of detection reagents (antibodies, enzymes), rather than non-specific binding of probe.

Similar to the nylon-based membranes are the Immobilon-N membranes (Millipore), which are made from PVDF, an extremely hydrophobic fluorocarbon with a charge-modified surface to enhance the ionic interaction with the phosphate backbone of nucleic acids. This membrane has an even higher retention of DNA than the charged nylon membranes. It is also more easily blocked during prehybridization giving rise to lower background signals than nylon membranes with both isotopic and non-isotopic probes. Like the nylon-based membranes, this membrane is very durable and flexible and can be used for multiple hybridization experiments.

SPOT BLOT HYBRIDIZATION

One of the simplest and most effective filter hybridization methods is to spot crude or purified mixtures of nucleic acids directly onto the surface of a membrane, such as nitrocellulose, where they are immobilized by baking (Kafatos *et al.*, 1979). Spot blot procedures are rapid, semi-quantitative and can be used to detect the presence of specific nucleic acid in many samples simultaneously on the same filter. In order to apply specific volumes of nucleic acid onto well defined surface areas, convenient manifolds, such as the Minifold I and II (Schleicher & Schuell), Bio-Dot (Bio-Rad) and Hybri-Dot (Bethesda Research Laboratories) are commercially available. These manifolds consist of multiple wells into which the sample is applied and allowed to flow to the membrane as discrete 'spots' or 'slots' under gentle vacuum. The wells are then repeatedly rinsed with wash solutions, the membranes removed and baked or irradiated to fix the nucleic acids. The filter can then be hybridized with a specific probe as described in Procedure 5.12 or 5.15. Unbound probe is washed off and spots containing the DNA or RNA of interest are detected by autoradiography, scintillation counting or reaction with enzyme substrates, for example. When non-radioactive probes are used, the membranes must be incubated after hybridization, with horse serum, BSA, or casein to block protein-binding sites which would contribute to non-specific signals.

The following procedure demonstrates the use of a slot-blot apparatus (Minifold II, Schleicher & Schuell) to detect viral DNA sequences in cultured cells. Up to 2 µg of purified DNA or extracts from up to 2×10^5 cultured cells can be applied per well. The DNA should be denatured and adjusted to 6x SSC before applying to filters. If very small amounts of DNA are present in the sample, the addition of 200 ng of carrier DNA, such as salmon sperm DNA, will assure quantitative binding to the filter. For quantitation studies, it is desirable to make serial dilutions of the DNA to be tested in 6x SSC containing 200 ng carrier DNA.

PROCEDURE 5.1

SLOT BLOTTING OF DNA

Reagents and Equipment:
a) TE Buffer
    10 mM Tris-HCl, pH 7.6
    1 mM EDTA
b) 6x SSC
c) 15x SSC
d) Minifold II manifold (Schleicher & Schuell)
e) Nitrocellulose (Schleicher & Schuell)

Procedure:
1. Wear gloves when handling the membrane or the manifold. Pre-wet the nitrocellulose filter in water (precut membranes for the Minifold apparatus are available from the manufacturer). When the filter is completely hydrated, transfer it to 15x SSC.
2. Separate the top and bottom halves of the Minifold apparatus Apply 2

sheets of the blotter paper (Schleicher & Schuell #470) to the top of the bottom half of the well section of the plates, being careful to align the notches properly. Do not pre-wet the blotter paper.

3. Turn the top half of the Minifold apparatus upside down and lay the wet nitrocellulose filter carefully into position, avoiding any air bubbles.

4. Assemble the two plates together and clamp firmly.

5. Denature the DNA sample (in water or TE) by boiling for 5 minutes and quick cooling on ice. Adjust the volume to 200 µl in 6x SSC and centrifuge in a microfuge for 1 minute to bring down insoluble material which may clog the filter.

6. Apply up to 200 µl of the clarified sample into each well. The sample will be drawn into the nitrocellulose by the wicking action created by the blotting paper. To avoid getting haloes instead of sharp slots, apply the sample at a steady rate directly into the center of well. Avoid getting air bubbles trapped in the wells.

7. Attach a vacuum hose and apply gentle suction.

8. After the samples had completely entered the wells, wash each well twice with 100 µl of 6x SSC under gentle vacuum.

9. Remove the nitrocellulose and bake it in a vacuum oven for 2 hours at 80°C. The baked filters can be stored in heat-seal bags until they are ready for use in hybridization experiments (Procedures 5.12 and 5.15)

PROCEDURE 5.2

SLOT BLOTTING OF RNA

A similar procedure can be used for the slot-blot analysis of RNA. Up to 10 µg of total RNA (purified by phenol/chloroform or guanidinium thiocyanate extraction) can be loaded in each well.

Reagents and Equipment:

a) Formaldehyde/SSC Buffer
    6.15 M formaldehyde in 10x SSC

b) Minifold II manifold (Schleicher & Schuell)

c) Nitrocellulose (Schleicher & Schuell)

Procedure:

1. Prepare the Minifold apparatus as described in Procedure 5.1, Steps 1-4.

2. To denature the RNA, combine 50 µl of RNA in water with 150 µl of formaldehyde/SSC buffer.

3. Apply the sample to the slot-blot manifold and process as described in Procedure 5.1, Steps 6-9.

CYTOPLASMIC DOT HYBRIDIZATION

Rapid methods for RNA extraction have been designed to allow the screening of multiple biological samples for the presence of specific transcripts quickly and conveniently. The demonstration by Thomas (1980) that denatured RNA binds effectively to nitrocellulose in high salt permitted not only the dot-blot analysis of RNA, but also the size analysis of RNA species on northern blots (Procedures 5.8 and 5.9). However, the purification procedure for RNA is time-consuming, making routine screening of multiple samples difficult. Moreover, the variable recovery rates of the RNA,using complex isolation techniques, make quantitation of the RNA in the samples unreliable.

Simplified sample processing techniques not involving extraction and purification of RNA from cells have overcome some of these difficulties. Cellular cytoplasmic extracts can be prepared from a variety of animal cells by brief treatment with a hypotonic buffer containing 0.5% Nonidet P40 (White and Bancroft, 1982). Nuclei and cell debris are removed by centrifugation, leaving a cytoplasmic extract which is enriched for cytoplasmic RNA and is relatively free of genomic DNA. This crude RNA can be denatured with formaldehyde in the presence of high salt and loaded directly onto nitrocellulose without additional processing. This method permits the rapid analysis of large numbers of samples and requires only small amounts of cells ($5x10^4$) or tissue. In all work with RNA, precautions must be taken to ensure that endogenous RNase activity is inactivated. One method is to add a ribonucleoside vanadyl complex (RVC) to the samples. All other precautions for maintaining RNase-free conditions must also be followed (Section 2). The following procedure is for the extraction of RNA from cultured cells.

PROCEDURE 5.3

CYTOPLASMIC DOT HYBRIDIZATION

Reagents:
a)   Phosphate buffered saline (PBS, Appendix A)
b)   SSC/RVC
     3 parts: 20x SSC (Appendix A)
     2 parts: 200 mM ribonucleoside vanadyl complex (Procedure 2.9)
c)   Nonidet P40
d)   Formaldehyde/SSC
     3 parts: 20x SSC
     2 parts: 37% formaldehyde

Procedure:
1.   Wash the harvested cells with PBS and pellet them by centrifugation at 1,000 x g for 10 minutes.

2. Resuspend the cells in a small volume of PBS ($1-10 \times 10^8$ cells/ml) and transfer them to microfuge tubes. Centrifuge for 3 minutes to pellet the cells.
3. Resuspend the cell pellet using 45 µl of ice-cold SSC/RVC per $1-10 \times 10^6$ cells.
4. Lyse the cells by the addition of 10 µl Nonidet P-40. Vortex and incubate the tube on ice for 5 minutes. (Note: The cells should be thoroughly resuspended before the addition of the NP40 to avoid the formation of clumps.)
5. Pellet the nuclei and cell debris for 3 minutes in a microfuge.
6. Remove the supernatant containing the cytoplasmic extract and add to it 50 µl of the SSC/formaldehyde solution (freshly prepared).
7. Denature the RNA by heating at 60°C for 15 minutes.
8. Apply the sample to the Minifold apparatus as described in for Procedure 5.1. Extracts from up to 2×10^5 cells can be loaded into each well. Extracts from more than 5×10^5 cells tend to clog the well and give decreased hybridization signals.

DOT BLOTTING OF INTACT CELLS

Cell cultures can be rapidly screened for the presence of specific DNA sequences by a method analogous to the bacterial colony screening procedure (Grunstein and Hogness, 1975). Whole cells are spotted onto nitrocellulose filters and their DNA is released, denatured and fixed to the filter by treatment with NaOH. The resulting spots are then hybridized and detected by standard methods. Using this method, Brandsma and Miller (1980) detected as little as 5 pg of Epstein-Barr viral DNA per 10^5 cultured cells.

Dot blotting of intact cells is suitable for screening large numbers of samples, since the cells are lysed directly on the filter, the recovery of DNA is very high, equal to or higher than that obtained through conventional extraction methods. The presence of impurities in the DNA does not affect hybridization with ^{32}P-labeled probes, but this method may not be suitable for use with non-radioactive probes, since the impurities can result in high non-specific background signals.

PROCEDURE 5.4

RAPID SCREENING OF CELL CULTURES FOR DNA SEQUENCES BY DOT BLOTTING

Reagents and Equipment:
a) Phosphate buffered saline (PBS) (Appendix)
b) Minifold II apparatus (Schleicher & Schuell)
c) 0.5 N NaOH

d) Neutralization Buffer I
   0.6 M NaCl
   1.0 M Tris-HCl, pH 6.8
e) Neutralization Buffer II
   1.5 M NaCl
   0.5 M Tris-HCl, pH 6.8
f) 0.3 M NaCl
g) 95% ethanol
h) Chloroform:isoamyl alcohol (24:1)
i) Nitrocellulose (Schleicher & Schuell)

Procedure:

1. Wash the cells with PBS (10 ml per 10^8 cells) and pellet the cells at 2,000 x g for 10 minutes.
2. Resuspend the cells in PBS at 1×10^6 cells/ml.
3. Load up to 2×10^5 cells (200 µl) per well under a gentle vacuum using the Minifold II or similar apparatus (Procedure 5.1, Steps 1-6). At the higher cell concentrations, it may be necessary to allow a few minutes for the buffer to be pulled completely through the filter.
4. Carefully remove the filter from the apparatus using forceps. Lyse the cells and denature the DNA by laying the filter with the cell-side up on top of a piece of Whatman 3 MM filter saturated with 0.5 M NaOH, for 10 minutes. It is helpful to hold the nitrocellulose filter at both ends with forceps. Apply the nitrocellulose filter from the middle and gradually lower it onto the 3 MM paper, being careful to avoid air bubbles. This operation is analogous to preparing colony lifts of bacterial cells (Procedure 5.10 and 5.11).
5. Neutralize the filter by transferring it to a second Whatman 3 MM filter saturated with neutralization buffer I as described above and incubate for 5 minutes.
6. Transfer the filter to a third Whatman 3 MM filter saturated with neutralization buffer II and incubate again for 5 minutes.
7. Air-dry the filter for 20 minutes.
8. Dehydrate the nitrocellulose filter by floating it on 95% Ethanol. Remove the filter and allow it to air-dry for 5 minutes.
9. Wash the filter twice by immersing it in chloroform:isoamyl alcohol (24:1)
10. Air-dry for 15 minutes.
11. Rinse the filter in 0.3 M NaCl with gentle agitation to wash off the surface debris. Loose debris can also be *gently* rubbed off with gloved fingers.
12. Air-dry the filter and bake it at 80ºC for 2 hours.
13. The filter is ready for prehybridization and hybridization (Procedure 5.12)

SOUTHERN BLOT HYBRIDIZATION

The transfer of DNA restriction fragments from an agarose gel to a membrane is an essential technique in the analysis of genome organization and expression. This technique, known as Southern blotting, also has important applications in the study of genetic diseases, DNA fingerprinting and the analysis of polymerase chain reaction products (Figure 5.1). The DNA fragments are first separated by agarose gel electrophoresis. The DNA is then denatured in the agarose gel by soaking the gel in a NaOH solution and neutralizing it in Tris buffer (Southern, 1975). The DNA is then blotted onto the nitrocellulose filter by capillary action in the presence of high salt. The DNA is transferred as sharp bands which are fixed onto the filter by baking and are ready for hybridization. The main drawback of this procedure is that small fragments of less than 200 base pairs in length do not transfer efficiently to nitrocellulose and may be underrepresented. For efficient transfer of small nucleic acids, use nylon membranes (see discussion at the beginning of this Section).

AGAROSE GEL ELECTROPHORESIS

Restriction fragments of DNA (0.3-25 kb) can be conveniently separated on the basis of size by electrophoresis in agarose gels. In general, for separation of large molecular weight (800-12,000 bp) fragments, low-concentration agarose (0.7%) should be used. For separation of smaller fragments (500-10,000 bp), use a higher concentration of agarose (1.0%); for fragments of 300-5,000 bp, use 1.3% agarose. Electrophoresis chambers are available in various sizes, depending on the amount of sample to be separated and the speed of separation and the

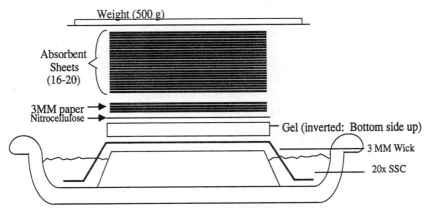

FIGURE 5.1 Southern Transfer. A simple set-up for Southern transfer of DNA from agarose gels to nitrocellulose is shown. The equilibrated gel is inverted onto the paper wick so that the DNA side is closest to the nitrocellulose.

resolution required. Consult the instructions provided with the electrophoresis
unit or refer to Maniatis *et al.* (1982). The following instructions are for running
a midi-gel, 11x14 cm and 1 cm thick.

PROCEDURE 5.5

AGAROSE GEL ELECTROPHORESIS

Reagents and Equipment:
a)   Tris-Acetate-EDTA (TAE) Buffer
     40 mM Tris base, pH 8.1
     2 mM acetic acid
     0.2 mM EDTA
b)   10x Loading Buffer
     20% Ficoll 400
     0.1 M EDTA, pH 8.0
     1% SDS
     0.25% bromophenol blue
c)   10 mg/ml ethidium bromide
d)   DNA molecular weight markers
     (1 *Hind* III digest or fX174 *Hae* III digest, BRL)
e)   Electrophoresis chamber and tray for an 11x14 cm agarose gel
f)   Constant voltage power supply
g)   Agarose (Seakem GTG, FMC)

Procedure:
1.   Prepare a gel cast by taping the open ends of the gel tray with masking
     tape.
2.   Prepare the appropriate percent (w/v) agarose solution in 100 ml of TAE
     buffer, based on the DNA fragment sizes to be separated.
3.   Melt the agarose by boiling on a hot plate or in a microwave, stirring
     occasionally. Allow the agarose to cool below 60°C.
4.   Pour the agarose into the gel tray and insert the comb into position.
     Allow the gel to solidify for about 30 minutes.
5.   Remove the tape and comb, then place the gel tray in the electrophoresis
     chamber. Add TAE buffer to the chamber until the gel is covered by
     about 0.5 cm of buffer.
6.   Mix the DNA sample with 1/10 volume 10x loading buffer and load it
     into the wells of the gel. The maximum sample volume will be 15-30 μl,
     depending on comb thickness. Load DNA molecular weight markers into
     adjacent wells for subsequent determination of the size of the sample
     DNA. We normally electrophorese overnight at a constant voltage of
     20V.

7. Stain the gel by immersing it in TAE buffer containing 0.5 mg/ml ethidium bromide for 30 minutes. Ethidium bromide can also be added directly into the electrophoresis buffer or into the agarose just before pouring it into the gel tray. Caution: Ethidium bromide is a suspected carcinogen - handle with care and dispose of properly.

8. The gel can be photographed on a short-wave (254 nm) transilluminator using an orange (Wratten) photographic filter. We normally use a high-speed Polaroid film (Type 55), an exposure time of 20-40 seconds and a lens setting of f 4.5.

PROCEDURE 5.6

SOUTHERN BLOT TRANSFER TO NITROCELLULOSE

Reagents:
a) Denaturing Buffer
   1.5 M NaCl
   0.5M NaOH
b) Neutralization Buffer
   1 M Tris HCl, pH 8.0
   1.5 M NaCl
c) 2x SSC
d) 6x SSC
e) 10x SSC
f) 3 MM paper (Whatman)
g) Blotting paper (pre-cut blotting paper is available from BRL or Sigma)
h) Pyrex baking dishes
i) Nitrocellulose (Schleicher & Schuell)

Procedure:
1. Trim the gel to the desired size. Make a notch in the upper left-hand corner of the gel to help in subsequent orientation.
2. Immerse the gel in a Pyrex dish filled with denaturing buffer and gently agitate for 15 minutes.
3. Immerse the gel in a Pyrex dish filled with neutralization buffer and gently agitate for 30 minutes.
4. While the gel is equilibrating, cut a nitrocellulose filter to the size of the gel. Wear rubber gloves when handling the gel or the membrane. Immerse the filter in water and then in 10x SSC. Also cut Whatman 3 MM paper (2-4 pieces) and blotting paper to the size of the gel. (Note: The nitrocellulose and the blotting paper must not be larger than the gel so that the 10x SSC cannot by-pass the gel and nitrocellulose to be absorbed directly by the blotting paper.)

5. In a flat Pyrex dish, prepare a platform (an inverted gel tray works well) just larger than the gel and place a piece of Whatman 3 MM paper wick over it (Figure 5.1). Add a small volume of 10x SSC buffer (one inch deep) to pan such that buffer does not rise above the platform. The Whatman 3 MM paper should be well saturated.
6. Place the gel on top of the paper with the underside of the gel facing up.
7. Place the pre-cut and wetted nitrocellulose carefully over the gel, aligning it exactly. Start at one end and lay the filter down gradually, avoiding any trapped air bubbles. With a gloved hand, use a pipette to roll out any air bubbles. The nitrocellulose should not come in contact with the wicking paper.
8. Position the pre-cut Whatman 3 MM paper on top of the nitrocellulose. The Whatman 3 MM paper should not come in direct contact with the gel.
9. Place the blotting paper on top of the 3 MM paper and cover it with a flat weight (such as a Plexiglass plate with a small weight).
10. The buffer in the bottom of the pan will be drawn through the gel and transfer the DNA to the nitrocellulose filter by the wicking action of the blotting paper. Allow the transfer to proceed overnight at room temperature. Be certain that a sufficient volume of buffer is present in the bottom of the pan. Replace blotting paper when saturated with buffer.
11. Remove the blotting paper and peel the nitrocellulose from the gel with forceps. Briefly rinse nitrocellulose filter in 6x SSC (optional).
12. Air-dry the filter, then bake it at 80°C for 2 hours.
13. The filter is ready for hybridization or it can be stored dry in a heat-sealed bag at room temperature.

SOUTHERN TRANSFER TO NYLON MEMBRANES

As discussed previously, nylon membranes have various advantages over nitrocellulose in terms of durability, stability to acids and bases, binding of low molecular weight DNAs and reprobing capacity (see discussion at the beginning of this section). Transfer of DNA to nylon filters does not require high salt, so the transfer can be done directly in 0.5 M NaOH (Reed and Mann, 1985). This permits less handling of the gel and filter and more rapid transfer. An added advantage is that it is not necessary to bake the filter, since the DNA can bind tightly to the nylon under alkaline conditions. Brief exposure to UV irradiation can be used to bind the DNA covalently to the membranes and is particularly useful for enhancing the binding of short DNA fragments. The covalent binding of the DNA, coupled with the durability of the membranes, allows the hybridized probes to be completely stripped by stringent washing, permitting multiple rehybridizations of the same target DNA with different probe preparations. An additional advantage of the alkaline transfer technique is that the strong binding of the DNA minimizes diffusion of the bands, resulting in sharper, more highly resolved bands. The following procedure illustrates the relative ease of using nylon membranes for Southern blotting. To aid in the transfer of large molecular weight DNA, an acid treatment (depurination) step is included in this procedure.

PROCEDURE 5.7

TRANSFER OF DNA FROM AGAROSE GELS TO NYLON MEMBRANES

Reagents:
a) Denaturing Buffer
    1.5 M NaCl
    0.5M NaOH
b) 0.25 M HCl
c) 0.50 M NaOH
d) 3 MM paper (Whatman)
e) Blotting paper (pre-cut blotting paper is available from BRL or Sigma)
f) Pyrex baking dishes
g) Charged nylon membrane (Schleicher & Schuell; Bio-Rad; DuPont)

Procedure:
1. Prepare agarose gels and electrophorese the sample as described in Procedure 5.5. Photograph the gel under UV light, if desired.
2. Wear gloves when handling the gel or the membrane. Transfer the gel to a tray containing 0.25 M HCl for 15 minutes. The gel should be free-floating and agitated gently at room temperature during the treatments in Steps 2 and 3.
3. Transfer gel to a tray containing 0.5 M NaOH, 1.5 M NaCl for 30 minutes.
4. The transfer system described in Procedure 5.6, steps 4-8 is used. The DNA is transferred directly to the membranes by using 0.5 M NaOH as the transfer buffer instead of 10x SSC.
5. The gel is laid with the bottom side facing up, on top of the 3 MM wicking paper. A sheet of nylon membrane, cut to size, is wetted with 0.5 M NaOH and laid on top of the gel. With some nylon papers (such as Gene Screen Plus), the concave side should be in contact with the gel (check instructions provided by the manufacturer).
6. Place additional sheets of dry 3 MM paper on top of the nylon membrane. Place the blotting paper on top of the 3 MM paper and cover it with a flat weight (such as a Plexiglass plate with a small weight).
7. Allow transfer to take place overnight.

8. Remove the nylon filter using forceps. Baking is not required, but is effective in enhancing binding of the DNA to the filter. It may also be exposed to UV light from a transilluminator for 5 minutes to covalently bind the DNA to the filter.

NORTHERN BLOTTING OF RNA

The transfer of RNA from agarose gel to nitrocellulose (northern blot) is similar in principal to the transfer of DNA (Southern blot). Instead of using NaOH which would hydrolyze the 2'-hydroxyl group of RNA, it must be denatured with either methyl mercury hydroxide, glyoxal, or formaldehyde before loading onto a gel (Thomas, 1980; Lehrach et al., 1977). Denaturation promotes the binding of RNA to nitrocellulose during the transfer process. The transfer takes place in high salt in a format similar to Southern blotting, except that RNA is not firmly bound to the filter until after baking. The filter therefore must not be washed with low-salt buffer after transfer or the RNA may be eluted. Agarose gels that are to be used for the transfer of RNA should not be stained with ethidium bromide, since the dye interferes with binding of RNA to nitrocellulose. For sizing of the RNA, RNA molecular weight markers should be run in a lane of the same gel. The lane containing the markers can then be cut off the gel, stained and photographed, while the lanes containing the samples are processed separately for the northern transfer. To stain the markers in the gel, immerse the gel for 10 minutes in 0.1 M ammonium acetate containing 5 μg/ml ethidium bromide in the dark. Gels can be de-stained in water. Photograph the gel under UV light using a Polaroid camera (Procedure 5.6) The ethidium-stained RNA should be exposed to UV light only for the time required to take the photograph. Longer exposure to UV or prolonged exposure to incandescent light will cause the RNA signal to fade. Radiolabeled RNA ladders are also commercially available for use as markers. All procedures for running RNA gels and handling RNA should follow the RNase free conditions described in Section 2.

For isolation of functionally intact mRNA from agarose gels, methyl mercury hydroxide provides a strong, yet readily reversible denaturant (Procedure 5.8) Because of the toxicity of methyl mercury hydroxide, many researchers prefer to use formaldehyde to denature RNA gels for northern Blotting (Procedure 5.9).

PROCEDURE 5.8

RNA ELECTROPHORESIS IN METHYL MERCURY HYDROXIDE GELS AND TRANSFER CONDITIONS

Warning: Methyl mercury hydroxide is a neurotoxin. Avoid inhalation and contact. All procedures using methyl mercury hydroxide must be performed in a fume hood and gloves must be worn. Ammonium acetate or other complexing agents should be added to all solutions containing methyl mercury hydroxide prior to disposal (Bailey *et al.*, 1976).

Reagents:
a) BSE Buffer
    50 mM boric acid
    5 mM sodium borate
    10 mM sodium sulfate
    1 mM disodium EDTA, pH 8.2
b) Loading Buffer
    BSE buffer
    10% glycerol
    0.01% bromophenol blue
c) Methyl mercury hydroxide (Caution: Toxic)
d) 3 MM paper (Whatman)
e) Blotting paper (pre-cut blotting paper is available from BRL or Sigma)
f) Pyrex baking dishes
g) Nitrocellulose (Schleicher & Schuell) or
    charged nylon membrane (Schleicher & Schuell, Bio-Rad, DuPont)
h) 20x SSC
i) 20 mM ammonium acetate

Procedure:
1. Prepare a 1% agarose gel in BSE Buffer (Procedure 5.5).
2. Dilute the RNA sample in loading butter and add methyl mercury hydroxide to a final concentration of 10 mM.
3. Pipette the sample into the well. Electrophorese at a constant 60 V overnight or until the tracking dye is halfway to the bottom of the gel. Do not include ethidium bromide during electrophoresis. The marker lanes can be stained later.
4. Transfer gel immediately following electrophoresis. Wear gloves when handling gels or membranes.
5. Pre-wet 2 sheets of 3 MM paper with 20x SSC and place in gel transfer chamber to be used as wicking paper as described in Procedure 5.6.
6. Place the gel bottom-side up on top of the 3 MM paper.
7. Pre-wet a nitrocellulose or nylon membrane with water, then with 20x SSC. Lay it over the gel, being careful to eliminate all air bubbles. The membrane must not come in contact with the wicking paper.
8. Place two sheets of dry 3 MM paper on top and cover with blotting paper. Apply a weight to the paper and transfer overnight.
9. Remove the filter. If using nitrocellulose, do not wash the blot before baking or the RNA may come off.
10. Bake at 80°C for 2 hours in a vacuum oven for nitrocellulose membranes, bake or cross-link with UV light for nylon membranes.

11. To remove residual methyl mercury hydroxide, soak the membrane in 20 mM ammonium acetate twice for 20 minutes each time prior to hybridization.
12. The filter is ready for hybridization or it can be stored dry in heat-sealed bags.

PROCEDURE 5.9

RNA ELECTROPHORESIS IN FORMALDEHYDE GELS AND TRANSFER CONDITIONS

Reagents:
a) 10x MSE Buffer
   0.2 M morpholino propane sulfonic acid (MOPS), pH 7.0
   50 mM sodium acetate
   1 mM EDTA, pH 8.0
b) 5x Loading Buffer
   50% glycerol
   1 mM EDTA
   0.4% bromophenol blue
c) Formaldehyde: 37% solution in water (12.3 M)
   Formaldehyde should be stored and handled in a chemical hood. The pH of the concentrated solution should be above 4.0.
d) 3 MM paper (Whatman)
e) Blotting paper (pre-cut blotting paper is available from BRL or Sigma)
f) Pyrex baking dishes
g) Nitrocellulose (Schleicher & Schuell)
h) 20x SSC
i) Deionized formamide (Appendix A)
j) 50 mM NaOH containing 10 mM NaCl
k) 0.1 M Tris, pH 7.5

Procedure:
1. Combine 7 g of agarose and 40 ml of water. Heat to boiling to dissolve the agarose and allow the solution to cool to about 60°C. Add 7 ml 10x MSE buffer, 11.5 ml of formaldehyde and adjust the volume to 70 ml with water. Mix and pour into a prepared gel tray (Procedure 5.5).
2. When the gel has solidified, remove the comb and tape, place into a gel chamber and cover with 1x MSE buffer.
3. Denature RNA (up to 20 µg) in denaturation buffer containing:

RNA	4.5 µl
10x MSE buffer	2.0 µl
formaldehyde	3.5 µl
deionized formamide	10.0 µl

4. Heat at 55°C for 15 minutes. Chill on ice.
5. Add 2 µl of sterile 5x loading buffer.
6. Load samples into wells. Molecular weight markers for RNA (BRL) should also be loaded in separate wells for subsequent determination of the size of the RNA species.
7. Electrophorese at a constant 60V overnight.
8. Following electrophoresis, remove the gel from chamber and soak it in water two times for 5 minutes each.
9. (Optional) Hydrolyze any high molecular weight RNA (to enhance transfer) by soaking the gel in 50 mM NaOH, 10 mM NaCl for 45 minutes at room temperature.
10. Neutralize the gel by soaking it in 0.1 M Tris-HCl, pH 7.5, for 45 minutes at room temperature.
11. Wash the gel for 1 hour in 20x SSC.
12. Transfer the gel overnight in 20x SSC to nitrocellulose as described in Procedure 5.6.
13. Remove the nitrocellulose and bake it for 2 hours at 80°C in a vacuum oven.

Colony and Plaque Screening

The colony or plaque screening method allows the screening of a large number of bacterial colonies or phage plaques for the presence of specified DNA sequences or genes. This method allows the detection of a particular recombination event, even if this event occurs at extremely low frequencies and as such is particularly useful for screening recombinant DNA libraries (Grunstein and Hogness, 1975). The bacterial colonies to be screened are lifted from agarose plates onto nitrocellulose filters making an exact replica of the distribution of colonies on the original plate. The original plates can be stored refrigerated, while the replicas of the plates on the filters are processed for hybridization. Marking or notching the filters and plates prior to the lift permits subsequent alignment with the original plates allowing identification and isolation of the original colonies containing the sequences in question. To prevent movement of the DNA from its original site on the filter during lysis, denaturation and fixation procedures, the solutions used for these procedures are applied from the underside of the filter and allowed to diffuse into the colony. Once the DNA is deposited on the filters and the debris is washed away, the DNA is baked onto the filter and remains firmly bound through subsequent hybridization, washing and detection steps. A similar procedure can be used to select phage plaques containing a sequence of interest. Nylon-based filters may also be used and do not require baking to fix the DNA to the filters.

This procedure is suitable for screening up to 1,000 bacterial colonies per 100 mm plate. To screen larger numbers of colonies (up to 100,000 per 100 mm plate), up to 10^5 colony-forming bacteria are spread on an agar plate and incubated to establish small colonies. A replica is lifted onto a nitrocellulose filter, which is then applied to another agarose plate (cell side up) and incubated in medium containing chloramphenicol to allow amplification of the number of plasmid copies per bacteria. The filters are then processed and hybridized as described above. The areas of positive hybridization are keyed back to the original plate and a few colonies corresponding to the region of the hybridization signal are removed and re-spread on another agarose plate to give 100-200 colonies per filter. The enriched population can then be replicated and probed to allow isolation of individual clones containing the hybridizing DNA (Hanahan and Meselson, 1980).

PROCEDURE 5.10

LIFTING COLONIES FROM PLATES

Reagents:
a)   Prepared agar plates containing antibiotic (Maniatis *et al.*, 1982)
b)   100 mm nitrocellulose circles (Schleicher & Schuell)

Procedure:
1.   Plate bacteria onto agarose plates containing the appropriate antibiotic and incubate to allow the bacterial colonies to grow to visible size. Do not allow the colonies to overgrow each other so that individual colonies can be identified. Use a bacterial dilution expected to produce approximately 1,000 colonies per 100 mm plate.
2.   Incubate plates at 4°C for 15 minutes to harden the agarose prior to the lift.
3.   Make alignment marks on the 100 mm nitrocellulose discs using indelible ink or pencil.
4.   Starting at the middle and using forceps, carefully lay the membrane onto the agarose plate, making sure to avoid air bubbles. Once the filter has made contact with the agarose, do not readjust or move the filter so as not to smudge the colonies.
5.   Mark the plate at the location of the alignment marks with India ink for later orientation.
6.   Hold the filter on the plate for about 2 minutes to allow transfer of the colonies.
7.   Carefully lift out the nitrocellulose replica from the agarose plate using a slow continuous motion, being careful not to smudge the colonies. Process filters as described in Procedure 5.11.

8. The plates should be sealed with Parafilm and stored inverted at 4°C (for up to a month) until the results of the hybridization are obtained.

9. By matching the hybridized colonies back to the original plate, the colonies containing the sequence of interest can be isolated with a toothpick and regrown.

PROCEDURE 5.11

LYSING CELLS AND FIXING DNA ONTO FILTERS

Reagents:
a) Lysing/Denaturation Buffer
   0.5 M NaOH/1.5 M NaCl
b) Neutralization Buffer
   0.5 M Tris HCl, pH 7.4/1.5 M NaCl
c) Wash Buffer
   2x SSC
d) Pyrex dishes

Procedure:
1. (Optional) To improve the lysing/transfer step and thus increase sensitivity, prior to immersion of the filter in dish No. 1, place the filter on top of a Whatman 3 MM paper saturated with 0.5 M NaOH/1.5 M NaCl in a Pyrex dish. The open Pyrex dish can then be placed above boiling water in a covered kettle and steamed for 3 minutes (Maas, 1983). The filter can then be processed from dish No. 1 through to dish No. 3 as described.

2. Prepare three Pyrex baking dishes for processing the filters:
   a) Dish No. 1: Saturate a couple of layers of Whatman 3 MM paper with lysis/denaturation buffer (0.5 M NaOH, 1.5 M NaCl). The filter should be well saturated, but without large amounts of excess floating liquid on top.
   b) Dish No. 2: Saturate a couple of layers of Whatman 3 MM paper with neutralization buffer (0.5 M Tris HCl, pH 7.4/1.5 M NaCl) as in a).
   c) Dish No. 3: Fill dish with 2x SSC wash buffer.

3. Place the nitrocellulose filter, with the cells facing up onto the 3 MM paper in dish No. 1, being careful to avoid air bubbles. Incubate for 15-30 minutes at room temperature. This step lyses the cells and denatures the DNA.

4. Remove the nitrocellulose filter from dish No. 1 and transfer cell side up onto 3 MM paper in dish No. 2 to neutralize the NaOH. Incubate 15-30 minutes at room temperature.

5. Transfer the nitrocellulose filter to dish No. 3. Using clean gloved hands, gently rub the cellular debris off of the filter. Caution: Nitrocellulose is

fragile - be careful not to tear it. The filter should be free of surface debris for best results. When processing multiple filters, change the 2x SSC solution frequently or re-rinse in a fresh 2x SSC wash to ensure clean filters. The presence of excess debris interferes with hybridization and when using non-isotopic probes can lead to high backgrounds and false positive signals.

6.   Allow the filters to air-dry, then bake for 30 minutes at 80°C in a vacuum oven to fix the DNA.

7.   The filters are ready for hybridization or can be stored dry in sealed bags.

Filter Hybridization Procedures

DNA sequences immobilized on filters by the slot blot, Southern blot, northern blot, or lift procedures are hybridized in basically the same way. The filters are first prehybridized with hybridization buffer minus the probe. Non-specific DNA binding sites on the filter are thus saturated with carrier DNA and synthetic polymers. The prehybridization solution is then replaced with the hybridization buffer containing the labeled probe and incubated to allow hybridization of the probe to the target nucleic acid. Following hybridization, unhybridized probe is removed by a series of washing steps. The stringency of the washes must be adjusted for the specific probe used (Section 1). To increase sensitivity, use low stringency washing conditions (higher salt and lower temperature). Low stringency, however, can give rise to non-specific hybridization signals and high backgrounds. By using higher stringency washes (lower salt and higher temperature), the background can be reduced and only the specific signal will remain. The signal-to-noise ratio can also be effected by probe length, purity, concentration, sequence and target contamination.

Pre-hybridization, hybridization and washing are usually carried out in trays or in sealed plastic bags. Use 10-15 ml of solution for a 11 x 14 cm blot. Sealed bags are very convenient since they need only very small hybridization volumes, allowing the use of high probe concentrations for maximum sensitivity. There should be enough buffer in the bag so that the filter does not stick, but is free to move. After adding solution to the bag, partially seal it, leaving a small outlet to permit the air bubbles to be removed. Hold the bag vertically, with the outlet at the top and bring all air bubbles to the top. Carefully lay the bag down on absorbant paper on the bench top, placing the section with the outlet (and air bubbles) down last. Remove all air bubbles. Rolling a pipette over the bag towards the outlet works well, but be sure to allow any solution pushed up by the pipette to flow back into the bag before the bubbles are extruded. Seal the bag with a heat sealer and place horizontally in a water bath during each incubation.

PROCEDURE 5.12

HYBRIDIZATION OF FILTERS WITH RADIOLABELED PROBES

Reagents:
a) Hybridization Buffer
   50% deionized formamide
   5x SSC
   1x Denhardt's solution
   31 mM KH_2PO_4
   0.25% SDS
   30 µg/ml sheared, denatured salmon sperm DNA
   5% dextran sulfate (Pharmacia)
   The preparation of the stock reagents is described in Appendix A. Store at 4°C for up to 2 months or at -20°C for up to six months.
b) Salmon sperm DNA (Appendix A)
c) 20x SSC
d) 10% SDS

Procedure:
1. Place the dry filter containing target nucleic acid into a heat-seal bag (BRL) and pre-wet the filter with a small volume of 2x SSC. Remove excess buffer from the bag.
2. Separately aliquot enough hybridization buffer for prehybridization and hybridization steps. Warm the buffer to 42°C to redissolve the SDS. Add enough carrier DNA to a microfuge tube to give a concentration of 100 µg/ml in the prehybridization. Boil the DNA for 5 minutes and chill it on ice for 10 minutes.
3. Add the denatured carrier DNA to an aliquot of hybridization buffer, mix and add this prehybridization solution to the bag (about 15 ml for a 11 x 14 cm filter), remove air bubbles and seal the bag. Incubate at 42°C for 2 hours with shaking.
4. Denature the radiolabeled DNA probe by boiling for 5 minutes and cooling on ice for 10 minutes. Use at least 1×10^6 cpm of ^{32}P-labeled probe per ml of hybridization buffer. The probe should have a specific activity of at least 1×10^8 cpm/µg.
5. Add the denatured probe to the other aliquot of hybridization buffer and mix. Cut off a corner of the bag and drain the prehybridization solution. Add the hybridization buffer plus probe to the bag, remove air bubbles and reseal. Incubate at 42°C overnight with shaking.
6. Cut off a corner of the bag and drain the buffer into radioactive waste. Add back 2x SSC-0.1% SDS solution, agitate briefly to rinse out radioactivity and drain to radioactive waste.

7. Cut away the sides of the bag and transfer the filter to a tray containing about 200 ml of 2x SSC/0.1% SDS. Wash the filter for 15 minutes at room temperature with agitation. Additional washes can be carried out. The tray is placed in a shaker bath equilibrated to the desired temperature.

8. a) For high stringency washes:

    1. Wash 2 times with 2x SSC/0.1% SDS for 15 minutes each at room temperature.
    2. Wash 2 times with 0.1x SSC/0.1% SDS for 15 minutes each at room temperature.
    3. Wash 2 times with 0.1x SSC/0.1% SDS for 30 minutes each at 55°C.

    b) For low stringency washes:

    1. Wash 2 times with 6x SSC/0.1% SDS for 15 minutes each at room temperature.
    2. Wash 2 times with 2x SSC/0.1% SDS for 15 minutes each at room temperature.
    3. Wash 2 times with 1x SSC/0.1% SDS for 15 minutes each at 50°C.

9. Refer to Procedure 5.13 for performing autoradiography.

AUTORADIOGRAPHY

Radiolabeled compounds are conveniently detected by autoradiography on film. As radioactive emissions strike a film emulsion containing silver halide, they form a latent image that is visible after photographic processing. In typical applications, the low-energy ß-emitter, ^{35}S, or the high-energy ß-emitter, ^{32}P, is used in biological research. The low-energy ß- and g-emitter, ^{125}I, can also be used (refer to discussion in Section 3).

The time required to expose X-ray film to visualize radiation is directly dependent on both the type and amount of radioisotope present in the sample. The level of resolution obtainable by autoradiography is determined by the emission type and energy of the radionuclide (Cunningham and Mandy, 1987). The highly energetic ß-particles emitted by ^{32}P have a long mean path length and expose silver grains over a relatively large area on both sides of double-sided film. This leads to a strong signal but with a somewhat fuzzy image and therefore low resolution. Detection efficiency and therefore sensitivity, is even higher if an intensifying screen is used to generate light from the ß-particles that pass through the film. The lower energy ß-particles emitted by ^{35}S, on the other hand, cannot penetrate through the plastic backing of standard X-ray film to the opposite emulsion. Although this results in longer exposure times for comparable sensitivity to ^{32}P, the resolution of ^{35}S-labeled probes is sharper. The g-radiation emitted by ^{125}I readily penetrates the film, leading to high sensitivity with a screen. The low-energy electrons from ^{125}I are stopped entirely within the emulsion , providing high resolution without a screen. The very weak ß-emissions of ^{3}H yield the highest resolution, but provide low sensitivity and require a long exposure time.

An approximate exposure time for ^{32}P-labeled filters can be made by running a Geiger-Mueller counter across the filter prior to placing it in the cassette. A strong signal on the counter at a 0.1x setting usually requires 2-3 hours of autoradiography at -70°C, whereas a weak signal will require an overnight exposure. Exposures are performed at low temperature (-70°C) because it enhances the sensitivity of the X-ray film. The use of ^{35}S-labeled probes may require several days of exposure. Exposure times can be reduced by using intensifying screens such as Cronex Lightning Plus (DuPont). These screens contain inorganic phosphorus which becomes activated to emit light by emitted radiation passing through the X-ray film. The use of two screens, one on top of and one underneath the filter further intensifies the signal. Intensifying screens, however, do tend to diffuse the signal compared with longer exposures without screens.

PROCEDURE 5.13

AUTORADIOGRAPHY

Reagents and Equipment:
a) Clear plastic wrap
b) X-ray film (Kodak X-OMAT AR)
c) X-ray film cassette
d) Kodak liquid X-ray developer
   Kodak stop bath solution
   Kodak rapid fixer
   Or an automatic X-ray film processor

Procedure:
1. Following hybridization and washing, blot excess moisture from the filter and wrap it in clear plastic wrap. Smooth out the wrinkles. Use only a single layer of plastic on each side of the filter. This is to prevent radioactive contamination of the film or film cassette.
2. In the dark or under a safe light, place the filter against a sensitive X-ray film (Kodak X-OMAT AR) in a film cassette. When using intensifying screens, place the X-ray film between the screen and the filter. If a second screen is used, it should be placed underneath the filter. Close the cassette.
3. Expose the film at -70°C for the chosen amount of time.
4. Remove the cassette from the freezer and allow it to equilibrate to room temperature. If the film is frozen against the filter or screen, peeling it

away can produce static which can cloud the film or produce artifactual spotting. Remove the film in the dark or under a safe light.

5. Process the film using standard X-ray development methods:
   a) Develop the film in Kodak liquid X-ray developer for 1-5 minutes.
   b) Rinse the film in Kodak stop bath solution for 1 minute with gentle agitation.
   c) Fix the film in Kodak rapid fixer for 5 minutes with gentle agitation.
   d) Wash the film in a tray under running tap water for about 10 minutes. Air dry.

REPROBING OF FILTERS

Following hybridization and autoradiography, the filters can be stripped of the original probe with a high stringency wash and rehybridized with a different probe to allow examination of more than one sequence within the same nucleic acid sample. Because of their flexibility, durability and higher retention properties, nylon of PVDF-based filters should be used if multiple reprobing is required. These membranes can be successfully reprobed up to 12 times, saving on time, material and labor costs (Gatti *et al.*, 1984). Although nitrocellulose membranes can also be reprobed if handled carefully, these membranes are quite fragile and may fall apart during processing. Membranes to be reprobed must not be allowed to dry out completely after hybridization, since this may permanently bind the labeled probe to the filter. Stripped filters should again be prehybridized to block non-specific DNA binding sites. They can be conveniently stored moist in heat-sealed bags at 4°C until reprobed.

PROCEDURE 5.14

STRIPPING RADIOLABELED PROBES FROM MEMBRANES

Reagents:
a) High Stringency Wash Buffer
   0.1x SSC/0.1% SDS
b) Prehybridization buffer (Procedure 5.12)

Procedure:
1. Following hybridization and autoradiography, immerse the blotting membrane in 500 ml high stringency wash buffer and incubate at 95°C on a oscillating platform for 15-20 minutes.
2. Pour off buffer and replace with another 500 ml of fresh buffer preheated at 95°C and continue incubation and shaking for an additional 15-20 minutes at 95°C.

3. Place the stripped membrane in a plastic sealing bag containing 20 ml prehybridization buffer. Seal bag and incubate overnight at 42°C.
4. Remove membrane from prehybridization buffer, blot off excess fluid and rehybridize. A stripped, blocked filter can be stored moist in a sealed bag at 4°C for many months.

NON-RADIOACTIVE FILTER HYBRIDIZATION CONDITIONS

Non-radioactive DNA probes require modified hybridization conditions in order to avoid high background signals. The major differences are substitution of glycine for BSA in the hybridization buffer and limiting the dextran sulfate concentration to 5%. Since the following conditions have been optimized for non-radioactive probes, they are somewhat different from the conditions in Procedure 5.12, but they also work well with radioactive probes.

PROCEDURE 5.15

GENERAL FILTER HYBRIDIZATION CONDITIONS
FOR NON-RADIOACTIVE PROBES

Reagents:

a) 50x FPG
    1% Ficoll 400
    1% polyvinylpyrrolidone 360
    1% glycine
    Filter-sterilize and store in aliquots at -20°C.

b) 1M Potassium Phosphate
    136 g KH_2PO_4 per liter
    Adjust pH to 7.0, autoclave and store at room temperature.

c) Deionized Formamide
    Stir 200 ml of formamide with 20 g of Bio-Rad AG501-X8 resin, H⁺ form. After 1 hour, filter through Whatman #1 paper. Aliquot and store at -20°C.

d) 2x SSC/0.1% SDS:
    50 ml of 20x SSC
    5 ml of 10% SDS
    Dilute to 500 ml
    Autoclave. Store at room temperature

e) 0.1x SSC/0.1% SDS
    2.5 ml of 20x SSC
    5 ml of 10% SDS
    Dilute to 500 ml.
    Autoclave. Store at room temperature.

f) 50% Dextran Sulfate
    Gradually add 25 g of dextran sulfate (Pharmacia) to 15 ml of water in a
    50 ml screw-cap tube. Dissolve by shaking and heating to 50°C. Adjust
    the final volume to 50 ml. Store in aliquots at -20°C.

g) Hybridization Buffer
    These volumes are for minigel blots (about 5x7 cm) or dot blots of about
    the same size.

Deionized formamide	2.5 ml (50%)
20X SSC	1.25 ml (5x)
50X FPG	100 µl (1x)
1M K Phosphate	125 µl (25 mM)
10% SDS	100 µl (0.2%)
Carrier DNA* (10 mg/ml)	12.5 µl (25 µg/ml)
50% dextran sulfate	500 µl (5%)
Water	313 µl
Total volume	4.9 ml

(*Appendix A)

Procedure:
1. Prehybridize in the above solution minus probe for 2 hours at 42°C.
2. Combine 20 µl of probe (50 µg/ml) and 320 µl of sterile water. Denature
    by boiling for 5 minutes and chilling on ice for 10 minutes. Add it to the
    prehybridization solution (200 ng/ml final concentration) and hybridize at
    42°C for 18 hours, with shaking.
3. Wash blot in 20 ml of 2x SSC/0.1% SDS in a tray at room temperature, 2
    times for 5 minutes each, shaking slowly. The top from a package of
    micropipette tips works well as a disposable washing tray.
4. Transfer blot to a heat-seal bag and wash in 20 ml of 0.1x SSC/0.1% SDS
    at 55-65°C (depending on desired stringency), 2 times for 15 minutes
    each.
5. (Optional) Wash blot in a tray with 20 ml of 2x SSC for 5 minutes at room
    temperature, then begin detection procedure.

Note: Do not let the blot dry out. It must remain wet throughout detection and
color development. FPG and Denhardt's solution (Denhardt, 1966) are essentially
interchangeable, but the use of FPG results in lower backgrounds in our experience.
Best results are obtained with nitrocellulose. The use of nylon membranes is not
recommended, because they give high non-specific backgrounds. A probe
concentration of 200 ng/ml is suggested, but lower concentrations may result in
lower non-specific background signals. We use minigels whenever possible
instead of 11x14 cm gels, because the smaller transfers are easier to handle, are
less likely to dry between steps and require smaller buffer volumes.

HAPTEN DETECTION

Hapten-labeled probes (i.e., photo-DNP-labeled) are usually detected by incubation with an anti-hapten first antibody, followed by an enzyme-conjugated, species-specific, anti-IgG second antibody (Keller *et al.*, 1988). The optimum concentration of antibody in the detection solutions must be determined empirically. The optimum is the minimum concentration that gives the maximum signal. Incubation with each antibody is for 30-60 minutes; shorter times result in lower signals, but longer times (up to 2 hours) may result in a stronger signal.

      Anti-hapten antibodies are commercially available (Chemicon, Accurate, Kirkegaard & Perry), but keep in mind that the polyclonal (i.e., rabbit, goat) antibodies will usually exhibit stronger detection signals (because of their higher affinity constants) than their monoclonal counterparts. A wide selection of enzyme-conjugated second antibodies is also commercially available (Kirkegaard & Perry, Jackson Immunoresearch).

PROCEDURE 5.16

COLORIMETRIC DETECTION OF
HAPTEN-LABELED PROBES ON FILTERS

Reagents:

a) 20x Wash Buffer   1x:

1 M Tris base	121 g	50 mM
4 M NaCl	233 g	200 mM
6% Tween-20	60 ml	0.3 %
0.2% thimerosal	2 g	0.01%

Adjust pH to 7.4 with concentrated HCl and dilute to 1 liter.
Store at 4°C for up to 9 months.

b) 1x Wash Buffer
Prepare about 500 ml of 1x wash buffer by adding 25 ml of 20x wash buffer to 475 ml of deionized water. Store at 4°C for up to 2 weeks.

c) Blocking Buffer

Non-fat dry milk	2 g
1x wash buffer	to 20 ml

Store at 4°C for up to three days.

d) First Antibody Solution (usually 5 µg/ml, range: 1-20 µg/ml)

Blocking buffer	10 ml
Rabbit anti-hapten	50 µg

Prepare fresh and store at 4°C for up to 8 hours.

e)   Enzyme-Labeled Second Antibody Solution (usually 2 µg/ml, range: 1-20 µg/ml)

Blocking buffer	10 ml
Alkaline phosphatase anti-rabbit IgG	20 µg

Prepare fresh and store at 4°C for up to 8 hours.

f)   Substrate Buffer
Add 20 ml of 10x alkaline phosphatase substrate buffer (Appendix A) to 180 ml of deionized water. Store at 4°C up to 1 week.

g)   Alkaline Phosphatase Substrate Solution
To 8 ml of 1x substrate buffer add 1 ml of 10x NBT substrate concentrate (Appendix A) and mix gently. Add 1 ml of 10x BCIP substrate concentrate (Appendix A) and mix again. Prepare within 2 hours of use and store at room temperature in the dark.

Procedure:

1.   After hybridizing the prelabeled probe to your target nucleic acid, wash the filter at the desired stringency and leave wet in 2x SSC. Do not let the nitrocellulose dry out during any of the following steps. Use nitrocellulose filters only. This procedure results in a high background with nylon filters.

2.   The following incubations should be performed in heat-seal bags which are cut to be slightly larger than the filter. All incubations are performed at room temperature with shaking.

3.   Incubate the blot in 10 ml of diluent buffer for 15 minutes to block the filter.

4.   Pour off the diluent buffer and add 5 ml of the anti-hapten (first antibody) solution to the same bag. Incubate for 30 minutes.

5.   Pour off the first antibody solution and be sure to squeeze out residual liquid. Add 5 ml of the enzyme-labeled second antibody solution. Incubate for 30 minutes.

6.   Remove the filter from the bag and place in a small tray containing 1x wash buffer. Use a small plastic tray. The top from a tray of blue or yellow micropipette tips works well. Wash the blot 3 times for 5 minutes each with 1x wash buffer.

7.   Place the blot in a new heat-seal bag containing 5 ml of alkaline phosphatase substrate solution (NBT/BCIP). The solution must be changed promptly if its yellow color fades or turns purple. Develop in the dark until the desired bands or spots appear (usually 15 minutes-2 hours), but do not overdevelop. If the background is light after 2 hours and more development is needed, it can be continued.

8.   Stop development by washing the blot with deionized water and dry it on filter paper in the dark or in a vacuum oven at 80°C for 5 minutes. Store

developed blots dry in heat-sealed bags in a notebook or box, out of direct light.

Note: When using heat-seal bags, be sure to use 5 ml of blocking buffer or antibody solution in bags of up to 4x4 inches (10x10 cm). The use of smaller volumes will result in a high background due to sticking of the nitrocellulose to the inside of the bag. Do not re-use the antibody solutions, in order to avoid high background signals.

BIOTIN DETECTION

Biotin detection with streptavidin is easier and faster than hapten detection because it usually requires only one ten-minute binding step (Leary *et al*,.1983), in contrast to two 30 to 60-minute antibody binding steps. However, some lots of enzyme-streptavidin conjugate can give high backgrounds, so we included a second procedure that employs two ten-minute binding steps and eliminates the direct conjugate. This procedure gives very low backgrounds on filters and in *in situ* hybridization (Procedure 5.27).

PROCEDURE 5.17

ONE-STEP COLORIMETRIC DETECTION OF BIOTIN-LABELED PROBES ON FILTERS

Reagents:
a) 3% BSA dissolved in 1x wash buffer (Appendix A)
b) 1x wash buffer (Appendix A)
c) Alkaline phosphatase-streptavidin conjugate (BRL)
d) NBT/BCIP substrate solution (Procedure 5.17)

Procedure:
1. After hybridizing the prelabeled probe to your target nucleic acid, wash the filter at the desired stringency and leave wet in 2x SSC. Do not let the nitrocellulose dry out during any of the following steps. The following incubations should be performed in heat-seal bags. All incubations are performed at room temperature with shaking.
2. Incubate the blot in a heat-seal bag with 10 ml of 3% BSA dissolved in 1x wash buffer for 15 minutes to block the filter.
3. Pour off the diluent buffer and add 5 ml of 1 µg/ml alkaline phosphatase-streptavidin conjugate dissolved in 3% BSA/1x wash buffer to the same bag. Incubate for 10 minutes. Also see the alternate protocol (Procedure 5.18).

4.   Pour off the conjugate solution and wash the blot 3 times for 5 minutes each with 1x wash buffer. Use a small plastic tray.

5.   Place the blot in a new heat-seal bag and add 5 ml of NBT/BCIP substrate solution. The solution must be changed promptly if its yellow color fades or turns purple. Develop in the dark until the desired bands or spots appear (usually 15 minutes-2 hours), but do not overdevelop. If the background is light after 2 hours and more development is needed, it can be continued.

6.   Stop development by washing the blot with deionized water and dry it on filter paper in the dark or in an 80°C vacuum oven for 5 minutes. Store developed blots dry in heat-seal bags in a notebook or box, out of direct light.

In both detection protocols (5.17 and 5.18), peroxidase-conjugated second antibody or streptavidin may be substituted for its alkaline phosphatase counterpart, if desired. Commercial substrate stock solutions are also available from companies such as Kirkegaard and Perry: NBT and BCIP for alkaline phosphatase and precipitable tetramethylbenzidine (TMB) for horseradish peroxidase.

ALTERNATIVE PROTOCOL

In most cases, the non-specific background obtained with biotinylated DNA probes may be decreased, without sacrificing detection sensitivity, by using streptavidin and biotinylated alkaline phosphatase instead of a direct conjugate.

PROCEDURE 5.18

TWO-STEP COLORIMETRIC DETECTION OF BIOTIN-LABELED PROBES ON FILTERS

Reagents:

a)   Streptavidin

Dissolve 1.5 mg of streptavidin (BRL) in 1.5 ml of 50% glycerol (redistilled). Store in aliquots at -20°C.

b)   Biotinylated Alkaline Phosphatase

1) Add 100 μl of alkaline phosphatase (1 mg) (Boehringer-Mannheim #567 752) to 900 μl of PBS. Prepare a 10 mg/ml solution of sulfo-N-hydroxysuccinimide-long chain biotin (Pierce) in water, about 5 mg in 500 μl (use dimethylsulfoxide if it does not readily dissolve in water). Prepare fresh and use immediately.

2) Add 7 μl of the NHS-biotin solution (70 μg, 15-fold molar excess) to the diluted alkaline phosphatase. Incubate in the dark at room temperature for one hour.

   3) Dialyze against 4 changes of 500 ml of 3 M NaCl, 20 mM Tris, pH 8.0.
   Store in aliquots at 4°C.
c)   3% BSA dissolved in 1x wash buffer (Appendix A)
d)   1x wash buffer (Appendix A)
e)   NBT/BCIP substrate solution (Procedure 5.17)

Procedure:
Follow Steps 1 and 2 in Procedure 5.17.
3.   a) Pour off the diluent buffer and add 5 ml of 1 µg/ml streptavidin
        dissolved in 3% BSA/1x wash buffer to the same bag. Incubate for 10
        minutes.
3.   b) Pour off the streptavidin solution and add 5 ml of 5 µg/ml biotinylated
        alkaline phosphatase in 3% BSA/1x wash buffer to the same bag.
     Incubate for 10 minutes.

Follow Steps 4-6 for washing and color development.

CHEMILUMINESCENT DETECTION

Chemiluminescent substrate systems are available for the visualization of
peroxidase.and alkaline phosphatase. The peroxidase system, which uses luminol
and an enhancer (Matthews *et al.*, 1985), is equal to or less sensitive than the
colorimetric detection of alkaline phosphatase, but the results can be conveniently
recorded on X-ray film. This system is available from Amersham as part of a
labeling and detection kit. The alkaline phosphatase system, which uses a
dioxetane-based substrate and can be enhanced, is reportedly 10-30 times more
sensitive than NBT/BCIP, partly because the light emission is relatively constant
for up to six hours (Bronstein and McGrath, 1989). This signal can also be
recorded on X-ray film.

PROCEDURE 5.19

CHEMILUMINESCENT DETECTION ON FILTERS

DETECTION OF PEROXIDASE
Develop the filter as above (Procedure 5.17), but use peroxidase-conjugated
streptavidin (Kirkegaard & Perry) as the conjugate. Proceed through the wash
steps, then develop as described below.

   Reagents:
      Luminol (3-aminophthalhydrazide; Aldrich)
      30% hydrogen peroxide (Aldrich)
      p-Hydroxycinnamic acid (pHCA; Aldrich)

a)   Luminol Stock
     Water   90 ml
     Luminol   0.022 g   (1.25 mM final)
     Hydrogen peroxide   30 µl   (2.70 mM final)
     Tris   10 ml of 1 M (0.1 M, pH 8.6 final)

     Total   100 ml

b)   Enhancer Stock
     pHCA   0.011 g   680 µM (68 µM final)
     Water   100 ml

     Total   100 ml

The luminol and enhancer stock solutions are stable for about 2 weeks at 4°C.

Procedure:
1.   To prepare a working solution, combine 9 ml of luminol stock solution
     and 1 ml of enhancer stock solution. Prepare enough to thoroughly wet
     the filter.
2.   Soak filter in the working solution for less than 1 minute, wrap in plastic
     wrap and expose to X-ray film at room temperature for up to 1 hour.

DETECTION OF ALKALINE PHOSPHATASE

Chemiluminescent detection of alkaline phosphatase can be accomplished by
using a specially modified dioxetane (AMPPD) available from Tropix, Inc.
Protocols are supplied with the substrate.

For stripping off non-isotopic probes visualized by colorimetric development,
the filters must be decolorized with dimethyl formamide and treated with
Proteinase K before stripping off the probe (Gebeyehu *et al.*, 1987). A method
for stripping nylon membranes from biotin-labeled probes detected by
streptavidin-alkaline phosphatase and visualized with BCIP/NBT is described
below.

PROCEDURE 5.20

STRIPPING BIOTIN LABELED PROBES FROM NYLON MEMBRANES

Reagents:
a)   N,N-dimethylformamide (DMF)
b)   2x SSC/0.1 % SDS
c)   2x SSC/0.1% SDS containing 500 µg/ml Proteinase K
d)   50% (v/v) formamide containing 10 mM sodium phosphate, pH 6.5

Procedure:

1. Decolorize filter by washing in N,N-dimethylformamide (DMF) at 65°C in a glass tray with gentle agitation. Replace with fresh DMF every 15 minutes until the color completely disappears (about 3-4 changes). (Do not use DMF on nitrocellulose membranes.)
2. Wash filter two times in 2x SSC/0.1 % SDS for 15 minutes each at room temperature.
3   Pour off buffer and replace with 2x SSC/0.1% SDS containing 500 µg/ml Proteinase K. Incubate at 65°C for 1 hour.
4. Wash filter with 2x SSC -0.1% SDS at 65°C two times for 15 minutes each.
5. Strip off probe by incubation in 50% (v/v) formamide, 10 mM sodium phosphate, pH 6.5 at 65°C for 1 hour.
6. Wash filter with 2x SSC - 0.1% SDS for 15 minutes at room temperature. The filters are ready for rehybridization.
7. Stripped filters can be stored moist in heat-sealed bags at 4°C, if desired, until ready for rehybridization.

In Situ Hybridization

In situ hybridization methods allow the examination of specific sequences in specimens fixed on microscope slides. Following hybridization and development of the hybridized signal, the slides are examined by light microscopy. This hybridization method is well suited for cytology and histology laboratories and is finding applications in other settings as well.

A major problem in the detection of virus nucleic acid in clinical specimens by filter hybridization is that typically only a small percentage of cells are actually infected. Since uninfected cells usually outnumber infected cells in a sample, the viral DNA or RNA is significantly diluted by the non-viral sequences, decreasing the sensitivity of the assay. *In situ* hybridization circumvents this problem by identifying the viral sequences concentrated within infected cells. The microscopic examination of the specimen allows detection of small amounts of hybridization signal in a well defined area.

The *in situ* hybridization assay also offers additional information that is not available from filter hybridization methods. By localizing specific sequences within the cells, *in situ* hybridization can identify the intracellular distribution of these sequences. Estimating the percentage of cells actually infected with a virus and even the relative number of viral sequences per cell can contribute to understanding the pathogenesis of that virus.

The results of *in situ* hybridization have been often compared with those obtained by immunocytochemistry with specific antibodies.

FIGURE 5.2 Moisture Chamber. The bottom of the chamber is lined with paper soaked in 2x SSC to generate moisture and maintain sample hydration. A foil cover is used to prevent condensation from dripping onto the slides. Slides should lie flat in the chamber.

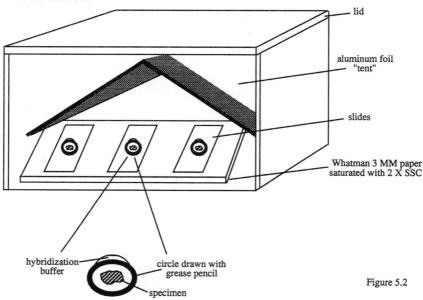

lid

aluminum foil "tent"

slides

Whatman 3 MM paper saturated with 2 X SSC

hybridization buffer

circle drawn with grease pencil

specimen

Figure 5.2

Immunocytochemistry is usually easier to perform and in many cases may be superior in sensitivity, due in part to the fact that the number of a specific viral protein molecules in a cell usually far exceeds the number of RNA molecules coding for those proteins. In certain applications , probes may have a clear advantage over antibodies since specific DNA probes are easier to produce and characterize and can be used to type viruses or bacteria. The technology for *in situ* hybridization is still relatively new and undergoing significant improvements in sensitivity, specificity and reproducibility.

A variety of radioactive and non-radioactive probes are suitable for use in *in situ* hybridization. The choice of probes depends on the specific application desired. Tritium and ^{35}S-labeled probes are most commonly used when radioactive detection is desired. For many applications ^{3}H-labeled probes are appropriate, since they have a long half-life and shelf-life, and the hybridization signal can readily be localized by autoradiography. However, ^{3}H-labeled probes usually have low specific activities and are suitable only for examination of multi-copy (100-1,000 copies per cell) or large (>10 kb) genes. Probes labeled with ^{35}S, on the other hand, achieve a high specific activity (> 10^9 cpm/μg) and generate a sharp image on autoradiographs (Rogers, 1979). Probes labeled with ^{32}P have high specific activities, but the isotopic emission gives rise to very diffuse grains, making localization of the site of hybridization difficult. Probes labeled with ^{125}I can give high resolution and high specificity resulting from its low energy secondary b-emissions (Allen *et al.*, 1987). The non-radioactive biotin and hapten-labeled probes discussed in Section 4 can also be adapted for use in *in situ* hybridizations.

Probes for *in situ* hybridization can be radioactively labeled by standard methods of nick translation, primer extension, or end labeling (Section 3). Specific activities of more than 10^9 cpm/µg can be achieved by using one or more [^{35}S]dNTP. The length of a probe is a critical consideration for use in *in situ* hybridization. Probes with an average length of 400 nucleotides appear to be optimal. Longer probes are not as effective, presumably because of their slower diffusion into the fixed cells. To reduce the size of long probes, they can be cut with restriction endonucleases, subjected to limited DNase I digestion, or sonicated prior to labeling. Sample fixation conditions also play a major role in determining hybridization efficiency (Section 2). The rate of probe diffusion can be increased by removing some of the proteins from the sample. This can be achieved by treatment of the slides with 0.2 N HCl, digestion with Proteinase K and dehydration in graded alcohols (50%, 70%, 95%). The concentration of probe required depends on the number of sequences per cell that are to be detected. These concentrations should be adjusted proportionately for detection of targets of greater or lesser complexity.

It is useful to circle the area surrounding a specimen with a grease pencil before beginning hybridization. This helps to locate the specimen and to confine the hybridization buffer in a small area conserving the amount of probe used per specimen. To prevent evaporation of the hybridization buffer during incubation, the specimen can be covered with a coverslip and the edges sealed with rubber cement. Placement of the slides in a moisture chamber during hybridization also helps to minimize evaporation. For a moisture chamber we use a closed plastic box in which the slides are placed on top of several layers of paper towel or Whatman 3 MM paper saturated with 2x SSC (Figure 5.2). A small tent of aluminum foil is placed over the slides to prevent condensation from dropping directly on slides. The boxes are closed and incubated at the appropriate temperature. We have found that when such a moisture chamber is used, it is not necessary to cover specimens with cover slips. The hybridization solution is applied over the sample, so that a small dome of buffer forms over the specimen. The circle drawn with the grease pencil defines the area in which the buffer is confined. It will not spread out over the rest of the slide if care is taken not to jar the chamber during incubation.

Prior to hybridization, several optional pre-treatments can be used to reduce background signals, or to better fix the specimens. Pretreatment of the slides with Denhardt's solution and acetic anhydride helps to limit non-specific binding of probes (Gendelman *et al.*, 1985). This is particularly important when targets of low copy number are to be detected.

When formalin-fixed, paraffin-embedded tissues are to be examined, particularly for RNA targets, pretreatment with 0.2 N HCl and Proteinase K helps to make the tissue more permeable to probe and thus give stronger signals. Be aware that these pre-treatments can be harsh and may damage cell morphology. Post-fixation with paraformaldehyde can help to retain morphology and nucleic acid integrity through the *in situ* hybridization and detection steps.

PROCEDURE 5.21

PRE-TREATMENT OF SLIDES WITH DENHARDT'S SOLUTION

Reagents:
a)   1x Denhardt's Solution
      50x Denhardt's solution   1 ml
      20x SSC   5 ml
      Water   44 ml
      Stock solutions are described in Appendix A.
b)   Buffered Acetic Anhydride
      0.25% (v/v) acetic anhydride
      0.1 M triethanolamine
      Adjust pH to 8.0
c)   Ethanol Solutions
      95% in water (v/v)
      70% in water (v/v)
      50% in water (v/v)
d)   Ethanol/acetic acid (3:1)

Procedure:
1.   Immerse the slide in 95% ethanol for 30 minutes.
2.   Transfer to 1x Denhardt's solution and incubate at 65°C for 3 hours.
3.   Rinse the slide in deionized water for 1 minute.
4.   Incubate the slide in ethanol-acetic acid for 20 minutes.
5.   Air-dry.
6.   Immerse the slide in buffered acetic anhydride for 20 minutes.
7.   Dehydrate through graded ethanol solutions (50%, 70% and 95%), for 5 minutes in each solution.
8.   Air-dry. Store the slide desiccated at -70°C.

PROCEDURE 5.22

PRETREATMENT OF FORMALIN-FIXED PARAFFIN-EMBEDDED SLIDES FOR USE WITH NON-RADIOACTIVE PROBES

For the detection of RNA sequences, all solutions must be treated with DEPC and RNase-free conditions must be maintained throughout the procedure (Section 2).

Reagents:

a)   100% ethanol

b)   <u>5 mM Levamisole Solution</u>
    50 mM levamisole (Appendix A)   5 ml
    Water   45 ml

c)   0.2 N HCl
d)   1x PBS (Appendix A)
e)   0.2% glycine in 1x PBS
f)   4% paraformaldehyde (Procedure 2.22)
g)   Xylene

h)   <u>Proteinase K Solution</u>
    Dissolve Proteinase K (Boehringer-Mannheim) to 25 µg/ml in DEPC-treated water.

Procedure:

1. De-wax tissue by incubation in xylene for 30 minutes at room temperature.
2. Incubate the slide in 100% ethanol for 10 minutes.
3. Incubate in a 5 mM levamisole solution for 30 minutes.
4. Wash the slide with 1x PBS for 5 minutes.
5. Wash with water for 5 minutes.
6. Incubate the slide in 0.2 N HCl for 20 minutes, then rinse in water for 5 minutes.
7. Incubate in the Proteinase K solution for 60 minutes at 37°C. (The optimal digestion time and enzyme concentration should be determined by the investigator).
8. Wash the slide in 0.2% glycine two times for 5 minutes each.
9. Wash in 1x PBS for 10 minutes.
10. Post-fix in 4% paraformaldehyde for 1 minute.
11. Wash slide in 1x PBS two times for 5 minutes each.

PROCEDURE 5.23

IN SITU HYBRIDIZATION USING ^{35}S-LABELED PROBES

Note: For the detection of RNA targets, all solutions should be DEPC-treated and RNase conditions maintained prior to and through the hybridization steps (Section 2).

Reagents:
a)   2x SSC
b)   0.25% acetic anhydride (Procedure 5.22)
c)   Tris-Glycine Buffer
     0.1 M Tris
     0.1 M glycine
     Adjust the pH to 7.4
d)   Ethanol Solutions
     95% in water (v/v)
     75% in water (v/v)
     50% in water (v/v)

Procedure:
PREHYBRIDIZATION
1.   Rinse slide two times for 1 minute each in 2x SSC.
2.   Acetylate in 0.25% acetic anhydride for 10 minutes with gentle agitation.
3.   Rinse slide in 2x SSC two times for 1 minute each.
4.   Incubate in Tris-glycine buffer for 30 minutes.
5.   Rinse slide in 2x SSC two times for 1 minute each.
6.   Dehydrate through graded ethanol solutions (50%, 70% and 95% ethanol), for 1 minute each.

HYBRIDIZATION

Reagents:
a)   Hybridization Buffer (per ml)

Deionized spectral grade formamide	500 µl
20x SSC	100 µl
10 mg/ml sheared, salmon sperm DNA	100 µl
20 mg/ml *E. coli* t RNA	50 µl
20 mg/ml bovine serum albumin	40 µl
1 M dithiothreitol (in water)	10 µl

Refer to Appendix A for stock solution protocols.
b)   Labeled Probe
     [35S]RNA probe (5×10^8 cpm/µg)   200 µl
     Final concentration is 500 ng/ml

Procedure:
1. Before use, heat hybridization buffer to 90°C for 10 minutes and place at 50°C. Optimum hybridization temperature varies with G+C content and should be determined by the investigator (Section 1).
2. Apply hybridization buffer (from step 1) to the slide. Use approximately 100 µl of hybridization buffer per cm^2 of sample area. Apply buffer to the specimen (circled with grease pencil) and incubate in a moisture chamber (Figure 5.2).
3. Incubate at 50°C for 3 hours.

POST-HYBRIDIZATION STEPS

Reagents:
a) <u>50% Formamide</u>
    Deionized formamide
    20x SSC
    Water
b) 2x SSC
c) <u>Ethanol Solutions</u>
    95% in water (v/v)
    75% in water (v/v)
    50% in water (v/v)
d) <u>RNase Solution</u>
    RNase A (Sigma)   100 µg/ml
    RNase T1 (Boehringer-Mannheim)   5 units/ml
    Dissolve in 2x SSC

Procedure:
1. Rinse slides in 50% formamide at 56°C with gentle agitation for 5 minutes.
2. Transfer slides to fresh 50% formamide for 20 minutes at 56°C. Wash temperature may be varied depending on stringency required (Section 1).
3. Rinse slide in 2x SSC three times for 1 minute each.
4. Dehydrate slide through graded ethanol solutions (50%, 70%, 95%) for 1 minute each.
5. Add about 100 µl (per cm^2) of RNase solution. Incubate at 37°C for 30 minutes.
6. Rinse slide with 50% formamide at 56°C for 5 minutes.
7. Rinse in 2x SSC for 1 minute. Wash in fresh 2x SSC for 10 minutes with gentle agitation.
8. Dehydrate slide in graded ethanol solutions (50%, 70% and 95%) for 1 minute each with gentle agitation. Air-dry.

AUTORADIOGRAPHY

Reagents:
a)   NTB2 nuclear track emulsion (Kodak
b)   Dektol developing solution (Kodak)
c)   Stop bath (Kodak)
d)   Fixative bath (Kodak)
e)   Hematoxylin stain (Procedure 5.24)

Procedure:
1.   Work in a dark room, using a safe light. Apply emulsion, diluted 1:1 with water, over specimen.
2.   Allow emulsion to flood the surrounding area. Turn the slide on its side to permit excess to drain off, but do not wipe off the excess. Allow the slide to air-dry in the dark for 1-2 hours. Place the slide in a black slide box which contains desiccant. Double-wrap the slide box with aluminum foil and place in a -70°C freezer. The autoradiography exposure time depends on the number of target copies per cell. Using a probe labeled with ^{35}S to 5×10^8 cpm/μg:
     a) For more than 1,000 copies per cell, incubate overnight at -70°C.
     b) For 50-500 copies per cell, incubate 5 days at -70°C.
     c) For less than 10 copies per cell, incubate 10 days - 1 month at -70°C.
3.   Work in a dark room, using a safe light. After exposure, remove slide from box and allow it to equilibrate to room temperature. Place slide, emulsion side up, in a small tray containing developing solution for 1-2 minutes.
4.   Transfer the slide to a tray containing stop bath for 30 seconds.
5.   Transfer the slide to fixative bath for 1-2 minutes.
6.   Rinse the slide for 15 minutes in running tap water. Blot excess water from around the wells. Stain the sample with hematoxylin.
7.   View the slide under a light microscope. Use the oil immersion lens (400x) and count individual silver grains to quantitate the signal.

STAINING OF SLIDES

Following autoradiography, slides can be stained to allow visualization of the cells. Various stains have been used in conjunction with *in situ* hybridization, with hematoxylin and eosin being very effective and widely used. The method of rapid progressive hematoxylin staining allows staining through the photographic emulsion without stripping it (Gowans *et al.*, 1989). Following staining, the emulsion must be dehydrated gradually to retain its integrity.

PROCEDURE 5.24

STAINING SLIDES WITH HEMATOXYLIN
AFTER *IN SITU* HYBRIDIZATION

Reagents:
a) Hematoxylin solution (Sigma, HHS-2-16)
b) Eosin solution (Sigma, HT110-3-16)
c) Permount or glycerol gelatin (Sigma)
d) Xylene
e) Ethanol Solutions
    95% in water (v/v)
    75% in water (v/v)
    50% in water (v/v)

Procedure:
1. Immerse slide in hematoxylin solution for 1 minute.
2. Wash slide in 0.1x SSC, for 1 minute.
3. Wash in 2x SSC, for 15 minutes.
4. Dehydrate through graded ethanol solutions (50%, 70%, 95%), for 1 minute each.
5. Immerse in eosin solution for 1 minute.
6. Wash three times in 95% ethanol, for 1 minute each.
7. Soak in xylene, 2 times for 10 minutes each.
8. Mount sample in Permount or glycerol gelatin.

PROCEDURE 5.25

IN SITU HYBRIDIZATION WITH HAPTEN
OR BIOTIN-LABELED PROBES

For detection of RNA targets, all solutions should be DEPC-treated and RNase conditions must be maintained prior to and throughout the hybridization steps.

Reagents:
a) Hybridization Buffer
    50% deionized spectro-grade formamide
    4x SSC
    10% dextran sulfate
    0.5 mg/ml denatured salmon sperm DNA
    1x Denhardt's solution
    0.25 mg/ml yeast tRNA
b) 20x SSC
    The required stock solutions are described in Appendix A.

Procedure:

1.   Prehybridize slides in pre-hybridization buffer (same as hybridization buffer, but without probe) for 60 minutes.

2.   Remove prehybridization buffer and replace with hybridization buffer (containing 100-500 ng/ml of probe). For detection of DNA targets, denature probe and target DNA by incubating the slide at 90°C for 4 minutes and quick cooling on ice for 5 minutes. For detection of RNA targets, denature the probe DNA prior to applying to the slide. The probe should be 100-500 bp long for optimum results.

3.   Hybridize overnight at 45°C. The optimal hybridization temperature and probe concentration should be determined by the investigator.

4.   Following hybridization, wash the slide with gentle agitation in the following solutions:

    a) 2x SSC for 60 minutes.
    b) 1x SSC for 60 minutes.
    c) 0.2x SSC for 30 minutes.

(Stringency of washes should be determined by investigator. Over-stringent washes can decrease or obliterate the probe signal).

5.   Visualize the hybridized probe as described below. Do not let the slide dry out prior to detection.

PROCEDURE 5.26

VISUALIZATION OF HAPTEN-LABELED PROBES

Reagents:

a)   Blocking Buffer
    2.0% horse serum
    0.3% Tween-20
    0.1 M Tris-HCl, pH 7.4
    0.15 M NaCl

b)   Antibody Diluent
    1.0% horse serum
    0.3% Tween-20
    0.1 M Tris-HCl, pH 7.4
    0.15 M NaCl

c)   TE Buffer
    10 mM Tris-HCl, pH 7.6
    1 mM EDTA

d)   Anti-hapten antibody

e)   Alkaline phosphatase conjugated second antibody

f)   NBT/BCIP substrate solution containing 1 mM levamisol
     (Appendix A)
g)   1x NBT/BCIP substrate buffer (Appendix A)
h)   0.003% acridine orange in water

Procedure:
1.   All procedures are performed at room temperature. Block the sample
     with blocking buffer for 60 minutes.
2.   Dilute the anti-hapten antibody to about 5 µg/ml in antibody diluent and
     apply 100 µl to the sample. Incubate 1-18 hours at room temperature in a
     moisture chamber.
3.   Wash the sample in 0.1 M Tris pH 7.4/0.15 M NaCl for 15 minutes.
4.   Incubate sample for 1 hour in the appropriate anti-IgG antibody conjugated
     with alkaline phosphatase. Prepare a solution containing 1-2 µg/ml in
     antibody diluent. (Omit this step when using an anti-hapten antibody
     directly conjugated with alkaline phosphatase). *The actual first and
     second antibody concentrations will vary and must be empirically
     determined.*
5.   Wash sample in 1x substrate buffer for 2 minutes.
6.   Develop signal with BCIP/NBT substrate solution for up to 24 hours.
7.   Stop development by rinsing slide in TE buffer.
8.   Counterstain sample with acridine orange for 1-2 minutes.
9.   Rinse off counterstain with water and examine sample under the
     microscope. Positive cells will exhibit purple staining against a yellow
     background.

PROCEDURE 5.27

VISUALIZATION OF BIOTIN-LABELED PROBES

Reagents:
a)   Blocking Buffer
     3.0% BSA
     0.3% Tween-20
     1x TBS (Appendix A)
     Use acetylated BSA (Appendix A) when detecting RNA targets.
b)   Streptavidin (1 mg/ml, Procedure 5.18)
c)   Biotin-conjugated alkaline phosphatase (1 mg/ml, Procedure 5.18)
d)   NBT/BCIP substrate solution containing 1 mM levamisole (Appendix A)
e)   0.003% acridine orange in water
f)   TE Buffer
     10 mM Tris-HCl, pH 7.6
     1 mM EDTA

Procedure:

1. All procedures are carried out at room temperature. Block slide in blocking buffer for 30 minutes.
2. Wash slide with 0.3% Tween-20 in 1x TBS for 10 minutes with gentle agitation.
3. Incubate with 1 µg/ml streptavidin in blocking buffer for 10 minutes.
4. Wash slide as in Step 2.
5. Incubate with 5 µg/ml biotin-conjugated alkaline phosphatase in blocking buffer for 10 minutes.
6. Wash slide as in Step 2.
7. Incubate with BCIP/NBT substrate solution for 15 minutes to 4 hours, depending on the target DNA copy number, or until non-specific background staining begins to appear.
8. Stop development by rinsing slide in TE Buffer.
9. Counterstain with acridine orange for 1-2 minutes.
10. Rinse off counterstain with water and examine sample under the microscope. Positive cells will exhibit purple staining against a yellow background.

Hybridization Formats for Detection of Soluble Target

Solution hybridization was introduced in Section 1 because it was the earliest and simplest hybridization format. It has seen sporadic use over the past 30 years, but has not been as popular as formats using immobilized nucleic acid. Detection of labeled probe in *soluble* hybrids in the presence of excess soluble probe is more difficult than detection of labeled probe in *insoluble* hybrids in the presence of soluble excess probe. New developments in hybrid detection have again popularized solution hybridization for some potential commercial applications.

AFFINITY CAPTURE

The earliest affinity capture technique for quantification of hybrids was hydroxyapatite chromatography. DNA:DNA hybrids will specifically bind to the insoluble powder under low salt conditions and the bound, hybridized probe can be measured by centrifuging the hydroxyapatite (HAP), washing and counting the pellet for a radioactively-labeled probe. This approach was used by Gen-Probe in their early products for the detection of mycoplasma and pathogenic bacteria (Wilkinson *et al.*, 1986). A ^{3}H or ^{125}I-labeled DNA probe was hybridized in solution for about 1 hour (Figure 5.3), then a suspension of HAP in a buffer of

FIGURE 5.3   Capture of Double-Stranded Hybrids from Solution using Hydroxyapatite. Excess radioactively-labeled probe is hybridized in solution to its target nucleic acid. Hybrids are captured on hydroxyapatite, pelleted, washed and counted to determine the amount of bound probe.

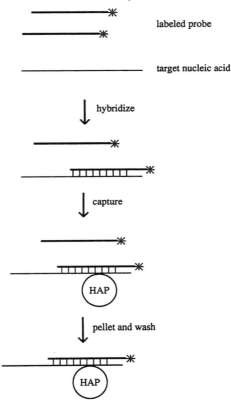

the appropriate salt concentration was added. After centrifugation and washing, the radioactivity in the pellet was proportional to the amount of target in the original sample. Another modification of this approach is currently in use in some Gen-Probe products. The DNA probe is labeled with an acridinium ester, which provides for sensitive chemiluminescent detection (Granato and Franz, 1989). The probe:target hybrids are captured on magnetized beads (cationic magnetic microspheres) which have the DNA binding properties of HAP. Instead of centrifugation, the beads are removed from solution by magnets, simplifying the washing steps. Bead-bound probe is measured by its chemiluminescence.

An example of a novel solution hybridization format for RNA detection was described by Yehle *et al.* (1987). A biotinylated DNA probe was hybridized

FIGURE 5.4 Affinity Capture of DNA:RNA Hybrids and Immunochemical Detection. A biotinylated DNA probe is hybridized in solution to its RNA target. The hybrids, as well as the unreacted probe, are captured an immobilized anti-biotin antibody. Hybridized is distinguished from unhybridized probe by binding of an enzyme-labeled anti-hybrid antibody and use of a fluorescent enzyme substrate.

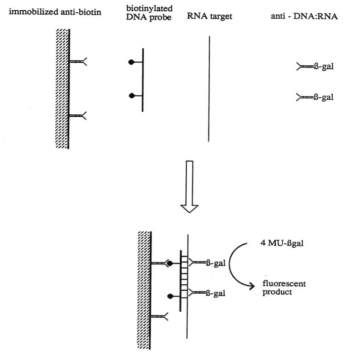

in excess in solution to target bacterial rRNA (Figure 5.4). Resulting hybrids as well as free probe were captured on succinylated avidin-coated beads while an enzyme-labeled monoclonal antibody specific for DNA:RNA hybrids was used to quantify the bead-bound hybrids. Using a colorimetric enzyme substrate, this system allowed rapid (2 hours) detection of RNA, with a sensitivity of about 10^7 copies.

This format was modified by Viscidi *et al.* (1989) to detect HIV-1 RNA in cultured cells. Hybrids of biotinylated probe and RNA target were captured in microtiter wells coated with goat anti-biotin antibody. The captured hybrids were detected using the same ß-galactosidase-labeled mouse antibody to DNA:RNA hybrids and a fluorescent substrate, 4-methylumbelliferyl-ß-D-galactoside. Sensitivity was 1 pg/ml using a model system consisting of poly(I) target and biotinylated poly(dC) probe.

FIGURE 5.5   A Homogeneous Hybridization Assay using Non-Radiative Energy Transfer. Two adjacent probes are labeled with different, light-emitting labels. After hybridization to the specific target, these labels are close enough to interact. The chemiluminescent moiety is chemically activated and emits light which can be absorbed and re-emitted at a different wavelength by the other moiety. The detector is tuned to only register the second wavelength and no light is emitted at this wavelength unless target is present, bringing the probes in proximity to each other.

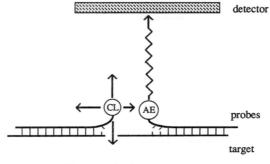

CL = chemiluminescent
AE = absorber/emitter

HOMOGENEOUS SOLUTION HYBRIDIZATION ASSAYS

The idea of a single-step hybridization reaction, with all components in solution, has been tempting and elusive. Tempting because a homogeneous system would not require immobilization or washing; elusive because specific detection of hybrids, without capture, is very challenging. The three systems described below illustrate some of the approaches that are being tested.

The phenomenon of nonradiative energy transfer was explored by Heller and Morrison (1985) to develop a homogeneous assay system. Their idea was to use two adjacent probes, one labeled with a chemiluminescent group (donor), the other labeled with a moiety capable of fluorescence only when both are in proximity (absorber / emitter). This scheme is illustrated in Figure 5.5. The two probes and the two detectable moieties are in proximity only when both are hybridized to target nucleic acid. On paper this is a clever and straightforward approach to the homogeneous assay puzzle. In practice, although feasibility experiments have been reported, it is not clear whether this type of system has yet achieved practical sensitivity which may be arbitrarily defined as detecting less than 10^7 copies of target nucleic acid. Morrison (1988) has described an improved application of the energy transfer principle using pyrene butyrate as the donor, ß-phycoerythrin as the absorber/emitter along with pulsed-laser excitation and electronic gating of the detection signals. Even with this improved

FIGURE 5.6 A Homogeneous Assay Format Based on Strand Displacement. A short RNA signal sequence is prehybridized to a longer DNA probe sequence. After hybridization to the target DNA, the RNA is displaced and enzymatically converted to NDPs. The ADP residues are subsequently used in an enzymatic reaction to produce light, which is quantitated.

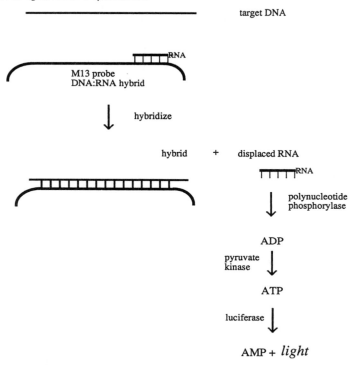

signal-to-noise ratio, the actual sensitivity of energy transfer-based hybridization reactions may still be far inferior to current assays. Another group (Cardullo *et al.*, 1988) has examined other exciter-emitter configurations, but they present no data that would allow sensitivity comparisons with other systems.

Strand Displacement. Another novel hybridization format which can be employed in a homogeneous format is the strand displacement assay. In a version developed by Vary (1987) a short RNA signal strand is pre-annealed to a single-stranded M13 DNA molecule containing a sequence homologous to the target sequence (Figure 5.6). When target DNA is present, it anneals to the homologous M13 insert, displacing the signal RNA by virtue of its longer sequence homology. The target:M13 hybrid is favored over the signal RNA:M13 hybrid because more bases (bonds) are involved, making it energetically more stable.

FIGURE 5.7   A Homogeneous Assay Format Based on an Acridinium Ester-Labeled Probe. Acridinium ester conjugated probes are hybridized in solution to their target nucleic acid. Next a developer solution is added which hydrolyzes the label from unhybridized probe, inactivating it. Finally the total luminescence is measured and is proportional to the amount of hybridized probe.

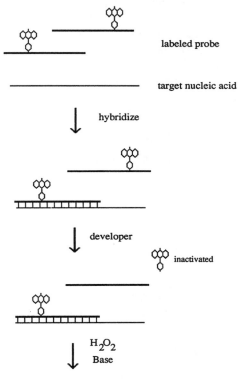

labeled probe

target nucleic acid

hybridize

developer

inactivated

H_2O_2
Base

measure luminescence

The displaced RNA was detected by a three-step enzymatic process:

1. The RNA was degraded to NDPs by polynucleotide phosphorylase. Since the enzyme is specific for single-stranded nucleic acid, only displaced RNA is degraded.
2. The ADP in the degradation products was converted to ATP by pyruvate kinase.
3. The ATP serves as a substrate for luciferase to produce light, which was quantified.

Two problems with this system were sensitivity and background. Detection sensitivity was limited to about 1 μg of target DNA. This amount is six orders of magnitude less sensitive than required for a practical assay. The background problem was due to sample and reagent contaminants such as RNA and nucleotides. Efficient removal of these contaminants appears to be tedious, as does the preparation of the M13:RNA probe hybrid. Much refinement is required before this format can be practical.

Acridinium Esters. Weeks *et al.* (1983, 1986) have employed certain acridinium esters as chemiluminescent tags in immunoassays. They developed an activated N-hydroxysuccinimide derivative which could be easily coupled to the primary amines on antibodies or antigens. These compounds can be induced to produce a short burst of light in the presence of alkaline hydrogen peroxide. Ligands labeled with such esters can be detected at lower concentrations (8×10^{-19} mole) than those labeled with [125]I , illustrating the sensitivity obtainable with these compounds. The use of acridinium esters in a heterogeneous assay was described earlier in this section (affinity capture). Nelson *et al.* (1988) of Gen-Probe Corp. described the application of this detectable group to develop a homogeneous assay system of useful sensitivity. This homogeneous hybridization assay is illustrated in Figure 5.7. After hybridization of the acridinium ester-labeled probe to its target nucleic acid, the acridinium moieties on the unhybridized probe molecules are selectively cleaved from the probe (and thus inactivated) by a proprietary process. The only chemiluminescence which remains is that associated with hybridized probe, so the remaining chemiluminescence is proportional to the amount of target nucleic acid. A drawback of the assay is detection sensitivity (about 1 ng of target), which makes this assay suitable only for the detection of amplified targets such as rRNA or PCR amplification products. Refer to Section 6 for further discussion of amplified targets.

SANDWICH HYBRIDIZATION

Solid Phase Sandwich Hybridization. The sandwich hybridization format was originally described by Dunn and Hassell (1977) and adapted by Ranki *et al.* (1983) and Ranki and Soderlund (1984). It was developed to avoid the tedious purification and immobilization of sample nucleic acid required in most solid phase hybridization formats. Sandwich hybridization has two main advantages over direct filter hybridization, sample immobilization is not required and crude samples can be assayed reliably. In addition, sandwich hybridization is potentially more specific than direct hybridization because two hybridization events must occur in order to generate a signal. Solid phase sandwich hybridization requires two adjacent, non-overlapping probes; an immobilized capture probe and a labeled detection probe. Figure 5.8 illustrates a typical sandwich hybridization scheme consisting of an immobilized capture sequence cloned into M13 and an adjacent detection sequence cloned into pBR322. A sandwich structure can form only if the sample contains nucleic acid which spans the original junction

FIGURE 5.8 General Diagram of Sandwich Hybridization. Two adjacent DNA fragments from the genome of interest are cloned into non-homologous vectors. Here, the capture fragment (B) is cloned into M13 and immobilized, while the probe fragment (A) is cloned into pBR322, linearized and labeled. Probe is specifically bound to the support only in the presence of target nucleic acid that spans the junction between fragments A and B.

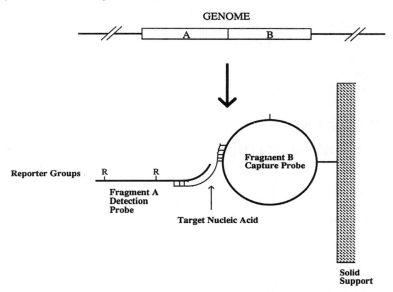

between the two fragments in genomic nucleic acid. Note that the two probes must be subcloned into separate, non-homologous vectors to avoid high background signals. Gel purification of the two adjacent fragments from the same clone is not suitable because, regardless of the care taken, each band will be contaminated with DNA from the other band.

Sandwich hybridization formats have utilized filters (Ranki *et al.*, 1983) and also utilized beads (Polsky-Cynkin *et al.*, 1985; Langdale and Malcolm, 1985) to immobilize the capture probe. The use of beads resulted in better standardization of the assays and easier handling of small numbers of samples. For large numbers of samples, however, beads can be difficult to handle and wash. Dahlen *et al.* (1987) have conducted sandwich hybridization in microtiter wells, which are more appropriate for handling large numbers of samples. They absorbed the capture DNA to the well, then fixed it to the plastic using UV light. Keller *et al.* (1989) used sandwich hybridization in microtiter wells to detect amplified nucleic acid fragments with a covalently coupled capture probe.

Sandwich hybridization in microtiter wells has a number of advantages over other hybridization formats. The use of sandwich hybridization provides specific signals using aliquots of the polymerase chain reaction (PCR) directly, even when the reaction contains crude cell lysate. This specificity is partly a result of the sample being *soluble* during the hybridization rather than being immobilized as with direct filter hybridization. This specificity is also due to the use of *two probes*, because two hybridization events must occur in order to generate a signal. The sensitivity of PCR product detection, using a photobiotinylated probe, is equivalent to Southern blotting with a ^{32}P-labeled probe (3×10^8 cpm/μg) and a 16 hour autoradiography exposure. Other advantages of using microtiter wells include the handling of 8-96 samples at a time, as well as multiple blocks of 96 samples, easy quantitation of the results and potential automation of the pipetting, washing and reading steps.

PROCEDURE 5.29

SANDWICH HYBRIDIZATION IN MICROTITER WELLS

Reagents:

a) <u>DNA Binding Buffer</u>

25 mM KH_2PO_4, pH 7.2	0.25 ml of 1 M
200 mM $MgCl_2$	2.00 ml of 1 M
Water	7.75 ml
	10.00 ml total

b) <u>DNA Binding/Wash Buffer</u>

25 mM KH_2PO_4, pH 7.2	1.25 ml of 1 M
200 mM $MgCl_2$	5.00 ml of 1 M
Water	43.75 ml
	50.00 ml total

c) <u>DNA Binding/Blocking Buffer</u>

1x PBS/K	5.0 ml of 10x
100 mM $MgCl_2$	5.0 ml of 1 M
Water	40.0 ml
BSA (Sigma)	0.5 g
	50.0 ml total

d) <u>10x PBS/K</u>

$Na_2HPO_4.7H_2O$	21.44 g
KH_2PO_4	2.04 g
NaCl	80.06 g
KCl	2.01 g

Dilute to 1 liter adjust pH to 7.2 with 10 N NaOH.

e) 1x TE
0.5 ml 1 M Tris, pH 8.0
0.2 ml 0.25M EDTA, pH 8.0
Water to 50 ml
f) TE/carrier DNA
10 µl of 10 mg/ml carrier DNA per 10 ml TE
g) Positive Control
Linearized target plasmid at 200 pg/µl in TE/carrier DNA
h) Detection probe
Biotin-labeled pBR322 clone or insert
i) 2x SSC/0.1% SDS
Add 50 ml of 20x SSC and 5 ml of 10% SDS to 445 ml of water.
Autoclave in 100 ml bottles and store at room temperature.
j) 3% BSA/1x Wash Buffer
Dissolve 1.5 g of BSA (Sigma #A-8022) in 50 ml of 1x wash buffer (see
Appendix A for 10x wash buffer). Make fresh daily and store at 4°C.

Procedure:

MICROTITER WELL PREPARATION

1. Use Costar high-binding, flat bottom, 8-well microtiter strips.
2. Capture DNA (M13 clone) should be 100 µg/ml in water. If the DNA is
   double-stranded, it must be nicked or cut and denatured by boiling and
   chilling.

	1 Strip	2 Strips	3 Strips	4 Strips
Capture DNA (100 µg/ml)	27	54	81	108
DNA Binding Buffer	425	850	1,250	1,650
Total Volume	452µl	904µl	1,331µl	1,758µl

3. Add 50 µl per well (300 ng) and shake for 2 hr at room temperature.
4. Wash wells 3 times with 400 µl of DNA binding/wash buffer. Add 400 µl
   of fresh DNA binding/blocking buffer to each well and incubate 1 hour at
   room temperature.
5. Empty wells. Wash 3 times with 400 µl of water.
6. Dry on a lyophilizer for at least 10 minutes. Use immediately or store at
   room temperature in a heat-sealed bag.
   The hybridization and detection steps are presented below. These are
   graphically illustrated in Figure 5.9.

FIGURE 5.9 Flowchart of Sandwich Hybridization in Microtiter Wells. Capture DNA is bound to microtiter wells and prehybridized to reduce non-specific binding of the probe. After hybridization with the sample and biotin-labeled probe, the wells are washed, blocked and developed using peroxidase-streptavidin and a colorimetric substrate.

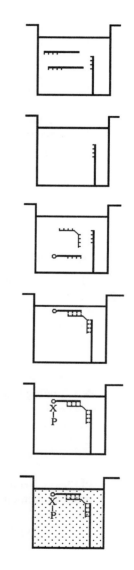

1. Bind capture DNA to multiwell strips.

2. Prehybridize 30 min at 42°C.

3. Add denatured sample + biotin-labeled probe. Hybridize 4 hrs at 42°C.

4. Wash wells and block with 3% BSA.

5. Add peroxidase-conjugated streptavidin to wells and incubate 10 min.

6. Wash wells and detect bound peroxidase with TMB.

PREHYBRIDIZATION (8 WELLS)

> 1,300 µl hybridization buffer (Procedure 5.15)
> 26 µl of 10 mg/ml denatured carrier DNA (200 µg/ml)
>
> ---
>
> 1,326 µl total

1. Add 150 µl per well. Cover wells with Mylar tape (Flow) and prehybridize for 30 min at 42°C. Empty wells using a multi-channel pipette just before adding hybridization reaction. Empty wells completely.

SANDWICH HYBRIDIZATION

2. Preparation of probe
    Combine: 18 µl biotinylated probe (50 µg/ml)   (1 µg/ml final)
    18 µl 10 mg/ml carrier DNA   (200 µg/ml final)

    ---

    36 µl total

3. Standard curve (in duplicate)

Well	Positive control (µl)	TE (µl)	Probe (µl)
A	5.0	5.0	4
B	5.0	5.0	4
C	2.5	7.5	4
D	2.5	7.5	4
E	1.0	9.0	4
F	1.0	9.0	4
G	0	10.0	4
H	0	10.0	4

Denature the reactions by boiling for 5 minutes and chilling on ice for 10 minutes. Centrifuge to recover the solution. Add 100 µl of hybridization buffer to each reaction, vortex and pipette entire reaction into the emptied, prehybridized wells. Cover the wells with Mylar tape and hybridize for four hours at 42°C.

4. Amplified samples:
    Thaw, if necessary, vortex and microtuge briefly. Combine 10 µl of amplified sample, with 4 µl of probe/carrier solution. Denature 5 minutes by boiling, cool on ice for 10 minutes and centrifuge to recover solution.

Add hybridization buffer (heated to 50°C), mix well and centrifuge again. Add reactions (110 µl) to empty, prehybridized wells. Mix for 1 minute on a microtiter plate shaker. Be sure that the solution is moving in all of the wells. Bubbles will prevent mixing. Incubate at 42°C until bubbles disappear and then again shake plate to mix wells.

5. Cover the wells with Mylar tape and hybridize for 4 hours at 42°C.
6. Wash 4 times with 200 µl of 2x SSC/0.1% SDS - shake each wash for 3 minutes, then shake out the buffer and blot the well strip on a paper towel. Incubate the final 2 washes at 42°C, then shake.

WELL STRIP DEVELOPMENT

7. Add 200 µl of 3% BSA/1x wash buffer - shake 10 minutes. Empty wells.
8. Add 100 µl of 1.0 µg/ml peroxidase-streptavidin (Kirkegaard & Perry) in 3% BSA/1x wash buffer and shake 10 min. Empty wells.
9. Wash wells 4 times with 200 µl of 1x wash buffer.
10. Develop wells with 100 µl of TMB reagent (Kirkegaard & Perry) for 30 minutes (up to 60 minutes if necessary).
11. If the blue color is strong, read the wells at 620 nm. Then add 100 µl of 2 N H_2SO_4 and read wells at 450 nm. The addition of acid stops the reaction and amplifies the signal up to fourfold.

Solution Phase Sandwich Hybridization. Sandwich hybridization can also be performed in solution, as is demonstrated by the next three examples. Syvanen *et al.* (1986) were the first to report such a format. They named it affinity-based hybrid collection and claimed that it allows more rapid hybridization kinetics because the capture probe is in solution and not immobilized. The assay retains the high specificity of solid phase sandwich hybridization, but uses affinity capture to separate hybridized from unhybridized detection probe. The scheme is illustrated in Figure 5.10. An excess of detection and capture probes are present in the hybridization reaction. The detection probe can be labeled with a radioactive isotope, a hapten, a fluorescent or a chemiluminescent group. The capture probe is labeled with an affinity label such as biotin, allowing later capture on an avidin-coated solid phase. Other useful affinity systems would be mercurated DNA with a thiol-substituted solid phase, or a poly(A)-tailed DNA with an oligo(dT)-substituted solid phase.

In the presence of target nucleic acid, both probes hybridize to the target, forming a sandwich structure. After hybridization is complete, the reaction is transferred to a new tube or well where hybridized and excess capture probe will bind to the affinity matrix. Only those capture probes that have hybridized to target nucleic acid will have detection probes attached, thus generating a signal. This system has a sensitivity limit of about 4×10^5 target molecules using a biotin-

FIGURE 5.10 Affinity-Based Hybrid Collection. This is a variant of sandwich hybridization in which hybridization occurs in solution and hybrids are subsequently captured from solution and detected. Two probes are simultaneously hybridized to the target nucleic acid, one for capture, the other for detection. In this example, the complex is captured in a streptavidin-coated microwell and quantified by radioactive detection techniques.

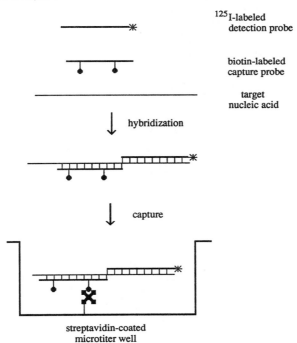

^{125}I-labeled
detection probe

biotin-labeled
capture probe

target
nucleic acid

hybridization

capture

streptavidin-coated
microtiter well

labeled capture probe and an ^{125}I-labeled detection probe. When ^{125}I was replaced with a direct europium conjugate, the limit of sensitivity was about 8×10^5 target molecules.

A similar approach has been used by Gene-Trak Systems in its tests for HIV-1 and CMV nucleic acids (Decker *et al.*, 1989). Their system is illustrated in Figure 5.11. They employed an ^{125}I-labeled RNA detection probe and a poly(dA)-tailed DNA capture probe. The affinity matrix consisted of poly(dT)-coated magnetic particles. Sample lysis and hybridization occur in 5 M guanidinium thiocyanate, which permits easy sample preparation and low-temperature (37°C) solution hybridization. Hybridization was chosen as the affinity capture system because it has an inherently lower background than protein-based interactions. The low complexity poly(dA):(dT) system was selected so that hybrids could be eluted from the magnetic particles and recaptured under conditions that would not disrupt the probe:target sandwich structure. This is usually accomplished by cycling the guanidinium thiocyanate concentration between 1M (capture) and 3M (elution).

These elution:recapture cycles ('target cycling') are performed 3-4 times with fresh magnetic particles each time. The cycles reduce the nonspecific background associated with the capture step; the background is discarded with the used particles. For detection, the magnetic particles with their sandwich hybrids attached are transferred to a filter on a dot blot manifold for autoradiography. Detection sensitivity was about 6×10^5 target molecules using a six-day exposure.

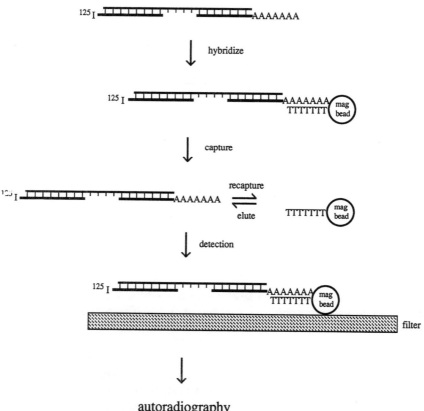

autoradiography

FIGURE 5.11 Hybridization Affinity Capture with Target Cycling. This is another example of solution-phase sandwich hybridization combined with affinity capture. In this case, hybridization between homopolymers is used as the affinity step. This allows conditions where the probe:target complex can be eluted and recaptured without disrupting the complex itself. In this way, the non-specific background associated with the capture beads can be discarded with the beads after each cycle, lowering the overall background of the assay.

While this format incorporates innovative features, its main advantage seems to be ease of sample preparation. In spite of the 'target cycling' steps to lower background, detection sensitivity is no better than that achieved by the format of Syvanen *et al.* (1986), in which no such cycling was employed. It may be that the background reduction achieved by 'target cycling' is offset by the loss of specific hybrids which are not recaptured in subsequent cycles.

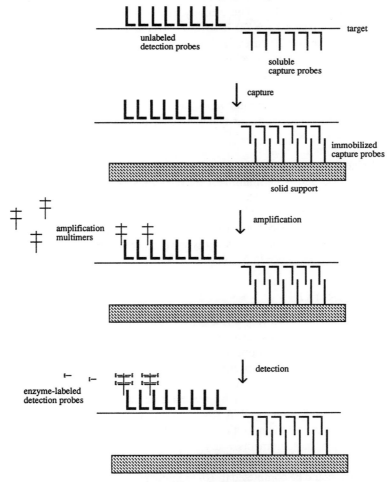

FIGURE 5.12 Schematic Diagram of Soluble Sandwich Hybridization using Multiple Synthetic Probes. a) Multiple oligomer capture and detection probes are hybridized to the target nucleic acid in solution. b) The complex is captured onto a solid support by hybridization to immobilized capture probes. c) Cross-linked secondary probes (amplification multimers) are hybridized to the primary probes to amplify the number of binding sites for the (d) tertiary, enzyme-labeled detection probes.

Perhaps the most original and sensitive variation on solution phase sandwich hybridization is that developed by Mickey Urdea and his colleagues at Chiron Corporation (Urdea *et al.*, 1987; Urdea, 1988; Sanchez-Pescador *et al.*, 1988). They have employed synthetic oligonucleotide probes and non-radioactive detection, a combination which usually provides a low detection sensitivity. However, by using multiple probes and chemiluminescent detection, they can detect as little as 5×10^4 molecules of double-stranded DNA. Their format is illustrated in Figure 5.12. The primary probes (unlabeled detection probes/ soluble capture probes) are 50 bases long containing 30 bases of organism-specific sequence and 20 bases of single-stranded tail to be used to capture the probe:target complex from solution or to bind the labeled detection probe. Typically, about 25 different detection probes and 10 different capture probes are used in an assay.

Both beads and microtiter wells have been used as solid supports. Each labeled detection probe contains many attached enzymes (alkaline phosphatase or peroxidase) to achieve amplification of the unlabeled detection probe (see Section 6 for more details). Only one type of labeled detection probe and immobilized capture probe is needed and these are common to all assays, regardless of target. Chemiluminescent enzyme substrates were used to gain improved sensitivity over colorimetric substrates. Enhanced luminol was used for peroxidase detection, while an enzyme-triggerable dioxetane was used for alkaline phosphatase detection. This assay format has been applied to tests for hepatitis B virus, *Chlamydia trachomatis* and *N. gonorrhoeae*, as well as plasmid-borne antibiotic resistance in *N. gonorrhoeae*.

OTHER FORMATS

Immobilized Probe. Two very unusual hybridization formats, which do not fall under the above definitions, have been described in the literature. The first uses an unlabeled immobilized probe to capture target RNA by hybridization (Miller *et al.*, 1988). A DNA probe specific for bacterial rRNA was covalently attached to diazotized latex particles and hybridized to the sample rRNA (Figure 5.13). Specific hybrids were detected by the binding of an alkaline phosphatase-conjugated antibody against DNA:RNA hybrids, collection and washing of the particles on filters and visualization of bound alkaline phosphatase using BCIP and reflectance measurements. By using latex particles, a hybridization temperature of 80°C and a theoretical probe concentration of 2 μg/ml, the hybridization could be completed in 10-15 minutes. Substrate development time was kept short (40-70 seconds) by measuring development rate rather than endpoint signal. Detection sensitivity was about 5×10^6 target copies with a minimal amount of manipulation.

The second assay employs labeled sample nucleic acid in combination with unlabeled, immobilized probe DNA and is known as 'reversed hybridization' (Dattagupta *et al*., 1989). The advantage of this format is that it provides a way to detect a number of different nucleic acid targets simultaneously in a sample in a single hybridization reaction. A new photoactivatable DNA biotinylation reagent, biotin-polyethylene glycol-angelicin (BPA), was developed for this

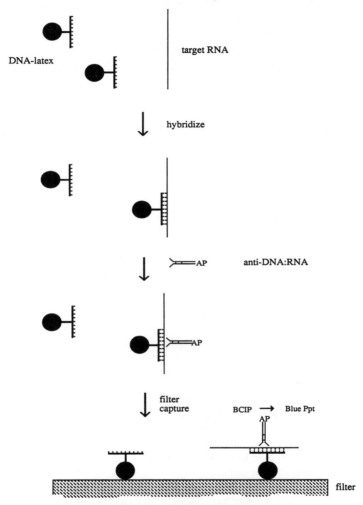

FIGURE 5.13 Hybridization Format using an Immobilized Probe and Anti-Hybrid Immunochemical Detection. Latex-bound probe DNA is hybridized in suspension to its target RNA and reacted with an enzyme-labeled anti-DNA:RNA hybrid antibody. The latex is captured on a filter, washed and wetted with a colorimetric substrate solution. The resulting color is proportional to the amount of target RNA.

procedure. BPA's DNA-binding moiety is a reactive furocoumarin derivative which forms covalent bonds with DNA bases in the presence of long-wave UV light. BPA's reactivity seems to be more specific for DNA than photobiotin and it does not react with nucleic acid under visible light. These properties allow the use of BPA to label nucleic acids in crude cell lysates without labeling proteins, polysaccharides or other cellular macromolecules. It is also unnecessary to remove unreacted BPA before hybridization since, in the absence of UV light, free BPA will not label the immobilized probe DNA during hybridization. The assay was demonstrated by using it to detect and identify bacterial infections in human urine. Urine samples were boiled under alkaline conditions, neutralized and labeled with BPA. The labeled samples were hybridized to filters containing eight DNA samples from various sources and accurate results were obtained. Using peroxidase-conjugated anti-biotin antibody and enhanced isoluminol detection, about 10^4 bacterial cells could be detected. This format is not rapid considering the labeling, hybridization and development times, but it is an interesting approach to the simultaneous screening of multiple pathogens.

References

1. Allen, J.M., Sasek, C.A., Martin, J.B. and Heinrich, G. (1987): Use of complementary ^{125}I-Labeled RNA for single cell Resolution by *in situ* hybridization 5, 774-777.
2. Alwine, J.C., Kemp, D.J. and Stark, G.R. (1977): Method for detection of specific RNAs in agarose gels by transfer to diazobenzlyoxymethyl paper hybridization with DNA probes, Proc. Natl. Acad. Sci. USA 74, 5350-5354.
3. Bailey, J.M. and Davidson, N. (1976): Methylmercury as a reversible denaturing agent for agarose gel electrophoresis, Anal. Biochem. 70, 75-85.
4. Brandsma, J. and Miller, G. (1980): Nucleic acid spot hybridization: Rapid quantitative screening of lymphoid cell lines for Epstein-Barr viral DNA, Proc. Natl. Acad. Sci. USA 77, 6851-6855.
5. Bresser, J. and Gillespie, D. (1983): Quantitative binding of covalently closed circular DNA to nitrocellulose in NaI, Anal. Biochem. 129, 357-364.
6. Britten R.J., Graham, D.E., and Neufeld, B.R. (1974): Analysis of repeating DNA sequences by reassociation, Methods in Enzymology 29, 363-418.
7. Bronstein, I. and McGrath, P. (1989): Chemiluminescence lights up, Nature 338, 599-600.
8. Cannon, G., Heinhorst, S., and Weissbach, A. (1985): Quantitative molecular hybridization on nylon membranes, Anal Biochem 149, 229-237.
9. Cardullo, R.A., Agrawal, S., Flores, C., Zamecnik, P.C. and Wolf, D.E. (1988): Detection of nucleic acid hybridization by nonradiative fluorescence resonance energy transfer, Proc. Natl. Acad. Sci. USA 85, 8790-8794.
10. Cunningham, M. and Mandy, C. (1987): Labeling nucleic acids for hybridization, Nature 236, 723-724.

11. Dahlen, P., Syvanen, A.C., Hurskainen, P., Kwiatkowski, M., Sund, C., Ylikoski, J., Soderlund, H. and Lovgren, T. (1987): Sensitive detection of genes by sandwich hybridization and time-resolved fluorometry, Molecular and Cellular Probes **1**, 159-168.

12. Dattagupta, N., Rae, P.M.M., Huguenel, E.D., Carlson, E., Lyga, A., Shapiro, J.A. and Albarella, J.P. (1989): Rapid identification of microorganisms by nucleic acid hybridization after labeling the test sample, Anal. Biochem. **177**, 85-89.

13. Decker, S., Logan, K., Aswell, J. and Lawrie, J. (1989): Hybridization assay for quantitative detection of viral nucleic acids: application to human immunodeficiency virus-1 and cytomegalovirus, American Society for Microbiology annual meeting abstract #C46.

14. Denhardt, D.T. (1966): A membrane filter technique for the detection of complementary DNA, Biochem. Biophys. Res. Commun. **23**, 641-646.

15. Dunn, A.R. and Hassell, J.A. (1977): A novel method to map transcripts: Evidence for homology between an adenovirus mRNA and discrete multiple regions of the viral genome, Cell **12**, 23-36.

16. Flavell, R.A., Birfelder, E.J., Sanders, P.M., and Borst, P. (1974): DNA-DNA hybridization on nitrocellulose filters. 1. General considerations and non-ideal kinetics, Eur J Biochem **47**, 535-543.

17. Gall, J. and Pardue, M.L. (1969): Formation and detection of RNA-DNA hybrid molecules in cytological preparations, Proc. Natl. Acad. Sci. USA **63**, 378-383.

18. Gowans, E., Jilbert, A. and Burrell, C. (1989): Detection of specific DNA and RNA sequences in tissues and cells by *in situ* hybridization, in *Nucleic Acid Probes*, (R. Symons, ed.), CRC Press, Boca Raton, FL.

19. Gatti, R., Concannon, P. and Salser, W. (1984): Multiple use of Southern blots, Biotechniques May/June, 148-155.

20. Gebeyehu, G., Rao, P. SooChan, P. Simms, D. and Klevan, L. (1987): Novel biotinylated nucleotide-analogs for labeling and colorimetric detection of DNA, Nucleic Acids Res. **15**, 4513-4534.

21. Gendelman, H., Moench, T., Narayan, O., Griffin, D. and Clements, J. (1985): A double labeling technique for performing immunochemistry and *in situ* hybridization in virus infected cell cultures and tissues, J. Virol. Methods **11**, 93-103.

22. Granato, P.A. and Franz, M.R. (1989): Evaluation of a prototype DNA probe test for the noncultural diagnosis of gonorrhea, J. Clin. Microbiol. **27**, 632-635.

23. Gross, D.S., Huang, S.Y. and Garrad, W.T. (1985): Chromatin structure of the potential Z-forming sequence (dT-dG)n-(dC-dA)n: Evidence for an alternating-B conformation, J. Mol. Biol. **183**, 251-265.

24. Grunstein, M. and Hogness, D.S. (1975): Colony Hybridization: A method for the isolation of cloned DNAs that contain a specific gene, Proc. Nat. Acad. Sci. USA **72**, 3961-3965.

25. Hanahan, D. and Meselson, M. (1980): Plasmid screening at high colony density, Gene **10**, 63-67.

26. Heller, M.J. and Morrison, L.E. (1985): Chemiluminescent and fluorescent probes for DNA hybridization systems, in *Rapid Detection and Identification of Infectious Agents*, pp. 245-256, Academic Press, San Diego, CA.

27. Johnson, D., Gautsch, J., Sportsman, R.and Elder, J. (1984): Improved technique: Utilizing nonfat dry milk for analysis of proteins and nucleic acids transferred to nitrocellulose, Gene Anal. Techn. **1**, 3-8.

28. Kafatos, F.C., Jones, C.W., and Efstratiadis, A. (1979): Determination of nucleic acid sequence homologies and relative concentrations by a dot hybridization procedure, Nucleic Acids Res **7**, 1541-1552.

29. Keller, G.H., Cumming, C.U., Huang, D.P., Manak, M.M. and Ting, R. (1988) A chemical method for introducing haptens onto DNA probes, Anal. Biochem. **170**, 441-450.

30. Keller, G.H., Huang, D.P. and Manak, M.M. (1989): A sensitive nonisotopic hybridization assay for HIV-1 DNA, Anal. Biochem. **177**, 27-32.

31. Leary, J.J., Brigati, D.J. and Ward, D.C. (1983): Colorimetric method for visualizing biotin-labeled DNA probes hybridized to DNA or RNA immobilized on nitrocellulose: Bio-blots, Proc. Natl. Acad. Sci. USA **80**, 4045-4049.

32. Langdale, J.A. and Malcolm, A.D.B. (1985): A rapid method of gene detection using DNA bound to Sephacryl, Gene **36**, 201-210.

33. Lehrach, H., Diamond, D., Wozney, J. and Boedtker, H. (1977): RNA molecular weight determinations be gel electrophoresis under denaturing conditions: a critical reexamination, Biochemistry **16**, 4743-4751.

34. Maas, R. (1983): An Improved Colony Hybridization Method with Significantly Increased Sensitivity for Detection of Single Genes, Plasmid **10**, 296-298.

35. Maniatis, T., Fritsch, E. and Sambrook, J. (1982): in *Molecular Cloning: A Laboratory Manual*, Cold Spring Harbor Laboratory, Cold Spring Harbor, New York

36. Matthews,J.A., Batki, A., Hynds, C. and Kricka, L.J. (1985): Enhanced chemiluminescent method for the detection of DNA dot hybridization assays, Anal. Biochem. **151**, 205-209.

37. Meinkoth, J. and Wahl, G. (1984): Hybridization of nucleic acids immobilized on solid supports, Anal Biochem **138**, 267-284.

38. Miller, C.A., Patterson, W.L., Johnson, P.K., Swartzell, C.T., Wogoman, Albarella, J.P. and Carrico, R.J. (1988): Detection of bacteria by hybridization of rRNA with DNA-latex and immunodetection of hybrids, J. Clin. Microbiol. **26**, 1271-1276.

39. Morrison, L.E. (1988): Time-resolved detection of energy transfer: theory and application to immunoassays, Anal. Biochem. **174**, 101-120.

40. Nelson, N.C., Hammond, P.W., Wiese, W.A and Arnold, L.J., (1988): Novel assay formats employing acridinium ester-labeled DNA probes, in abstracts of the Third San Diego Conference, "Practical Aspects of Molecular Probes."

41. Polsky-Cynkin, R., Parsons, G.H., Allerdt, L., Landes, G., Davis, G. and Rashtchian, A. (1985): Use of DNA immobilized on plastic and agarose supports to detect DNA by sandwich hybridization, Clin. Chem. **31**, 1438-1443.

42. Ranki, M., Palva, A., Virtanen, M., Laaksonen, M. and Soderlund, H. (1983): Sandwich hybridization as a convenient method for the detection of nucleic acids in crude samples, Gene **21**, 77-85.

43. Ranki, M. and Soderlund, H.E. (1984): Detection of microbial nucleic acids by a one-step sandwich hybridization test, U.S. patent #4,486,539.

44. Reed, K.C. and Mann, D.A. (1985) Rapid transfer of DNA from agarose gels to nylon membranes, Nucleic Acids Res. **13**, 7207-7221.
45. Rogers, A. (1979): *Techniques for Autoradiography*, Elsevier, North Holland, Amsterdam.
46. Sanchez-Pescador, R., Stempien, M.S. and Urdea, M.S. (1988): Rapid chemiluminescent nucleic acid assays for the detection of TEM-1 beta-lactamase-mediated penicillin resistance in Neisseria gonorrhoeae and other bacteria, J. Clin. Microbiol. **26**, 1934-1938.
47. Southern, E.M. (1975): Detection of specific sequences among DNA fragments separated by gel electrophoresis, J. Mol. Biol. **98**, 503-517.
48. Syvanen, A.C., Laaksonen, M. and Soderlund, H. (1986): Fast Quantification of Nucleic Acid Hybrids by Affinity-Based Hybrid Collection, Nucleic Acids Res. **14**, 5037-5048.
49. Thomas, P. (1980): Hybridization of denatured RNA and small DNA fragments transferred to nitrocellulose, Proc. Natl. Acad. Sci. U.S.A. **77**, 5201-5205.
50. Urdea, M.S., Running, J.A., Horn, T., Clyne, J., Ku, L. and Warner, B.D. (1987): A novel method for the rapid detection of specific nucleotide sequences in crude biological samples without blotting or radioactivity: application to the analysis of hepatitis B virus in human serum, Gene **61**, 253-264.
51. Urdea, M.S. (1988): Application of a rapid non-radioactive nucleic acid analysis system to the detection of sexually transmitted disease organisms and their associated antimicrobial resistances, in abstracts of the Third San Diego Conference, "Practical Aspects of Molecular Probes."
52. Vary, C.P.H. (1987): A homogeneous nucleic acid hybridization assay based on strand displacement, Nucleic Acids Res. **15**, 6883-6897
53. Viscidi, R.P., O'Meara, C., Farzadegan, H. and Yolken, R. (1989): Monoclonal antibody solution hybridization assay for detection of human immunodeficiency virus nucleic acids, J. Clin. Microbiol. **27**, 120-125.
54. Weeks, I., Sturgess, M., Brown, R.C. and Woodhead, J.S. (1986): Immunoassays using acridinium esters, Methods in Enzymology **133**, 366-390.
55. Weeks, I., Behesti, I., McCapra, F., Campbell, A.K. and Woodhead, J.S. (1983): Acridinium esters as high specific activity labels in immunoassay, Clin. Chem. **29**, 1474-1479.
56. White, B.A. and Bancroft, F.C. (1982): Cytoplasmic dot hybridization, J. Biol. Chem. **257**, 8569-8572.
57. Wilkinson, H.W., Sampson, J.S. and Plikaytis, B.B. (1986): Evaluation of a commercial gene probe for identification of *Legionella* cultures, J. Clin. Microbiol. **23**, 217-220.
58. Yehle, C.O., Patterson, W.L., Boguslawski, S.J., Albarella, J.P., Yip, K.F. and Carrico, R.J. (1987): A solution hybridization assay for ribosomal RNA from bacteria using biotinylated DNA probes and enzyme-labeled antibody to DNA:RNA, Molecular and Cellular Probes **1**, 177-193.

Section 6:
Probe and Target
Amplification Systems

Introduction

The future of nucleic acid hybridization as a research tool and as a commercial process lies in the ability to amplify target or probe. Amplification systems can increase the amount of probe or target by factors of 10^6 or more, allowing the detection of 1-10 molecules in a sample using current non-radioactive detection systems. Since there is currently no system for amplifying protein probes or targets to this degree, amplified hybridization assays are by far the most sensitive means of direct pathogen detection and even the most sensitive means of detecting biological molecules. These assays will find increasing commercial use in areas such as confirmation of retroviral infection, monitoring of anti-viral and anti-bacterial drug studies and treatment, vaccine testing and oncogene expression. The most outstanding and powerful means of amplifying hybridization assay signals are discussed in this section.

Target Amplification

POLYMERASE CHAIN REACTION

Currently, the most effective means of target amplification is the polymerase chain reaction (PCR) developed by Kary Mullis and his colleagues at Cetus (Mullis, 1987; Mullis *et al.*, 1987; Mullis and Faloona, 1987). Figure 6.1 illustrates how the PCR works. A pair of specific oligomer primers is used to initiate DNA synthesis in combination with a heat-stable Taq I DNA polymerase. Following this first round of 'primer extension' at 70°C, the reaction is heated to about 93°C to denature the product from its template. The temperature is then cooled to 37-55°C to permit annealing of the primer molecules to the original template DNA as well as the newly synthesized DNA fragments. Primer extension is then resumed at 70°C. By repeating these cycles of denaturation, annealing and extension, the original target DNA can be amplified exponentially

FIGURE 6.1 Schematic Diagram of Two Cycles of the Polymerase Chain Reaction (PCR). In cycle 1, a pair of primers is used with DNA polymerase to copy each strand of a specific DNA region for a total of four copies. After denaturation and reannealing of the primers, a second round of synthesis results in eight copies of the region. Thirty cycles result in about a 1×10^7-fold amplification of the target region.

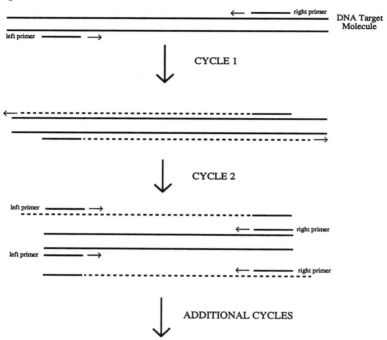

according to the formula: 2^n, where n is the number of cycles. In theory, 25 PCR cycles would result in a 3.4×10^7-fold amplification. However, since the efficiency of each cycle is less than 100%, the actual amplification after 25 cycles is about 1-3×10^6-fold. The size of the amplified region is generally 100-400 base pairs, although stretches of up to 2 kb can be efficiently amplified (Saiki *et al.*, 1988).

Messenger RNA can also be specifically amplified with some additional steps (Doherty *et al.*, 1989). Total nucleic acid may be isolated in crude form (cell lysate) or it can be purified by phenol-chloroform extraction. Residual DNA may be digested with RNase-free DNase so that it does not contribute to the final PCR product. A cDNA copy of the mRNA is synthesized using the PCR primers and reverse transcriptase; the one primer complementary to the mRNA serves to initiate cDNA synthesis. The use of the PCR primers is preferred over the standard oligo(dT) priming of cDNA synthesis. First, with PCR primers, more cDNA material will be synthesized since poly(A)⁻ as well as poly(A)+ RNA will be copied. Second, if the 3' poly(A) region is far from the stretch to be amplified, then the cDNA transcripts synthesized using an oilgo(dT) primer may not efficiently represent that stretch of RNA. On the other hand, the primer-initiated cDNA will span exactly the same region that will be amplified during the PCR. The single-stranded cDNA product can then be amplified by the PCR after heat inactivation of the reverse transcriptase and adjustment of the reaction to PCR conditions.

Identifying short stretches of sequence suitable for priming DNA synthesis is the initial step in performing the PCR. The major considerations for primer selection are listed below.

Primer Selection Guidelines

1.   The recommended primer length is 20-26 bases.
2.   Base composition should be 40-60% G-C.
3.   Avoid interstrand complementary regions at the 3' ends of the primers.
4.   Avoid intra-strand complementary regions.
5.   If a coding region is being amplified, avoid ending primers at the third (degenerate) position of the codon.
6.   Reject primer sequences that have homology with unwanted sequences of more than 70%, or 8 or more bases in a row.

1) The constraints on primer length are sufficient length (complexity) to provide specific priming, but short enough to allow rapid annealing to the template. For detection of sequences that are not well conserved, longer is better because a single base change is less likely to affect annealing as primer length increases. 2) The specified G-C content helps to assure the formation of stable and specific hybrids during and extension. 3) Interstrand 3' complementary regions allow the formation of primer hybrids (primer dimers) which can be extended by the polymerase. This artifactual product can interfere with interpretation of the PCR results. 4) Intra-strand complementary regions must be avoided to prevent formation of secondary structure which may interfere with the annealing of the primer to its template. 5) Since the third base position of a codon often can vary without affecting the specified amino acid, primers ending at this position are likely to have a primer:template mismatch at their 3' end. Since polymerase extension occurs from the 3' end of the primer, such mismatches will inhibit the polymerase reaction. 6) This 70%/8 rule must be followed to assure amplification of only the desired region. Failure to follow these rules will greatly reduce your chances of success, but conversely, they do not guarantee success. Each primer pair must be tested on various known templates before analysis of unknowns.

If priming is specific, then upon gel electrophoresis of the reaction products, a fragment will be observed corresponding in length to the distance between the ends of the primers. The identity can be further confirmed by Southern blotting and hybridization with a specific probe. Of course, no product should be detected when the template contains non-specific DNAs or no DNA. These controls not only test for primer specificity, but also for contamination which can be a serious problem with the PCR. Additional specificity can be obtained at the amplification level by amplifying more than one region per sample and by using more sophisticated strategies such as 'nested primers' (Mullis and Faloona, 1987). After amplifying a region of DNA with one set of primers, amplification is continued with a different pair of primers that are closer together and so are 'nested' within the original region. The idea is that any non-specific amplification products directed by the first primer set are very unlikely to serve as a template for the second primer set. Specificity can also be controlled at the detection level, as discussed below.

A number of detection formats have been used successfully with the PCR. One method, oligomer restriction (Saiki et al., 1985a; Saiki et al., 1985b), was originally developed to detect point mutations, but it is not the best choice for general PCR analysis. This technique is based on the design of short (20-40 nt) oligomer probes that generate a restriction site upon hybridization. However, this places additional limits on the choice of primer sequences and provides a detection system that is almost too specific. Point mutations in the probe region of the target sequence could affect hybrid stability and restriction cutting, resulting in false negatives. On the other hand, using a pair of specific primers and the above primer selection guidelines, target DNA present in more than 10^4 copies can be detected simply by gel electrophoresis and ethidium bromide staining (Chehab et al., 1987). The most straightforward approach for detection is traditional Southern blotting, using radioactive or non-radioactive probes, provided that the transfer and hybridization conditions are optimized for short DNA fragments. Detection by slot blotting has been reported (Higuchi et al., 1988), but this technique is probably not specific enough for all applications. Sandwich hybridization is another alternative which is both simple and specific (Ranki et al., 1983). In sandwich hybridization, sample immobilization is not required and it is potentially more specific than direct hybridization because two hybridization events must occur in order to generate a signal. Sandwich hybridization is an ideal system for incorporating non-radioactive probes and non-filter based hybridization formats (Keller et al., 1989). The principle of gel retardation has also been used to detect PCR products (Greenberg et al., 1989). Radiolabeled oligomer probes are hybridized in solution to aliquots of the PCR product, then electrophoresed on native agarose gels. The gels are autoradiographed to visualize the bands. Free probe runs much faster than probe:PCR product hybrids. A labeled primer (instead of a probe) was employed by Lee et al. (1989) to eliminate the hybridization step. Aliquots of the PCR reaction are loaded directly onto gels, separated and autoradiographed. Bands corresponding to the free primer, the specific PCR product and sometimes nonspecific PCR products can be observed with this technique.

The greatest, and perhaps only, drawback to PCR is the tendency of PCR products to contaminate negative samples, buffers, microliter pipettes and everything else in the laboratory, generating false positive results (Kwok and Higuchi, 1989). Our approach has been to perform sample preparation and amplification in a dedicated laboratory. After amplification, the reaction products are only opened and handled in a separate laboratory, to avoid spreading amplified products around the room. Plasmid DNA in quantities greater than a few picograms is also not allowed in the dedicated PCR laboratory. All reagents are aliquoted, separate pipettemen are used for each operation and they are disassembled and cleaned frequently. Three or four negative controls are run with each PCR reaction. If any are positive after analysis, the entire experiment is discarded and the contamination problem solved before continuing. These precautions are especially important in the detection of human retroviruses, where positive samples may contain only 5-10 target molecules in 10^6 cells.

Internal controls are also an important part of any PCR experiment. The most commonly used controls for human DNA are ß-globin and HLA DQa alleles. The control region may be amplified in the same reaction as the experimental region, but one must be certain that the control primers do not cause inhibition of the reaction. Such controls serve to confirm consistent DNA recovery from test samples and confirm the lack of any PCR inhibitors in the DNA preparations. Negative results cannot be relied upon unless the internal control is positive. Thermal cycling can be accomplished using three water or oil baths - either manually or with a robot arm (Zymark). There are also many automated thermal cyclers on the market (Perkin Elmer Cetus, Techne, Ericomp); most use drilled metal blocks to hold the reaction tubes, but at least one is an oven format (Biotherm) which would permit the use of reaction containers other than microfuge tubes.

PROCEDURE 6.1

SAMPLE PREPARATION METHOD FOR THE PCR

Reagents:
a)   Phenol:chloroform:isoamyl alcohol (25:24:1) saturated with 10 mM Tris, pH 8.0. (Appendix A)
b)   4 M sodium acetate (Appendix A)
c)   10 mM Tris, pH 8.0, containing 1.0% SDS
d)   Proteinase K (25 mg/ml)
e)   Isopropanol

Procedure:
1. DNA may be extracted from cultured cells or patient peripheral blood lymphocytes (PBLs) as follows. Suspend about 5×10^6 cells in 500 µl of 10 mM Tris, pH 8.0, containing 1.0% SDS. Heat at 95°C for 5 minutes.
2. Let sample cool and add 10 µl of Proteinase K (25 mg/ml) and incubate for one hour at 55°C or overnight at 37°C.
3. Extract the crude DNA twice for 20 minutes at room temperature with an equal volume of phenol:chloroform:isoamyl alcohol.
4. Precipitate the DNA by adding 1/5 volume of 4 M sodium acetate, 1 volume of isopropanol and incubate at -20°C from 1 hour to overnight. After centrifugation, dry and dissolve the pellet in 50 µl of water. Measure the UV absorbance of a 10 µl aliquot to determine the concentration.

PROCEDURE 6.2

RAPID PCR SAMPLE PREPARATION FROM WHOLE BLOOD
(modification of Buffone and Darlington, 1985)

Reagents:
a) Lysis Buffer
   0.32 M sucrose
   10 mM Tris-HCl, pH 7.6
   5 mM $MgCl_2$
   1% Triton X-100
b) 2 M KCl
c) Proteinase K
   25 mg/ml in water
d) 10 mM Tris, pH 8.0, containing 1% SDS

Procedure:
1. Mix 0.75 ml of blood with 0.75 ml of lysis buffer in a 1.5 ml microfuge tube.
2. Centrifuge at full speed for 30 seconds.
3. Remove supernatant with a micropipette and resuspend the pellet in 1.5 ml of lysis buffer by vortexing.
4. Repeat steps 2 and 3 twice.
5. The pink pellet is dissolved in 117 µl of 10 mM Tris, pH 8.0 containing 1% SDS. Heat at 70°C for 5 minutes. Cool to 55°C and add 3 µl of Proteinase K solution. Incubate at 55°C for 1 hour.
6. Heat the tube in a boiling water bath for 5-10 minutes.
7. Add 30 µl of 2 M KCl and incubate on ice for 5 minutes.

8. Centrifuge at full speed in a microfuge for 5 minutes. Aliquot the supernatant and store at -70°C until amplification. (Ten µl of sample is equivalent to 50 µl blood.)

Additional rapid sample preparation protocols have been developed and are described in Kogan *et al.* (1987) and Erlich (1989).

PROCEDURE 6.3

ENZYME AMPLIFICATION OF TARGET DNA USING THE PCR

Please note that these are typical conditions and are optimized for Taq DNA polymerase from specific sources. The reader must optimize $MgCl_2$ and enzyme concentrations for each *primer set* and each *source of enzyme*. The optimum annealing temperature between 37° and 55°C should also be determined.

Reagents:
a) 2x PCR buffer

Component	2x conc	1x conc
Tris, pH 8.8	140 mM	70 mM
$MgCl_2$	4-8 mM	2-4 mM
$(NH_4)_2SO_4$	40 mM	20 mM
BSA	300 µg/ml	150 µg/ml (BRL, nuclease-free)
DTT	16 mM	8 mM

b) 0.5 mM dNTPs
c) *Thermus Aquaticus* DNA polymerase (U.S. Biochemical, New England Biolabs)
d) Oligonucleotide primers

Procedure:
1. Two micrograms of DNA in about 10 µl of water (Procedure 6.1) or 10 µl of DNA from Procedure 6.2 are used in each PCR reaction.
2. Add 50 µl of 2x PCR buffer, followed by 10 µl of DMSO and adding each dNTP to 0.5 mM and each primer to 6.6 µg/ml. This gives a final primer concentration of 1 µM or 100 pmoles per 100 µl reaction. The actual working range is 10-100 pmoles and the minimum amount that gives a strong, specific signal should be determined for each target.
3. Denature the reaction at 98°C for 7 minutes, cool to room temperature and add 5-7 units of Taq DNA polymerase. The final reaction volume is 100 µl and it is overlaid with 50-100 µl of mineral oil to prevent evaporation.
4. The reaction is centrifuged for 10 seconds and elongation started at 70°C for 3 minutes. The reaction is taken through 25-30 cycles of alternating

temperature, with each cycle consisting of: 92°C for 1 minutes, 37°C for 1 minutes and 70°C for 3 minutes. The final 70°C incubation is for 10 minutes.

5. Amplified samples are stored at -20°C until analysis.

HYBRIDIZATION ANALYSIS OF PRODUCTS

Reagents:
a) Nusieve GTG and Seakem HGT agarose (FMC Bioproducts)
b) Nylon membrane (Zetaprobe, Bio-Rad)
c) 1 M Tris, pH 8.0

Procedure:
1. For Southern analysis, a 20 µl aliquot of the amplification reaction is separated on a 2.5% agarose gel consisting of 2% Nusieve GTG and 0.5% Seakem HGT (FMC Bioproducts). This combination results in a fairly rigid gel and gives good separation of small (100-1,000 bp) fragments. Be careful not to cross-contaminate sample wells. Gels should be loaded with no running buffer on top, then submerged after samples have run into the gel.
2. Transfer the DNA to a nylon membrane (Zetaprobe, Bio-Rad) according to Procedure 5.7, but with the following modifications. After transfer, bake the membrane in a vacuum oven at 80°C for 20 minutes. Neutralize the filter by dipping it into 1 M Tris, pH 8.0, and blot to remove excess buffer. *Be sure to test specific lot samples of Zetaprobe™ membrane before purchasing a large quantity. Some lots produce high non-specific backgrounds.*
3. The transfer is hybridized with a ^{32}P-labeled probe. Autoradiography (procedure 5.13) is for 4-16 hours at -70°C.

The degree of amplification to be expected from a PCR reaction is presented in Table 6.1.

PCR cycles	Theoretical (2^n)	Actual*
20	1×10^6	8×10^5
25	3×10^7	3×10^6
30	1×10^9	1×10^8

(*Using 10 pg of target DNA and the protocol described above)

TABLE 6.1 Approximate degree of amplification obtained with specific cycles of the PCR.

The reaction efficiency decreases with increasing cycles because 1) dNTPs and primers are rapidly incorporated into product, lowering their concentration; 2) as product increases, the ratio of enzyme to template decreases, and 3) the enzyme gradually loses activity because of the high denaturation temperature (93°C) and the temperature cycling. Although many publications cite PCR experiments where 50 or more temperature cycles are performed, in our experience very little additional amplification is observed beyond 30 cycles.

It is possible to use more than one primer set per PCR reaction. In fact, Chamberlain *et al.* (1988) simultaneously and successfully amplified nine regions in human genomic DNA. Amplifying more than one region in very rare targets, such as retroviral DNA in patient peripheral blood lymphocytes, is more difficult since the PCR is less efficient at amplifying 10-500 molecules of viral DNA than it is at amplifying 10^6 molecules of genomic DNA. Also, the reaction conditions must be chosen for efficient performance of the primer mixture, which means that any given target region may not be amplified as efficiently as it would be in an optimized reaction with one primer pair.

Try the above conditions initially then, with experience, you may want to try shorter cycle times, multiple primers, labeled primers, and many of the other PCR variations that are being reported. One good source of updated information is the free publication 'Amplifications' published by Perkin Elmer Cetus.

PCR has also been used to prepare ^{32}P-labeled DNA probes (Schowalter and Sommer, 1989) by including a [^{32}P]dNTP during amplification. The most powerful result of this PCR variation is the preparation of probes directly from genomic DNA without cloning or plasmid preps. Even minute amounts of template can provide an unlimited source of probe by performing non-radioactive PCR, aliquoting the product and using the aliquots as template for labeling reactions. When aliquots run low, one aliquot is used to prepare more unlabeled template and so on. This is also an efficient method of synthesizing and labeling short probes of 100-500 bp. Labeled RNA probes can also be generated by including the T7 RNA polymerase promoter sequence in one of the primers. After PCR amplification of the DNA template, T7 RNA polymerase and a [^{32}P]NTP are added to produce radioactive RNA transcripts.

TRANSCRIPTION-BASED AMPLIFICATION SYSTEM

A second method of target amplification, called transcription-based amplification system (TAS), has been described by Kwoh *et al.* (1989). Their approach uses transcription to amplify an RNA target rather than using DNA replication to amplify a DNA target. As with the PCR, oligonucleotide primers define the endpoints of the amplified region and enzymes and temperature cycles are used to sequentially amplify the original target. The TAS process is illustrated in Figure 6.2. The first cycle of TAS proceeds as follows.

FIGURE 6.2 Schematic Diagram of a Transcription-Based Amplification System (TAS)._TAS consists of repeating cycles in which RNA is converted to double-stranded cDNA, then each double-stranded cDNA serves as a template for the synthesis of multiple copies of RNA. Four such cycles result in a 2-5x10^6-fold amplification of the target RNA sequence.

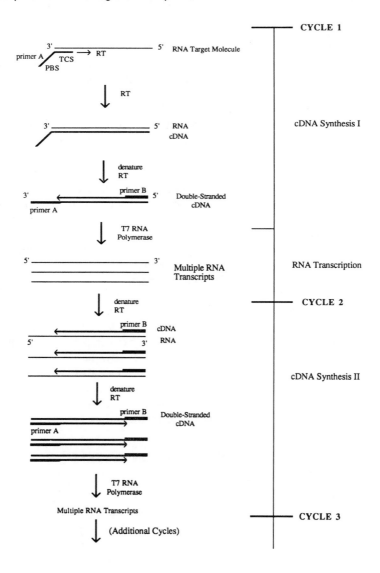

Cycle 1: (step 1) A cDNA copy of the RNA target is synthesized using reverse transcriptase and primer A. Primer A contains a target complementary sequence (TCS) and a polymerase binding site (PBS). (step 2) After denaturation and addition of more reverse transcriptase, a second cDNA strand is synthesized using primer B to yield double-stranded cDNA (step 3). In step 4, this double-stranded cDNA serves as a template for T7 RNA polymerase, resulting in 10-100 RNA transcripts per double-stranded cDNA, which is the actual amplification step.

Cycle 2: The new RNA transcripts, with additional reverse transcriptase, serve as templates to synthesize more double-stranded cDNA (steps 5 and 6) which with additional RNA polymerase, is used in turn to synthesize more RNA transcripts. After four cycles the original RNA target will be amplified $2-5 \times 10^6$-fold, with an average amplification of 38 to 47-fold per cycle. The total time required is about four hours.

Although TAS is an interesting process and it can amplify targets to about the same degree as the PCR, it seems to have no advantages over the PCR. Indeed, it is not even as simple and useful as the PCR. The TAS cycles are complex and require repeated additions of two different enzymes, because some or all of the enzyme activity is destroyed during the denaturation step. PCR can amplify RNA and DNA targets while TAS cannot be used for DNA amplification without incorporating one or two PCR steps at the beginning of the amplification.

Probe Amplification

In contrast to the PCR and TAS amplification systems, which amplify target nucleic acid, the next two approaches amplify the probe nucleic acid or the probe signal after hybridization.

Q-BETA REPLICASE SYSTEM

The RNA-dependent RNA polymerase from bacteriophage Qß has the ability to synthesize large amounts of product strand from a small amount of template strand (million to billion-fold increases). The reaction mechanism is exponential because each product strand can serve as a template strand following synthesis. RNA synthesis continues at an exponential rate until the number of RNA molecules equals the number of polymerase molecules. In order to take advantage of this property, RNA probes have been produced which can be replicated and thus amplified by Qß RNA polymerase (Lizardi *et al.*, 1988).

To synthesize these probes, a recombinant plasmid was constructed which carries the MDV-1 cDNA sequence (MDV-1 is a 'midivariant' of phage

FIGURE 6.3 Structure of the Plasmid used to Produce RNA Probes that are Replicatable with Qß Polymerase. RNA polymerase is used to produce RNA transcripts from cloned MDV-1 DNA, into which a probe sequence has been inserted at the polylinker site. The transcripts are hybridized to their complementary target and unhybridized probe is removed by washing. The bound probe is eluted, amplified with Qß replicase and detected, perhaps in a subsequent hybridization step. Billion-fold amplification in one 30-minute step is theoretically possible.

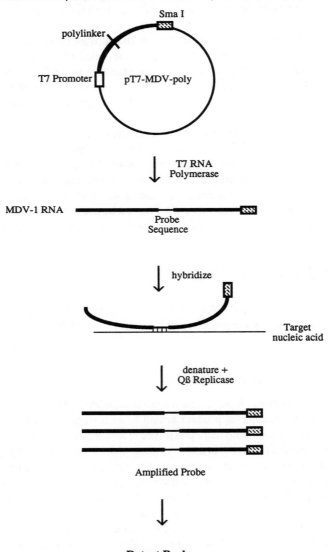

Qß RNA, 223 nt in length) attached to a T7 RNA polymerase promoter (Figure 6.3). The transcript, MDV-1 RNA, is a natural template for Qß replicase. A polylinker region in the middle of the cDNA was used to insert short probe sequences (20-30 bp). The presence of the extra nucleotides from the polylinker and probe sequences have no effect on the RNA replication rate.

The use of replicatable RNA probes in hybridization assays is expected to have the following unique advantages. 1) Speed and sensitivity: amplification of up to a billion-fold in one step in 30 minutes, compared with 30 steps and 3 hours for 10 million-fold with PCR. 2) Target quantitation: the amount of hybridized probe RNA is directly proportional to the final amount of amplified RNA, when incubation times are long enough for all amplification reactions to finish exponential synthesis and this relationship is valid over six orders of magnitude. For PCR, there is no simple relationship between starting and ending copy number.

The greatest drawback of these probes is the amplification of non-specifically as well as specifically hybridized probe, resulting in high backgrounds and low signal-to noise ratios. Thus, even though billion-fold amplification of probes can be achieved, the detection limit with replicatable RNA probes is presently 10^4 molecules in hybridization assays, because of background. Two solutions to this problem are being investigated: molecular switches and target-dependent replication.

RNA probes were constructed to contain a region that is partially double-stranded in the unhybridized probe, but is single-stranded in the target bound probe. The partially double-stranded region is disrupted in the hybrid because the hybrid double-stranded region is longer, thus the hybrid conformation is more stable than the native one. The region is termed a 'molecular switch' because the switch region is sensitive to ribonuclease III cleavage before hybridization and insensitive after hybridization. Unhybridized probe can be specifically degraded after hybridization and prior to detection to reduce non-specific background signals.

The target-dependent replication scheme is more complex and also requires two DNA probes (Figure 6.4). DNA probe 1 contains a T7 RNA polymerase promoter sequence, the left half of the MDV-1 DNA sequence and is complementary to the left half of a target sequence. After extension with DNA polymerase, the complex is denatured and a second DNA probe, containing the right half of MDV-1 and sequences complementary to the right half of the target sequence is hybridized. After extension with DNA polymerase, a double-stranded DNA results which contains a functional T7 promoter and the target sequence embedded in MDV-1 RNA. Replicatable copies are synthesized using T7 RNA polymerase and these copies are in turn amplified using Qß replicase.

It is clear from the information published to date that replicatable RNA probes will play an important role in the detection of rare nucleic acid targets.

These probes combine the amplification power of the PCR with speed and theoretical simplicity. If the background problems can be solved, these RNA probes will be found in a significant number of commercial diagnostic tests.

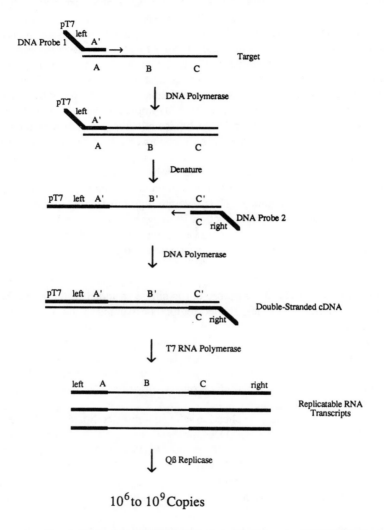

FIGURE 6.4 Target -Dependent Probe Replication Scheme. A pair of DNA primers are used to synthesize a double-stranded cDNA copy of the target region surrounded by MDV-1 sequences and a T7 RNA polymerase promoter. The promoter allows the synthesis of RNA copies of the cDNA which can then be amplified by Qβ replicase. No probe is synthesized in the absence of target, so the background after amplification should be very low.

PROBE NETWORKS

A number of research publications have described the formation of probe networks as a means of amplifying probe signals (Fahrlander, 1988), but the system described by Urdea *et al.* (1987) and Sanchez-Pescador *et al.* (1988) is the most successful example. As described in Section 5, this method includes a solution phase sandwich hybridization assay which uses multiple oligonucleotide probes as the first amplification step and polymerized secondary probes (amplification multimer) as the next amplification step (Figure 6.5). The tertiary probes are each conjugated to an enzyme for detection and bind to the arms of the amplification multimer. These multimer structures with their bound tertiary probes serve as a sort of polymerized enzyme reagent, but actually perform far better. Because all of the binding reactions involve hybridization rather than protein-protein reactions, the signal-to-noise ratio is much higher than that obtained with multiple antibodies, for instance.

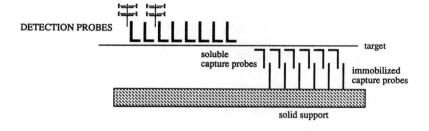

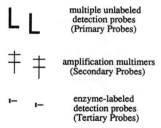

FIGURE 6.5 Probe Signal Amplification using Multiple Primary Probes and Amplification Multimers. A system of three probe types is used to achieve signal amplification. First, there are multiple primary probes, which bind to the target. Second, an amplification multimer binds to each primary probe and third, multiple enzyme-labeled probes bind to each amplification multimer. The degree of amplification, compared with using a single oligomer probe, is at least 100-fold.

The actual degree of amplification achieved with this system is about 100-fold, enough to extend the detection limit for an enzyme-labeled oligomer from 10 pg to 0.1 pg. The probe multimers were originally constructed by cross-linking monomers of amino-modified oligomers which contained multiple N^4-alkylamino deoxycytidine residues. Urdea and his colleagues have now developed techniques for synthesizing branched oligomers so these complex structures can be made reproducibly on a DNA synthesizer. This improvement may lead to assays which are yet another order of magnitude (10^3 molecules) more sensitive.

References

1. Buffone, G.J. and Darlington, G.J. (1985): Isolation of DNA from biological specimens without extraction with phenol, Clin. Chem. **31**, 164-165.
2. Chamberlain, J., Gibbs, R.A., Ranier, J.E., Nguyen, P.N. and Caskey, C.T. (1988): Deletion screening of Duchenne muscular dystrophy locus via multiplex DNA amplification, Nucleic Acids Res. **16**, 141-156.
3. Chehab, F.F., Doherty, M., Cai, S., Kan, Y.W., Cooper, S. and Rubin, E.M. (1987): Detection of sickle cell anemia and thalassaemias, Nature **329**, 293-294.
4. Doherty, P.J., Huesca-Contreras, M., Dosch, H.M. and Pan, S. (1989): Rapid amplification of complementary DNA from small amounts of unfractionated RNA, Anal. Biochem. **177**, 7-10.
5. Erlich, H. (1989): PCR technology: Principles and applications for DNA amplification, Stockton Press, New York, N.Y.
6. Fahrlander, P.D. (1988): Amplifying DNA probe signals: a 'Christmas tree' approach, Biotechnology **6**, 1165-1168.
7. Greenberg, S.J., Ehrlich, G.D., Abbott, M.A., Hurwitz, B.J., Waldmann, T.A. and Poiesz, B.J. (1989): Detection of sequences homologous to human retroviral DNA in multiple sclerosis by gene amplification, Proc. Natl. Acad. Sci. USA, **86**, 2878-2882.
8. Higuchi, R., von Beroldingen, C.H., Sensabaugh, G.F. and Erlich, H.A. (1988): DNA typing from single hairs, Nature **332**, 543-546.
9. Keller, G.H., Huang, D.P. and Manak, M.M. (1989): A sensitive nonisotopic hybridization assay for HIV-1 DNA, Anal. Biochem. **177**, 27-32.
10. Kogan, S.C., Doherty, M. and Gitschier, J. (1987): An improved method for prenatal diagnosis of genetic diseases by analysis of amplified DNA sequences, N. Engl. J. Med. **317**, 985-990.
11. Kwoh, D.Y., Davis, G.R., Whitfield, K.M., Chappelle, H.L., DiMichelle, L.J. and Gingeras, T.R. (1989): Transcription-based amplification system and detection of amplified human immunodeficiency virus type I with a bead-based sandwich hybridization format, Proc. Natl. Acad. Sci. USA **86**, 1173-1177.
12. Kwok, S. and Higuchi, R. (1989): Avoiding false positives with PCR, Nature **339**, 237-238.

13. Lee, H., Swanson, P., Shorty, V.S., Zack, J.A., Rosenblatt, J.D. and Chen, I.S.Y. (1989): High rate of HTLV-II infection in seropositive IV drug abusers in New Orleans, Science **244**, 471-475.

14. Lizardi, P.M., Guerra, C.E., Lomeli, H., Tussie-Luna, I. and Kramer, F.R. (1988): Exponential amplification of recombinant RNA hybridization probes, Biotechnology **6**, 1197-1202.

15. Mullis, K.B. and Faloona, F.A. (1987): Specific synthesis of DNA *in vitro* via a polymerase catalyzed chain reaction, Methods in Enzymology **155**, 335-350.

16. Mullis, K.B., Erlich, H.A., Arnheim, N., Horn, G.T., Saiki, R.K. and Scharf, S.J. (1987): Process for amplifying, detecting and/or cloning nucleic acid sequences, U.S. Patent No. 4,683,195.

17. Mullis, K.B. (1987): Process for amplifying nucleic acid sequences, U.S. Patent No. 4,683,202.

18. Ranki, M., Palva, A., Virtanen, M., Laaksonen, M. and Soderlund, H. (1983): Sandwich hybridization as a convenient method for the detection of nucleic acids in crude samples, Gene **21**, 77-85.

19. Saiki, R.K., Gelfand, D.H., Stoffel, S., Scharf, S.J., Higuchi, R., Horn, G.T., Mullis, K.B. and Erlich, H.A. (1988): Primer-directed enzymatic amplification of DNA with a thermostable DNA polymerase, Science **239**, 487-494.

20. Saiki, R.K., Scharf, S., Faloona, F., Mullis, K.B., Horn, G.T., Erlich, H.A. and Arnheim, N. (1985a): Enzymatic amplification of beta-globin genomic sequences and restriction site analysis for diagnosis of sickle cell anemia, Science **230**, 1350-1354.

21. Saiki, R., Arnheim, N. and Erlich, H.A. (1985b): A novel method for the detection of polymorphic restriction sites by cleavage of oligonucleotide probes: application to sickle-cell anemia, Biotechnology **3**, 1008-1012.

22. Sanchez-Pescador, R., Stempien, M.S. and Urdea, M.S. (1988): Rapid chemiluminescent nucleic acid assays for the detection of TEM-1 beta-lactamase-mediated penicillin resistance in *Neisseria gonorrhoeae* and other bacteria, J. Clin. Microbiol **26**, 1934-1938.

23. Schowalter, D.B. and Sommer, S.S. (1989): The generation of radiolabeled DNA and RNA probes with polymerase chain reaction, Anal. Biochem. **177**, 90-94.

24. Urdea, M.S., Running, J.A., Horn, T., Clyne, J., Ku, L. and Warner, B.D. (1987): A novel method for the rapid detection of specific nucleotide sequences in crude biological samples without blotting or radioactivity: Application to the analysis of hepatitis B virus in human serum, Gene **61**, 253-264.

Appendix A:
Reagents

Buffers and Reagents

Always use the highest purity reagents available.

Ammonium Sulfate Solution, saturated

Add 225g of ammonium sulfate to 200 ml of water. Adjust the volume to 500 ml and dissolve by stirring and gentle heating (40-60°C) for about 2 hours. Cool to room temperature and add another 50 g of ammonium sulfate. Adjust the pH to 7.5 and store at room temperature.

Carrier DNA

Dissolve 1g of salmon sperm DNA (Sigma) in 100 ml of 0.4 M NaOH and stir overnight at room temp. Boil 45 min to shear, chill on ice and neutralize with glacial acetic acid. Centrifuge to remove debris, add 2 volumes of ethanol to the supernatant, chill and centrifuge. Wash the pellet with 70% and 100% ethanol and dissolve in 50 ml of TE (10 mM Tris, pH 8.0, 1 mM EDTA). Determine the A_{260} and dilute to 10 mg/ml (1 OD = 40 μg/ml of denatured DNA). Store at -20°C in 1 ml aliquots.

Carrier tRNA

Dissolve yeast tRNA (Sigma R0128) to 10 mg/ml in water. Store in aliquots at -20°C.

Denhardt's Solution (50x) 1x

Ficoll	5 g	.02%
Polyvinylpyrrolidone	5 g	.02%
BSA, Sigma fraction V	5 g	.02%
Water to 500 ml.		

Filter sterilize and store in aliquots at -20°C.

EDTA, 0.25 M, pH 8.0

Dissolve 52.02 g of EDTA (dihydrate, MW=416.20) in 400 ml of water and adjust pH to 8.0. Dilute to 500 ml and autoclave in 100 ml bottles and store at room temperature.

Ethanol (200 proof)
Aliquot at 100% and 70% and store at -20°C.

Glycerol
(Mallinckrodt) Aliquot and store at room temperature.

Magnesium Chloride, 1 M
Dissolve 47.60 g of $MgCl_2$ (MW=95.21, Sigma #M-8266) in 500 ml of water. Autoclave in 100 ml bottles and store at room temperature.

PBS, 10x 1x
NaH_2PO_4	4.20 g	35 mM
Na_2HPO_4	4.20 g	30 mM
NaCl	87.5 g	0.15 M

Dilute to 1 liter and adjust the pH to 7.0. Autoclave and store at room temperature.

Peroxidase-Streptavidin
Add 1 ml of 50% glycerol to a 0.5 mg vial of lyophilized conjugate (Kirkegaard & Perry #14-30-00) and vortex gently to dissolve. Aliquot 250 µl per tube and store at -20°C for 6 months.

Phenol, buffered
Redistilled phenol must be used for purification of DNA, since oxidation products of phenol can cause nicks in DNA. Phenol can be distilled in the laboratory, or obtained in an already redistilled form from commercial sources. The redistilled phenol should be melted at 65°C in a water bath and 8-hydroxyquinoline (an antioxidant) added to 1 mg/ml phenol. An equal volume of 50 mM Tris-HCl, pH 7.6, is added and the two phases are mixed well and allowed to separate at room temperature. The aqueous phase (top) is drawn off, leaving a small layer of buffer on top of the phenol. The phenol should be stored at 4°C (liquid phase) in a brown bottle for up to 2 months or frozen at -20°C (crystalized) for up to 1 year. Phenol:chloroform:isoamyl alcohol solution for extraction of DNA can be prepared by mixing 25 parts phenol, 24 parts chloroform and 1 part isoamyl alcohol and stored at 4°C for up to 2 months in a brown bottle.

Phenol:Chloroform:Isoamyl Alcohol (25:24:1)
        50 ml phenol
        48 ml chloroform
         2 ml isoamyl alcohol
        10 ml 50 mM Tris HCl, pH 7.8
Mix well.
Allow to stand until phases separate.
Draw off aqueous layer and discard.

Store phenol:chloroform:isoamyl alcohol solution in an amber bottle (protected from direct light) at 4°C for up to 2 months. Note: Use only glass or polypropylene pipettes, bottles, etc. Polystyrene may dissolve in the phenol mixture!

Potassium phosphate, 1 M, pH 7.0

Dissolve 68.05 g of anhydrous KH_2PO_4 in 450 ml of water. Adjust pH to 7.0 and dilute to 500 ml. Autoclave in 100 ml bottles. Store at room temperature.

Sec-Butanol

Use as supplied.

Sodium acetate, 4 M

Dissolve 82 g of anhydrous NaOAc (82.04) in 200 ml of autoclaved water. Adjust pH to 6.5 with glacial acetic acid, dilute to 250 ml, autoclave, pass through a 0.45 µ filter and aliquot 10 ml per tube. Store at room temperature.

Sodium Bicarbonate, 1 M, pH 9.6 and 9.0

Dissolve 21 g of $NaHCO_3$ in 200 ml of autoclaved water and adjust pH to 9.6 or 9.0 with 10 N NaOH. Dilute to 250 ml, filter (0.45 µ) and store at room temperature.

Sodium Dodecyl Sulfate, 10%

Dissolve 10 g of SDS in 50 ml of autoclaved water. Dilute to 100 ml and aliquot. Store at room temperature.

Sodium Hydroxide, 10 N

Aliquot 10 N NaOH (Fisher SO-S-255) and store at room temperature.

SSC, 20x   1x

NaCl	175.3 g	0.150 M
Sodium citrate	88.2 g	0.015 M

Water to 1 liter
Adjust pH to 7.0 with 10 N NaOH
Autoclave and store at room temperature.

2x SSC/0.1% SDS

Add 50 ml of 20x SSC and 5 ml of 10% SDS to 445 ml of water. Autoclave in 100 ml bottles and store at room temperature.

SSPE, 20x   1x

NaCl	175.3 g	0.150 M
$NaH_2PO_4 \cdot H_2O$	30.5 g	0.011 M
EDTA	9.5 g	0.002 M

Water to 200 ml.
Adjust pH to 7.0.
Autoclave and store at room temperature.

Sulfuric Acid, 2N

Add 28 ml conc H_2SO_4 (18 M) to 222 ml water. Store at room temperature.

TBE Buffer, 10x1x

Tris base	108 g	89 mM
Boric acid	55 g	89 mM
0.5 M EDTA	40 ml	2 mM

Dissolve in 800 ml of water, adjust pH to 8.0 and dilute to 1 liter. Autoclave and store at room temperature.

TBS, 20x1x

1 M Tris, pH 7.4	121 g	50 mM
4 M NaCl	233 g	200 mM

dilute to 1 liter.

Autoclave and store at room temperature.

Tetramethylbenzidine (TMB) Reagent

Kirkegaard & Perry (#50-76-00), store at 4°C for 9 months.

Tris Acetate Buffer, 10x1x

Tris-base	48.5 g	40.0 mM
NaOAc	27.2 g	33.0 mM
EDTA	7.5 g	2.5 mM

Dissolve in 800 ml of water and adjust pH to 7.8. Dilute to one liter.

Autoclave and store at room temperature.

Wash buffer, 20x1x

1 M Tris, pH 7.4	121 g	50 mM
4 M NaCl	233 g	200 mM
6% Tween-20	60 ml	0.3 %
0.2% thimerosal	2 g	0.01%

Dilute to 1 liter.

Store at 4°C.

Water

Autoclave deionized water in 100-500 ml bottles. Discard open bottles weekly.

Procedures

PROCEDURE A.1

LARGE-SCALE PREPARATION OF HYBRIDIZATION BUFFER

This hybridization buffer is suitable for both radioactive and non-radioactive hybridizations using filters or microtiter wells.

Reagents:
a)   50x FPG
     1% ficoll 400
     1% polyvinylpyrrolidone 360
     1% glycine
     Add 2g of each to 150 ml of water and dissolve. Dilute to 200 ml.
     Filter-sterilize and store in 30 ml aliquots at -20°C.
b)   1 M Potassium Phosphate
     136 g of KH_2PO_4 per liter.
     Adjust pH to 7.0, autoclave and store at room temperature.
c)   Deionized formamide
     Stir 550 ml of formamide with 55g of AG501-X8 resin (Bio-Rad), H^+
     form.
     After 1 hour, filter through Whatman #1 paper. Store at -20°C.
d)   50% Dextran Sulfate
     Add 100 g of dextran sulfate slowly to a small beaker containing 100 ml
     of water. When dissolved, dilute to 200 ml total. Freeze in 40 ml aliquots.
e)   5% SDS
     Dissolve 50 g of sodium dodecyl sulfate in 700 ml of water. Dilute to 1
     liter. Store at room temperature.
f)   20x SSC
     351 g NaCl
     176 g sodium citrate
     Dissolve in 1,600 ml of water.
     Adjust pH to 7.0, dilute to 2 liters. Aliquot 100 ml per bottle, autoclave
     and store at room temperature.

Procedure:
Combine the following reagents:

Reagent	Final Conc.	Volume
Deionized Formamide	(50%)	536.0 ml
20X SSC	(5x)	268.0 ml
50X FPG	(1.25x)	26.8 ml
1M KH_2PO_4	(31 mM)	33.6 ml
10% SDS	(0.25%)	26.8 ml
Salmon sperm DNA (20mg/ml)		
	(31 µg/ml)	1.5 ml
50% Dextran Sulfate	(5%)	107.2 ml
Total		1,000.0 ml

Aliquot into 100 ml polypropylene bottles and store at -20°C for up to 1 year. During use it may be stored at 4°C for up to 2 months. Warm to 42°C and mix before use.

PROCEDURE A.2

NBT AND BCIP SUBSTRATE SOLUTIONS FOR ALKALINE PHOSPHATASE
(Leary et al., 1983)

NBT and BCIP are the most sensitive of the insoluble colorimetric substrates for alkaline phosphatase. Thus, for detection of the enzyme on filters or slides, no other colorimetric substrate provides a stronger signal. These substrates have the additional advantage that their stock solutions are quite stable. NBT and BCIP solutions are available from Kirkegaard & Perry as 10x concentrates and highly concentrated solutions are available from BRL as part of their Blugene biotin detection kit. NBT and BCIP produce a purple signal, but if a red signal is desired, refer to Procedures A.3 and A.4. A red signal is often preferred for use with *in situ* hybridization. The following protocols produce NBT and BCIP substrate solutions which are convenient to use and are stable at 4°C for 12 months. Described below are the substrate concentrates and buffer for preparing an 8:1:1 mixture.

Caution: Work in subdued light.

Reagents:
a) 10x NBT Concentrate(600 ml)
    Combine 60 ml of dimethylformamide (Aldrich 22,705,6 gold label) and 24 ml of water. Dissolve 2 grams of nitroblue tetrazolium (Sigma #N-6876) in this solvent, then add 516 ml of water. Final concentration is 3.3 mg/ml. Store at 4°C in a foil-wrapped glass bottle for up to 9 months. Aliquots can be packaged in brown polyethylene bottles (Nalgene) for 6-9 months.
b) 10x BCIP Concentrate(500 ml)
    Dissolve 1 gram of 5-bromo-4-chloro-3-indolyl phosphate (p-toluidine salt) (Biosynth International) in 100 ml of dimethylformamide. Gradually add 400 ml of deionized water. Final concentration is 2.0 mg/ml. Store at 4°C for 12-24 hours. Filter if necessary (if a precipitate forms) through Whatman #1 using a glass funnel. Store in a foil-wrapped glass bottle at 4°C for up to 9 months. Aliquots can be packaged in brown polyethylene bottles (Nalgene) for 6-9 months.

c)   10x Alkaline Phosphatase Substrate Buffer(500 ml)
        Tris-base   60.5 grams
        NaCl   29.2 grams
        $MgCl_2$ 5.1 grams
        Dilute to 400 ml with deionized water, adjust pH to 9.0 and dilute to 500 ml. Store at 4°C for up to 9 months.

d)   50 mM Levamisole Solution
        Levamisole   1.2 g
        1x substrate buffer   100 ml
        Store at 4°C for up to 9 months.

Procedure:
    Working solution
    1x substrate buffer   8 ml
    10x NBT concentrate   1 ml
    10x BCIP concentrate   1 ml
    50 mM levamisole   200 µl (optional)

The working solution is stable for at least 24 hours in the dark at room temp. Development times of up to 24 hours may be used. Levamisole inhibits the non-intestinal alkaline phosphatases found in many tissues. It is used during development of non-radioactive *in situ* hybridization experiments.

    Caution: Dimethylformamide is a strong irritant. Wear gloves when handling and avoid breathing fumes.

PROCEDURE A.3

INT AND BCIP SUBSTRATE SOLUTIONS
FOR ALKALINE PHOSPHATASE

If a red signal is desired, INT (p-iodo nitrotetrazolium violet) can be used in place of NBT. The sensitivity is about 2-3 fold less than NBT and BCIP and the stability of the INT stock solution is far less than NBT.

Reagents:
a)   10x INT Concentrate (25 ml)
        Dissolve 100 mg of p-iodo nitrotetrazolium violet (Amresco) in 4 ml of dimethyl formamide. Add 21 ml of water. Final concentration is 4 mg/ml in 16% DMF. This stock solution is stable at 4°C for about 1 month.
b)   10x BCIP concentrate (Procedure A.2)

Procedure:

To prepare the working solution, to 8 ml of 1x substrate buffer add 1 ml of 10x INT concentrate and 1 ml of 10x BCIP concentrate. Mix and use within 30 minutes. Development times up to 24 hours can be used. Also see the Fast Red substrate protocol below.

PROCEDURE A.4

FAST RED SUBSTRATE FOR ALKALINE PHOSPHATASE

As its name implies, fast red substrate, in the presence of alkaline phosphatase, produces a bright red insoluble signal at the site of the enzyme activity. It is especially useful for the detection of probes in *in situ* hybridization, where red signals can often be discerned better than signals of other colors. A disadvantage is that the stock solutions are not very stable.

Reagents:
a) 2x Fast Red
    (Fast red TR salt: Amresco P04403) Dissolve 250 mg in 50 ml of deionized water (5 mg/ml). Stable for 1 week when stored at 4°C in the dark.
b) 25x Napthol ASMX Phosphate
    (Sigma N-4875, free acid) Dissolve 12.5 mg of Napthol ASMX Phosphate in 50 ml of 1x substrate buffer (0.25%). Filter through a 0.45μ syringe filter. Stable for 2 months when stored at 4°C.
c) 1x Substrate Buffer
    100 mM Tris, pH 9.0
    100 mM NaCl
      5 mM $MgCl_2$
    Stable for 4 weeks when stored at 4°C in the dark.

Procedure:

Prepare the working solution as follows:

Reagent		1x conc.
Water	2.3 ml	
2x Fast Red	2.5 ml	2.5 mg/ml
25x N-ASMX-P	0.2 ml	0.01 %
	5.0 ml total	

Use immediately and discard unused solution. Within 5-60 min a red precipitate appears at sites of alkaline phosphatase activity. When used for *in situ* hybridization, slides can be mounted in Permount after air drying overnight.

PROCEDURE A.5

PREPARATION OF ACETYLATED BSA
(Gonzalez *et al.*, 1977)

Acetylation of BSA preparations is an effective procedure for inactivation of contaminating enzymes such as DNase, RNase and proteases.

Reagents:
a) Acetylation Buffer
    0.1 M Na_2HPO_4 7.1 g
    2.0 M sodium acetate   82.9g
    Dissolve in 500 ml of water. pH should be 8.5. Filter through Whatman #1 paper and store at room temperature for up to 1 week.
b) BSA (Sigma fraction V, A-8022)
c) Acetic anhydride (Aldrich 11,004-3, 99+%)

Procedure:
1. Dissolve 5 g of BSA in 100 ml of buffer. The final concentration is 5% or 50 mg/ml.
2. Slowly add 1.5 ml of acetic anhydride while stirring the solution at room temperature. Continue stirring for 45 minutes. Incubation on ice, as recommended in the reference, causes precipitation of the buffer.
3. Transfer the solution to dialysis bags. Leave no air space to avoid dilution. Dialyze against 4 changes of 4 liters of water at 4°C.
4. After dialysis, centrifuge in 50 ml polypropylene tubes at 5,000 xg (Sorvall RC3B) and store the supernatant in 10 ml aliquots at -20°C. Upon thawing, filter through a 0.45 μ syringe filter and do not re-freeze.

PROCEDURE A.6

PREPARATION OF 5X TAILING BUFFER

This buffer is used with terminal deoxynucleotidyl transferase (Tdt) to add polynucleotide 'tails' to the 3' ends of restriction fragments or oligomers.

Reagents:
a) Cacodylic acid (Sigma C-0125, free acid)
b) Chelex 100 (K^+ form) (BioRad, 200-400 mesh)
c) Dithiothreitol (DTT)
d) Cobalt chloride

Procedure:
1. Dissolve 13.8g of cacodylic acid in 35 ml of water.
2. Add solid KOH pellets until the pH is 7.25. Dilute to 88 ml.
3. Weigh out 50g of Chelex 100 (K^+). *If it is not in the K^+ form, wash the resin in a column as follows:*
    > 100 ml water
    > 200 ml 1N HCl
    > 300 ml water
    > 200 ml 1N KOH
    > 500 ml water

    This procedure converts the Chelex to the K^+ form. The resin is used to remove divalent metal ions from the buffer which can inhibit terminal transferase.
4. Let the column run dry. Pour the cacodylate solution into the column and collect the eluate in a 250 ml graduated cylinder. After all of the buffer passes through the column, add water to the column. Stop collecting at 176 ml. Check the pH at this point and adjust to 7.0 with solid KOH pellets. The pH after the column may be as low as 6.3. Mix and chill to 4°C.
5. To 44 ml of cold cacodylate solution add:
    > 500 µl of cold 0.1M DTT - mix thoroughly
    > 2.5 ml of cold 0.1M $CoCl_2$ - dropwise with stirring
    > Dilute to 50 ml.

    Filter-sterilize and store at -70°C in 1 ml aliquots.

1x buffer contains 100 mM cacodylate, pH 7.0, 1 mM $CoCl_2$, 0.2 mM DTT.

References

1. Gonzalez, N., Wiggs, J., and Chamberlin, M.J. (1977): A simple procedure for resolution of *Escherichia coli* RNA polymerase holoenzyme from core polymerase, Archives of Biochemistry and Biophysics **182**, 404-408.
2. Leary, J.J., Brigati, D.J. and Ward, D.C. (1983): Colorimetric method for visualizing biotin-labeled DNA probes hybridized to DNA or RNA immobilized on nitrocellulose: Bio-blots, Proc. Natl. Acad. Sci. USA **80**, 4045-4049.

DNA Conversion Tables

Avogadro's number: 6.02×10^{23} atoms or molecules/mole
Weight per DNA base pair (sodium salt): 660 Daltons
Abbreviations: ds, double-stranded; ss, single-stranded; kb, kilobase; bp, base pair; Da, daltons.

CONVERSION FACTORS

1 kb ds DNA (Na^+) = 6.6×10^5 Da
1 kb ss DNA (Na^+) = 3.3×10^5 Da
1 kb ss RNA (Na^+) = 3.4×10^5 Da
1 MDa ds DNA (Na^+) = 1.52 kb
1 pmol of a 1 kb DNA = 0.66 μg
1 μg pBR322 = 0.36 pmol DNA
1 pmol pBR 322 = 2.8 μg
Average mass of dNMP = 330 Da
Average mass of dNMP bp = 660 Da

CODING CAPACITY OF DNA

1 kb coding capacity = 333 amino acids = 40,000 Da protein
A 10,000 Da protein is coded for by about 270 bp of DNA
Average mass of an amino acid = 120 Da

QUANTITATION OF DNA AND RNA

Absorbance of double-stranded DNA: a 50 μg/ml solution has an A_{260} of about 1.0
Absorbance of single-stranded DNA: a 33 μg/ml solution has an A_{260} of about 1.0
Absorbance of single-stranded RNA: a 40 μg/ml solution has an A_{260} of about 1.0

	Length	*Weight*
l DNA	48.514 kb	30.8×10^6 Daltons
pBR322 DNA	4.363 kb	2.7×10^6 Daltons
Linker (ds: 8-mer)	0.008 kb	5.1×10^3 Daltons

METRIC PREFIXES

M	mega	10^6
k	kilo	10^3
m	milli	10^{-3}
μ	micro	10^{-6}
n	nano	10^{-9}
p	pico	10^{-12}
f	femto	10^{-15}
a	atto	10^{-18}

Nucleotide Extinction Coefficients

(Extinction Coefficients of Nucleoside Triphosphates at pH 7)

Triphosphate	λmax (nm) at pH 7-10	Absorbance at λmax for 100 mM solution
ATP	259	1540
CTP	280	1280
GTP	252	1370
TTP	262	1000
UTP	249	1270

CONVERSION FORMULA:

$$\frac{(100) \times (\text{observed absorbance at } \lambda max)}{\text{absorbance at lmax for 100 mM solution}} = \text{mM concentration of nucleotide}$$

Use these values to calculate exact concentrations for nucleotide solutions (deoxy, dideoxy, or ribonucleotides). Values are the absorbance measured in a cell with a 1 cm path length.

List of Abbreviations

BCIP	5-bromo-4-chloro-3-indolyl phosphate
bp	base pair
BSA	bovine serum albumin
Ci	Curie
cpm	counts per minute
Da	Dalton, the unit of molecular mass
DEPC	diethyl pyrocarbonate
DMSO	dimethyl sulfoxide
DNP	2,4-dinitrophenyl
ds	double-stranded (as in ds DNA)
DTT	dithiothreitol
EDTA	ethylenediaminetetraacetic acid
ELISA	enzyme-linked immunosorbent assay
IgG	immunoglobulin G
kb	kilobase: 1000 bases or base pairs, as appropriate
mA	miliamp
MDV	midivariant of bacteriophage Qβ RNA
MeV	million electron volts
mg	miligram
mmol	milimole: 10^{-3} mole
NBT	nitroblue tetrazolium
ng	nanogram: 10^{-9} gram
nm	nanometer
NHS	N-hydroxy succinimide
PBLs	peripheral blood lymphocytes
PBS	phosphate-buffered saline
PCR	polymerase chain reaction
pg	picogram: 10^{-12} gram
RVC	ribonucleoside vanadyl complex
SDS	sodium dodecyl sulfate
ss	single-stranded (as in ss DNA)
SSC	standard saline citrate
TBS	Tris-buffered saline
TE	Tris-EDTA buffer
μg	micorgram: 10^{-6} gram
V	volts

Appendix B:
Additional Protocols

Procedures

PROCEDURE B.1

PREPARATION OF RABBIT ANTI-DNP ANTIBODY
(Pohlit *et al.*, 1979; Becker and Makela, 1975; Keller *et al.*, 1988)

If you desire to label your DNA probes with a hapten for which no suitable antibody is commercially available, the following set of protocols can serve as an example of the steps required. In these examples, the hapten is 2,4-dinitrophenyl (DNP).

SYNTHESIS OF NHS-AMINOCAPROIC ACID-DNP

Reagents:
a)   e-Aminocaproic acid (Sigma)
b)   Dinitrobenzene sulfonic acid (Eastman, Na salt)
c)   Ethylene glycol dimethyl ether (EGD-ether, Sigma)
d)   Dimethyl formamide (Aldrich)
e)   N-hydroxysuccinimide (Sigma)
f)   N,N'-dicyclohexylcarbodiimide (DCC, Sigma)
g)   Methylene chloride (Aldrich)
h)   Sodium sulfate (Sigma)
i)   n-Hexane (Sigma)

Procedure:
(Preparation of the activated hapten)
Preparation of DNP-aminocaproic acid (MW = 297):
1.   Dissolve 6.55g of e-aminocaproic acid in 50 ml of 0.2 M NaHCO$_3$, 1 M NaOH (1M solution).   Add 15 g of dinitrobenzene sulfonic acid (10% molar excess).   Incubate overnight at 4°C in the dark.

2. Adjust the solution to pH 2 with conc. HCl (slowly with stirring) while on ice. Centrifuge out precipitate, discard supernatant and redissolve precipitate in NaOH/NaHCO$_3$ buffer. Repeat the precipitation.
3. The final pellet is dried under the hood for 1 hour, then lyophilized overnight or until dry. Store at 4°C.

Preparation of NHS-aminocaproic acid-dinitrobenzene (MW = 411):

4. Dissolve 2.7g of DNP-aminocaproic acid (0.009 mole) in 100 ml of ethylene glycol dimethyl ether (EGD-ether) containing 10% dimethyl formamide. Filter through filter paper. Add 2.25g of N-hydroxysuccinimide (0.015 mole) and 3.1g of N,N'-dicyclohexylcarbodiimide (DCC, 0.015 mole) dissolved in 5 ml of EGD-ether. Incubate overnight at 4°C.
    PERFORM SUBSEQUENT STEPS IN A FUME HOOD.
5. Filter out the N,N'-dicyclohexylurea precipitate. Pour filtrate into a Pyrex tray and evaporate in hood (takes about 3 hours). The residue should consist of an oily liquid and some crystals.
6. The residue is dissolved in 2 x 50 ml of methylene chloride (TOXIC) and transferred to a 250 ml bottle. It is extracted twice with an equal volume of 0.1M NaHCO$_3$, pH9. About 30 minutes are required for the phases to separate. Each time, the top aqueous layer and foamy interphase are pipetted off. After one more extraction with an equal volume of water, the emulsion is centrifuged in 50 ml plastic tubes and the top layer is removed.
7. The methylene chloride phases were poured into a 250 ml bottle containing 10g of Na sulfate and incubated from 2 hours to overnight at 4°C.
8. The material (100 ml) was next poured into 50 ml plastic tubes, 20 ml per tube (5 tubes). Each tube was then filled with n-hexane (2.5 vol) and chilled at -20°C for 1-2 hours. The tubes are then centrifuged in the tabletop unit at 3/4 speed for 5 minutes and the supernatant is poured off. Pellets are dried under the hood for 15 minutes. Dry on a lyophilizer overnight.

Checking product purity:

9. Samples are analyzed by TLC using the solvent system: chloroform/methanol (85:15). Use 170 ml of chloroform and 30 ml of methanol. Dissolve samples in EGD-ether and spot 1 microliter. Let plate develop 1 hour and dry. Desired material is fastest migrating yellow spot (least polar). Also check under short- and long-wave UV light. Plate may be sprayed with ninhydrin and heated to 50°C for 5 minutes to check for unreacted aminocaproic acid.

PREPARATION OF DNP-BSA

BSA (200 mg, 2.9×10^{-6} moles) is dissolved in 20 ml of 0.1M $NaHCO_3$, pH 9.0 (10 mg/ml). 20 mg of NHS-aminocaproic acid-DNP (17-fold molar excess) is dissolved in 1 ml of DMSO. The hapten solution is added slowly to the BSA solution and the reaction is incubated at room temperature overnight. Dialyze againtst five 1 liter changes of of PBS. Determine the A_{360}/ml. The molar extinction coefficient of DNP-lysine at 360 nm is 17,400. Use this factor to calculate the DNP/BSA molar ratio; it should be about 10. Store the conjugated BSA in 5 ml aliquots at -20°C.

IMMUNIZATION OF RABBITS

Use male New Zealand White rabbits weighing about 1 kg. Inject 500 μg per rabbit in a total volume of 1.5 ml (protein solution + adjuvant):

Combine: 50 μl DNP-BSA, 700 μl PBS and 750ul adjuvant according to the following schedule:

Week #		Adjuvant
0	inject	complete
2	boost	incomplete
6	boost	incomplete
7	bleed	
10	boost	incomplete
11	bleed	
14	boost	incomplete
15	bleed	

PROCESSING OF SERUM

Allow blood to clot at room temperature for 1 hour. Break up clots with a spatula and centrifuge in 30 ml Corex tubes at 12,000 xg, 4°C for 10 minutes. Keep on ice from this point. Remove supernatant to a new tube, break up pelleted clot and recentrifuge. Remove small supernatant, add to rest of serum and dispose of clot. Recentrifuge the pooled serum as above and transfer the supernatant to a new tube. The serum may be stored at -70°C. To precipitate the immunoglobulin fraction, add an equal volume of a saturated ammonium sulfate solution (pH 7.5) on ice with stirring. Incubate on ice for 30 minutes. Centrifuge at 12,000 xg, 4°C for 10 minutes. Pour off the supernatant, redissolve the pellet in the original serum volume of PBS and repeat the precipitation. Redissolve the pellet in the original serum volume of PBS and dialyze against PBS. Store in aliquots at -20°C. This fraction may be further purified by affinity chromatography on a protein A column. Refer to the directions supplied by the manufacturer.

PROCEDURE B.2

CONJUGATION OF ALKALINE PHOSPHATASE TO AN ANTIBODY
(Williams, 1984)

In the course of hapten detection, faster results can be obtained with an enzyme-conjugated first antibody, but with some sacrifice in sensitivity. In the following procedure, amino groups on the antibody are coupled to carbohydrate side chains on the enzyme. Purified IgG works well, but the use of Fab fragments usually results in lower backgrounds.

Reagents:
a)   1 M Sodium Carbonate, pH 9.5
       62 g/500 ml, of water
       Adjust pH to 9.5.
b)   Carbonate-Saline Buffer
       0.02 M Na carbonate 20 ml of 1M
       0.2 M NaCl   11.7 g
       Dilute to 1 liter.
c)   100 mM Sodium Acetate, pH 4.0
       5.3 g/500 ml of water.
       Adjust pH to 4.0.
d)   Antibody
       Protein A-purified or Fab fragment, 0.2 mg/ml in PBS. MW=140,000.
       Immobilized protein A and a kit for preparation of Fab fragments are
       available from Pierce.
e)   Alkaline Phosphatase
       Boehringer Mannheim #567752 supplied in 3M NaCl, 1 mM
       $MgCl_2$, 0.1 mM $ZnCl_2$, 30 mM triethanolamine, pH 7.6.
       MW=100,000.
f)   10x PBS (Appendix A)
g)   0.1 M Sodium Periodate (Aldrich)
       Dissolve 22 mg in 1 ml of sodium acetate buffer.
h)   1.6M Ethylene Glycol (Aldrich)
       Add 89 µl to 1 ml of water.
i)   Sodium Borohydride Solution (Aldrich)
       Dissolve 4 mg in 1 ml of water.

Procedure:
1.   Dialyze the antibody against carbonate-saline (4 changes of 1 liter) at
       4°C. Dialyze 5 mg of alkaline phosphatase (500 µl + 500 µl of 1 mM
       sodium acetate) against 1 mM sodium acetate, pH 4.0, overnight. Change
       the buffer once.

2. Add 0.2 ml of the sodium periodate solution to the alkaline phosphatase solution, stir for 20 minutes at room temperature.
3. Add 100 μl of the ethylene glycol solution to the alkaline phosphatase solution. Mix gently for 30 minutes at room temperature.
4. Dialyze against 1 liter of 1 mM sodium acetate, pH 4.0, overnight at 4°C. Change once. The final volume should be about 1.3 ml.
5. With stirring add 1 mg of antibody in 5.9 ml to the 5 μg of alkaline phosphatase. Stir for 3 hours at room temperature. The pH should be alkaline. Enzyme/antibody molar ratio is 7.0.
6. Add 100 μl of the sodium borohydride solution and incubate at 4°C for 2 hours without stirring.
7. Dialyze against 4 changes of 1 liter of PBS.
8. Store in 1 ml aliquots at -20°C.

PROCEDURE B.3

SYNTHESIS OF FITC-DIAMINOHEXANE

(McKinney *et al.*, 1964)

This compound can be used as a substitute for DNP-diaminohexane in the bromine mediated modification of DNA (Procedure 4.11) and in the synthesis of photo-DNP (Procedure 4.9). Like 2,4-DNP, fluoroescein isothiocyanate is another common hapten which elicits high affinity antibodies (Procedure B.4).

Reagents:
a) 1,6-diaminohexane (Aldrich)
b) Fluoroescein isothiocyanate (FITC, Sigma)
c) Dimethylsulfoxide (DMSO, Aldrich)
d) 1 N HCl
e) Chloroform
f) 100% methanol
g) Compressed nitrogen
h) Ninhydrin reagent (Sigma)

Procedure:
1. Add 60 μl of diaminohexane (5.1×10^{-4} moles) to 25 ml of water. Dissolve 100 mg of FITC (2.5×10^{-4} moles) in 2 ml of DMSO. Slowly add FITC solution to diaminohexane while vortexing to prevent precipitation. Incubate overnight at room temperature in the dark.
2. Final pH is about 6. Add 50 μl of 1 N HCl to precipitate all but the diaminohexane. Centrifuge at 12,000 xg for 10 minutes and pour off the supernatant.

3.   Dissolve the pellet in 10 ml of methanol and filter through a 0.45 μ filter if cloudy.
4.   Purify the desired product by preparative TLC using chloroform:methanol (170/190) as the solvent. Scrape off the lowest band (above the origin), elute the product from the silica by extraction with methanol, concentrate under a stream of N_2 and store at 4°C. Work in a fume hood with a mask to avoid inhaling silica dust.
5.   The material should run as a single spot on analytical TLC, and should darken after spraying with ninhydrin and heating. 0.64 OD = 3 μg/ml = 0.006 mM in 0.1 M phosphate, pH 6.8.

PROCEDURE B.4

CONJUGATION OF FITC TO BSA

In order to detect FITC-labeled DNA, a suitable antibody is required. This procedure is one method of antigen preparation. Another approach would be to synthesize NHS-aminocaproic acid-FITC and couple it to BSA by combining Procedures B.1 and B.3.

Reagents:
a)   Bovine serum albumin (BSA, Sigma fraction V, A-8022)
b)   Fluoroescein isothiocyanate (Sigma, MW = 389)
c)   10x PBS (Appendix A)
d)   0.1 N $NaHCO_3$, pH 9.0
e)   Dimethylsulfoxide (DMSO)

Procedure:
1.   200 mg of BSA is dissolved in 20 ml of 0.1 N $NaHCO_3$, pH 9.0.
2.   20 mg of FITC is dissolved in 1 ml of DMSO and added slowly to the BSA with stirring (15 fold molar excess). Incubate at 4°C for 2 hours.
3.   The reaction is dialyzed against five changes of 1 liter of PBS.
4.   Measure the UV absorbance of the solution to determine the number of moles of FITC bound per mole of BSA. The usual result is 5 moles FITC per mole of protein.
5.   Store in aliquots at -20°C. Innoculate rabbits as described in Procedure B.1.

Typical values:

Dilution	A_{280}	A_{495}	A_{280}/ml	A_{495}/ml
10/1010	0.363	0.397	36.7	39.6

$A_{280} - (0.35 \times A_{495}) / 0.66$ = protein concentration (mg/ml)
$2.87 \times A_{495} / A_{280} - (0.35 \times A_{495})$ = moles FITC/ mole protein

References

1. Becker, M. and Makela, O. (1975): Modification of bacteriophage with hapten-e-aminocaproyl-N-hydroxysuccinimide esters: Increased sensitivity for immunoassay, Immunochem. **12**, 329-331.

2. Keller, G.H., Cumming, C.U., Huang, D.P., Manak, M.M. and Ting, R. (1988): A chemical method for introducing haptens onto DNA probes, Anal. Biochem. **170**, 441-450.

3. McKinney, R.M., Spillane, J.T. and Pearce, G.W. (1964): Determination of the purity of fluorescein isothiocyanates, Anal. Biochem. **7**, 74-86.

4. Pohlit,H.M., Haas,W. and von Boehmer,H. (1979): in *Immunological Methods* (Lefkovits, I. and Pernis, B., eds) (Academic Press, New York) pp 181-195.

5. Williams, D.G. (1984): Comparison of three conjugation procedures for the formation of tracers for use in enzyme immunoassay, J. Immun. Meth. **72**, 261-268.

Appendix C: Suppliers

Accurate Chemical and Scientific Corp.
300 Shames Drive
Westbury, NY 11590
(800) 645-6264
(516) 433-4900
anti-hapten antibodies

Aldrich Chemical Co.
940 West Saint Paul Avenue
Milwaukee, WI 53233
(800) 558-9160
chemical reagents

Amersham
2636 South Clearbrook Drive
Arlington Heights, IL 60005
(312) 593-6300
radioactive nucleotides, non-radioactive labeling and detection kit

Amicon Division
W.R. Grace & Co.
24 Cherry Hill Drive
Danvers, MA 01923
(508) 777-3622
microconcentrators

Amresco
30175 Solon Industrial Parkway
Solon, OH 44139
(216) 349-1199
enzyme substrates

Applied Biosystems
800 Lincoln Centre Drive
Foster City, CA 94404
(415) 570-6667
DNA synthesizers and reagents

Beckman Instruments, Inc.
2500 Harbor Blvd.
Fullerton, CA 92634
(714) 871-4848
microfuges, ultracentrifuges

Bio-Rad Laboratories
Chemical Division
1414 Harbour Way South
Richmond, CA 94804
(415) 232-7000
nylon membranes, immunochemical detection systems, electrophoresis equipment

Biosynth International
P.O. Box 541
Skokie, IL 60076
(312) 674-5160
colorimetric and fluorescent enzyme substrates

Biotherm Corp.
3260 Wilson Boulevard
Arlington, VA 22201
(703) 522-1705
thermal cycling oven

255

**Boehringer Mannheim
  Biochemicals**
P.O. Box 50816
Indianapolis, IN 46250
(800) 428-5433
*restriction, polymerase and other
nucleic acid enzymes, hapten-based
DNA labeling and detection kit*

BRL/Life Technologies
P.O. Box 6009
Gaithersburg, MD 20877
(301) 258-8280
*restriction, polymerase and other
nucleic acid enzymes, DNA
biotinylation and detection reagents*

Chemicon International
100 Lomita Street
El Segundo, CA 90245
(800) 437-7500
(213) 322-2451
anti-hapten antibodies

Costar Corporation
One Alewife Center
Cambridge, MA 02140
(617) 868-6200
microtiter plates

Cruachem
460 Spring Park
Herndon, VA 22070
(800) 327-9362
oligonucleotide synthesis reagents

Clontech
4030 Fabian Way
Palo Alto, CA 94303
(800) 662-2566
(415) 424 8222
oligonucleotide synthesis reagents

DuPont
Barley Mill Plaza
Wilmington, DE 19898
(800) 551-2121
radioactive isotopes, DNA probes

Eastman Kodak
343 State Street
Rochester, NY 14652
(800) 225-5352
chemical reagents

Enzo Diagnostics
325 Hudson Street
New York, NY 10013
(212) 741-3838
*DNA biotinylation and detection
reagents; in situ hybridization kits*

Ericomp
10055 Barnes Canyon Road
Suite G
San Diego, CA 92121
(800) 541-8471
(619) 457-1888
thermal cycler

Fluka Chemical Corp.
980 S. Second Street
Ronkonkoma, NY 11779
(516) 467-0980
reagent chemicals

FMC Bioproducts
5 Maple Street
Rockland, ME 04841
*agarose, DNA labeling &
detection kit*

Hoefer Scientific
P.O. Box 77387
San Francisco, CA 94107
(415) 282-2307
electrophoresis equipment

IBI (International Biotechnologies, Inc.)
P.O. Box 9558
275 Winchester Avenue
New Haven, CT 06535
(800) 243-2555
molecular biology equipment & reagents

J.T. Baker
222 Red School Lane
Phillipsburg, NJ 08865
(800) 582-2537
chemical reagents

Jackson Immunoresearch
P.O. Box 9
West Grove, PA 19390
(800) 367-529
(215) 869-4024
enzyme-conjugated second antibodies

Kodak
Laboratory and Research Products Division
Rochester, NY 14650
(800) 225-5352
organic chemicals

Kontes
P.O. Box 729
Vineland, NJ 08360
(609) 692-8500
glassware

Kirkegaard & Perry Laboratories, Inc.
2 Cessna Court
Gaithersburg, MD 20879
(800) 638-3167
enzyme-conjugated antibodies and streptavidin

Mallinkrodt, Inc.
Science Products Division
675 McDonnell Blvd.
St. Louis, MO 63134
(314) 895-2333

Midland Certified Reagent Co.
3112-A West Cuthbert Avenue
Midland, TX 79701
(800) 247-8766
unlabeled and biotin labeled oligonucleotides

Millipore Corp.
80 Ashby Road
Bedford, MA 01730
(800) 225-1380
filtration products

MSI (Micron Separations, Inc.)
135 Flanders Road
Westborough, MA 01581
(508) 366-8212
filtration products

Nalge Corp.
P.O. Box 20365
Rochester, NY 14602
(716) 586-8800
plasticware

National Diagnostics, Inc.
1013-1017 Kennedy Blvd.
Manville, NJ 08835
(800) 526-3867
radioactivity detection products

New England Biolabs
32 Tozer Road
Beverly, MA 01915
(508) 927-5054
restriction enzymes and polymerases

Oncor
P.O. Box 870
Gaithersburg, MD 20877
(301) 963-3500
oncogene probes, biotin labeling
and detection reagents

Perkin Elmer Cetus
761 Main Avenue
Norwalk, CT 06859
(203) 834-6722
PCR thermal cycler

Pharmacia LKB Biotechnology
800 Centennial Avenue
Piscataway, NJ 08855
(800) 526-3618

Pierce Chemical Co.
P.O. Box 117
Rockford, IL 61105
(815) 968-0747
linker arms, biotinylation reagents

Promega
2800 S. Fish Hatchery Road
Madison, WI 53711
(800) 356-9526
enzymes, vectors and labeling kits

Schleicher & Schuell
10 Opitcal Avenue
Keene, NH 03431
(603) 352-3810
nitrocellulose and nylon membranes

Sigma Chemical Co.
P.O. Box 14508
St. Louis, MO 63178
(800) 346-6405
various reagents

Synthetic Genetics
10455 Roselle Street
San Diego, CA 92121
(619) 587-0320
PCR primers and probes,
biotinylated oligomer probes

Techne Inc.
3700 Brunswick Pike
Princeton, NJ 08540
(609) 452-9275
thermal cycler

Tropix
47 Wiggins Avenue
Bedford, MA 01730
(617) 271-0045
chemiluminescent enzyme substrates

United States Biochemical Corp.
P.O. Box 22400
Cleveland, OH 44122
(800) 321-9322
restriction enzymes and polymerases

Vector Labs
30 Ingold Road
Burlingame, CA 94010
(415) 697-3600
biotin/avidin reagents

Whatman LabSales
5285 N.E. Elam Young Parkway
Suite A-400
Hillsboro, OR 97124
(800) 942-8626
filter papers

**Worthington Biochemical
Corp.**
Freehold, NJ 07728
(800) 445-9603
enzymes

Zymark Corp.
Zymark Center
Hopkinton, MA 01748
(617) 435-9507
programmable robot arm